ENDOSCOPIC ENDONASAL SURGERY
SINUSES AND BEYOND

ENDOSCOPIC ENDONASAL SURGERY
SINUSES AND BEYOND

Editor

Milind V Kirtane MS (ENT) DORL
Professor Emeritus
Department of ENT
Seth GS Medical College and King Edward Memorial Hospital
Mumbai, Maharashtra, India

Senior Consultant ENT Surgeon
PD Hinduja National Hospital and Medical Research Centre
Breach Candy Hospital
Cumballa Hill Hospital
Saifee Hospital
Mumbai, Maharashtra, India

Foreword

MV Ingle

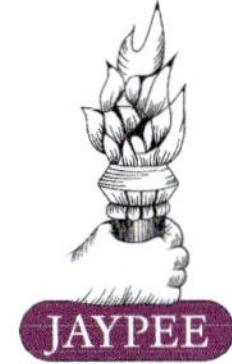

JAYPEE BROTHERS MEDICAL PUBLISHERS

The Health Sciences Publisher

New Delhi | London

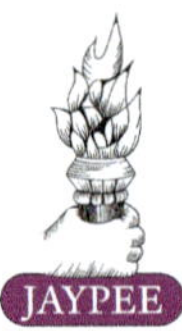 **Jaypee Brothers Medical Publishers (P) Ltd.**

Headquarters
EMCA House
23/23-B, Ansari Road, Daryaganj
New Delhi 110 002, India
Landline: +91-11-23272143, +91-11-23272703
+91-11-23282021, +91-11-23245672
E-mail: jaypee@jaypeebrothers.com

Overseas Office
JP Medical Ltd.
83, Victoria Street, London
SW1H 0HW (UK)
Phone: +44-20 3170 8910
E-mail: info@jpmedpub.com

Corporate Office
Jaypee Brothers Medical Publishers (P) Ltd.
4838/24, Ansari Road, Daryaganj
New Delhi 110 002, India
Phone: +91-11-43574357
Fax: +91-11-43574314
E-mail: jaypee@jaypeebrothers.com

EU GPSR Authorised Representative
Logos Europe, 9 rue Nicolas Poussin
17000, La Rochelle, France
Phone: +33 (0) 6 67 93 73 78
E-mail: Contact@logoseurope.eu

Website: www.jaypeebrothers.com
Website: www.jaypeedigital.com

Inquiries for bulk sales may be solicited at: jaypee@jaypeebrothers.com

Endoscopic Endonasal Surgery: Sinuses and Beyond

First Edition : 2015

Reprint: **2026**

ISBN 978-93-5152-150-1

Printed at Replika Press Pvt. Ltd.

Contributors

Abhijit A Raut   MD (Radiology)
Consultant Radiologist
Kokilaben Dhirubhai Ambani Hospital
Mumbai, Maharashtra, India

Abhineet Lall   MS (ENT)
Fellow
Dr Milind Kirtane Clinic
Mumbai, Maharashtra, India

Anagha Joshi   MBBS MS (ENT) DORL DNB (ENT)
Associate Professor
Department of ENT
Lokmanya Tilak Municipal Medical College
and General Hospital
Life Member, Association of Otolaryngologists of India
Life Member, Association of Phonosurgeons of India
Fellow, International College of Surgeons

Arpit Sharma   MS (ENT) DNB DORL
Assistant Professor
Department of ENT and Head Neck Surgery
Seth GS Medical College and King Edward
Memorial Hospital
Mumbai, Maharashtra, India

Bachi Hathiram   MBBS MS (ENT) DORL DNB (ENT)
Professor and Head
Department of ENT and Head Neck Surgery
Topiwala National Medical College and
BYL Nair Charitable Hospital
Mumbai, Maharashtra, India

Chandrashekhar E Deopujari   MS MCh
Consultant Neurosurgeon
Bombay Hospital
Mumbai, Maharashtra, India

Dhruv Satwalekar   MS (ENT)
Consultant ENT Surgeon
Cumballa Hill Hospital
Mumbai, Maharashtra, India

Gaurav Shankar Medikeri   MBBS MS (ENT)
Consultant ENT Surgeon
Co-Director
Medikeri's Superspecialty ENT Center
Bengaluru, Karnataka, India
Fellowship in Endoscopic Sinus Surgery
Fellowship in Rhinoplasty (Seoul, Korea)

Gauri Mankekar   MS (ENT) DNB PhD (Germany)
Former Consultant
Department of ENT
PD Hinduja National Hospital and
Medical Research Center
Mumbai, Maharashtra, India

Gauri M Kapre   MS (ENT)
Ex-Skull Base Fellow
Bombay Hospital
Mumbai, Maharashtra, India
Consultant
Neeti Clinics
Nagpur, Maharashtra, India

Hetal Marfatia Patel   MS (ENT) DORL DNB
Professor and Head, Unit II
Department of ENT
Seth GS Medical College and
King Edward Memorial Hospital
Mumbai, Maharashtra, India

JP Dabholkar   MS (ENT)
Professor and Head
Seth GS Medical College and
King Edward Memorial Hospital
Mumbai, Maharashtra, India

Kashmira Chavan   MBBS DNB (ENT)
Consultant ENT Surgeon
Dr LH Hiranandani Hospital
Mumbai, Maharashtra, India

Milind Navalakhe   MS (ENT) DORL
Associate Professor
Department of ENT
Topiwala Medical College and BYL Nair Charitable Hospital
Mumbai, Maharashtra, India

Milind V Kirtane   MS (ENT) DORL
Professor Emeritus
Department of ENT
Seth GS Medical College and King Edward
Memorial Hospital
Mumbai, Maharashtra, India
Senior Consultant ENT Surgeon
PD Hinduja National Hospital and Medical Research Center
Breach Candy Hospital
Cumballa Hill Hospital
Saifee Hospital
Mumbai, Maharashtra, India

Nishit J Shah   MS (ENT) DNB DORL
Consultant ENT Surgeon
Bombay Hospital
Mumbai, Maharashtra, India

Prashant S Naphade   MD DNB (Radiology)
Consultant Radiologist
ESIC Hospital, MIDC
Mumbai, Maharashtra, India

Prathamesh S Pai   MS (ENT) DNB DORL MNAMS
Professor and Surgeon
Department of Head & Neck and Surgical Oncology
Tata Memorial Hospital
Mumbai, Maharashtra, India

Rahul P Tejankar   MBBS MS (ENT)
Fellowship Endoscopic Sinus and Skull Base Surgery
Consultant ENT Surgeon
Tejankar Health Care and Research Institute
Ujjain, Madhya Pradesh, India

Renuka Bradoo   MS (ENT) DORL
Professor and Head
Department of ENT and Head & Neck Surgery
Lokmanya Tilak Municipal Medical College
and General Hospital
Mumbai, Maharashtra, India

Roshni Nambiar   MBBS DNB (ENT)
Junior Consultant
Dr Babasaheb Ambedkar Central Railway Hospital
Mumbai, Maharashtra, India

Samir Bhargava   MS (ENT) DLO (London) DORL DNB
Consultant ENT Surgeon
Hinduja Healthcare Hospital
Dr RN Cooper Hospital
Asian Heart Institute
Mumbai, Maharashtra, India

Satish Jain   MBBS MS (ENT) FRHS (London)
Consultant ENT Surgeon
Specialist in Endoscopic Skull Base and
Head & Neck Surgery
Jain ENT Hospital
Jaipur, Rajasthan, India

Sharmela Sondhi   MS (ENT)
Fellow
Dr Milind Kirtane Clinic
Mumbai, Maharashtra, India

Shraddha Deshmukh   MS (ENT) DNB
Assistant Professor
Government Medical College
Nagpur
Ex-Registrar
Seth GS Medical College and King Edward
Memorial Hospital
Mumbai, Maharashtra, India

Siddharth Chaudri   MS FCPS DORL DNB DLO (London)
Hon Consultant ENT Surgeon
Deenanath Mangeshkar Hospital
Pune, Maharashtra, India

Sujata Muranjan   MS (ENT) DNB DORL
Consultant ENT Surgeon
Bombay Hospital
Mumbai, Maharashtra, India

Sunita Kanojia   MS (ENT)
Ex-Skull Base Fellow
Bombay Hospital
Mumbai, Maharashtra, India

Swapna Patil   MS (ENT) DNB
Fellow
Dr Milind Kirtane Clinic
Mumbai, Maharashtra, India

TN Janakiram   MS (ENT) DLO
Director
Royal Pearl Hospital
Trichy, Tamil Nadu, India

Foreword

Endoscopic sinus surgery was introduced in India in 1986. Dr Milind Kirtane was one of the pioneers who started with this technique in King Edward Memorial Hospital, Mumbai, Maharashtra, India. This surgery was initially meant for chronic sinusitis refractory to medical treatment. The last three decades have seen a tremendous expansion in its indications. The nasal endoscopist now operates not only in the nose and sinuses but accesses also the surrounding areas such as the orbit, the infratemporal fossa and cranial cavity. Sophistication in instrumentation, advances in imaging techniques and introduction of intraoperative navigation have made this possible and relatively safe. Lesions of the skull base which were difficult to access can now be tackled under direct vision thanks to the endoscope.

The book addresses various aspects of endocopic endonasal surgery from the basic to the advanced. Starting with an elaborate chapter on surgical anatomy, the book deals with basic endoscopic techniques for the management of sinonasal diseases. The book also has well-illustrated chapters on imaging techniques and highlights the need for the endoscopist to have a comprehensive understanding of the same. Chapters deal with extended indications such as lesions of the pituitary, skull base tumors, orbital lesions, traumatic optic neuropathy, cerebrospinal fluid (CSF), rhinorrhea, etc. Pre- and postoperative care, which is of vital importance in optimizing outcomes, has also been addressed.

The illustrations complement the text for better comprehension. Dr Kirtane and his colleagues who have contributed to the book need to be congratulated for putting together the various aspects of endoscopic endonasal surgery so succinctly in the book.

I am confident that the book will be of great value to all practising nasal endoscopic surgeons.

MV Ingle
Former Honorary Professor
Department of ENT
Seth GS Medical College and
King Edward Memorial Hospital
Mumbai, Maharashtra, India

Preface

Functional endoscopic sinus surgery (FESS) was introduced as a treatment for intractable chronic sinusitis, which failed to respond to medical management. The concept was to re-establish the drainage and aeration of the paranasal sinuses so that the underlying mucosa, which was inflamed, could heal. Surgeons found that they could go beyond the scope of this indication and started operating on different conditions, including tumors within the nose and paranasal sinuses, and then expanded to the surrounding areas such as the orbit and the skull base.

Today, endoscopic endonasal sinus surgery has indications way beyond what it was originally designed for, and many skull-base lesions, which were thought to be unapproachable or inoperable are now being treated. This has been possible not only with improved surgical techniques, but also with ancillary aids such as the image guidance, powered instruments, and different techniques which have evolved to repair large defects that have been created, as also advancement in adhesive and sealing materials which help these repairs.

There are many surgeons in different parts of our country who have great expertise in endoscopic sinus surgery, and this book is an attempt to bring together their knowledge and experience in a handbook form, which may serve as a ready reference for the novice endoscopists as also to the experienced ones.

I would like to acknowledge the efforts of Dr Kashmira Chavan, Dr Harsh K Gupta, Dr Sujata Gawai, Dr Rachna Zaveri, and Dr Trishna Kakkad in the compilation of the book.

Milind V Kirtane

Contents

CHAPTER 1

Lateral Nasal Wall

Renuka Bradoo

INTRODUCTION

It is far easier to understand the endoscopic anatomy that we encounter intraoperatively and its surgical implications, if we have made a prior study of the lateral nasal wall as it appears in a cadaveric sagittal section of the head.

Viewing all the elevations and depressions that make up the lateral nasal wall from anterior to posterior together helps us understand the concept of the "layers" or "lamellae" that we transgress sequentially during endoscopic surgery.

OVERVIEW

The lateral nasal wall (Fig. 1.1) shows broadly two regions, an anterior one-third which is relatively featureless consisting of vestibule and atrium and a posterior two-thirds which shows three major elevations, i.e. the turbinates. Posterior to the turbinates is the region of sphenoid sinus and the nasopharynx. The posterior end of inferior turbinate is at the level of opening of the eustachian tube whereas the middle turbinate ends at the level of roof of posterior choana. The roof of nasal cavity, i.e. the skull base, slopes from above downwards starting anteriorly as the posterior wall of frontal sinus and ending posteriorly as the roof of sphenoid sinus. The part of skull base formed by the frontal and sphenoid bones is relatively thick while the central part which is formed by cribriform plate of ethmoid bone is thin and is perforated by a number of olfactory nerves.

VESTIBULE AND ATRIUM

The vestibule is skin lined and there is a clear line of demarcation between the skin and the mucosa of the atrium. This mucosa of the atrium is closely bound to the underlying bone, i.e. the nasal bone and frontonasal process of maxilla. A bulge is often seen in the atrium just anterior and a little superior to the anterior attachment of middle turbinate. This is due to the underlying agger nasi cell. An ill-defined ridge extends downwards from this bulge up to the inferior turbinate. This is the maxillary line and it overlies the nasolacrimal duct.

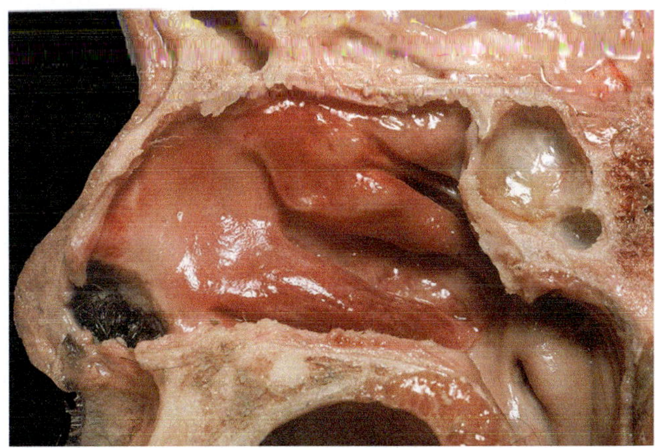

Fig. 1.1: Lateral nasal wall

TURBINATES

The inferior turbinate is a separate bone whereas the middle and superior turbinates are parts of the ethmoid bone. Although the inferior turbinate appears relatively straight, its attachment is in the form of an inverted "V". The maxillary line mentioned earlier ends at the apex of this "V" and the underlying nasolacrimal duct enters the inferior meatus at this point. The nasolacrimal duct travels submucosally for a few mm before opening in the lateral wall of the inferior meatus. This opening is guarded by a fold of mucosa called the Hasner's valve.

The middle turbinate is a convoluted structure bending in different planes similar to a dried leaf. It can be divided into three parts, depending on its attachment and its orientation in the three-dimensional space.

1. The anterior one-third is in the sagittal plane and is attached to the cribriform plate at the junction of the medial and lateral lamellae.
2. The middle one-third lies in the coronal plane and is attached to the lamina papyracea. It separates the anterior ethmoidal cells from the posterior ethmoidal cells. Since it stabilizes the middle turbinate, it is called the ground lamella or the basal lamella.
3. The posterior third lies in the horizontal plane and is attached to the lamina papyracea and the perpendicular plate of the palatine bone extending up to the roof of the posterior choana.

Besides these three attachments, there is also a relatively small but surgically significant fourth attachment which is often not mentioned in literature. The anterior most 2–3 mm of the middle turbinate is not attached to the cribriform plate but to the frontonasal process of maxilla. In doing so, it creates the axilla of the middle turbinate which is an important endoscopic landmark.

The superior turbinate is much smaller. It lies in the sphenoethmoidal recess and partially overhangs the anterior wall of sphenoid sinus and the sphenoid ostium.

OSTIOMEATAL UNIT

When the middle turbinate is trimmed to expose the middle meatus, we can see two important elevations, the anterior boomerang-shaped ridge is the uncinate process which consists of a vertical and a horizontal limb with an intermediate transitional part. Posterior to this is the well pneumatized and most constant anterior ethmoidal cell, namely the ethmoidal bulla. These structures are separated by a semilunar groove called the hiatus semilunaris. The hiatus semilunaris is two-dimensional and leads into a three-dimensional space called the infundibulum. The uncinate process, the bulla and the intervening infundibulum form the key area or the ostiomeatal unit (Fig. 1.2) into which the frontal, the maxillary and anterior ethmoidal sinuses drain.

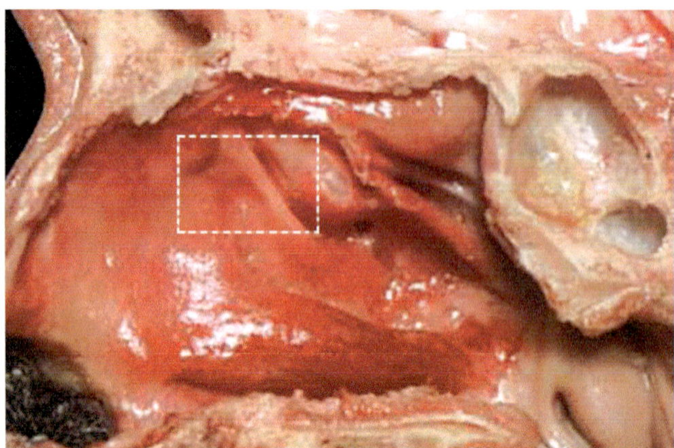

Fig. 1.2: Ostiomeatal unit (As shown by dotted rectangle)

Rarely (8%) the bulla may be rudimentary or absent. It is separated posteriorly from the ground lamella of the middle turbinate by a recess called the retrobullar recess. Occasionally, the bulla does not extend up to the base of the skull and is separated from it by the suprabullar recess. The retrobullar and suprabullar recesses together form a semilunar space above and behind the bulla called the sinus lateralis of Grunwald. This sinus opens into the middle meatus by a semilunar cleft which is opposite in orientation to the hiatus semilunaris and is called the hiatus semilunaris superioris. Thus the hiatus semilunaris inferioris leads into the infundibulum and the hiatus semilunaris superioris leads into the sinus lateralis of Grunwald.

MAXILLARY OSTIUM

The bony opening in the medial wall of the maxillary bone which leads into the maxillary sinus is called the maxillary hiatus. It is partially closed in the living by various processes of different bones as well as by mucosa. Hence the maxillary ostium itself is just a few mm in diameter. It lies deep to the intermediate/horizontal portion of the uncinate process. Since it lies deep within the infundibulum close to the attachment of the uncinate, it can therefore be seen only when the entire width of the uncinate process is removed. It is usually ovoid in shape and has a three-dimensional tunnel like configuration. It is related to two critical areas, superiorly to the lamina papyracea and the orbit, anteriorly to the nasolacrimal duct. A branch of the sphenopalatine artery runs along the lateral wall at a variable distance from the posterior margin of the foramen.

Some areas of the lateral nasal wall are covered by only two layers of mucosa, the mucosa of the lateral nasal wall and the mucosa of the maxillary sinus. These regions are called the fontanelles. The anterior fontanelle lies anteroinferior to the uncinate process. The posterior fontanelle lies just above and behind the posterior part of the uncinate process. The

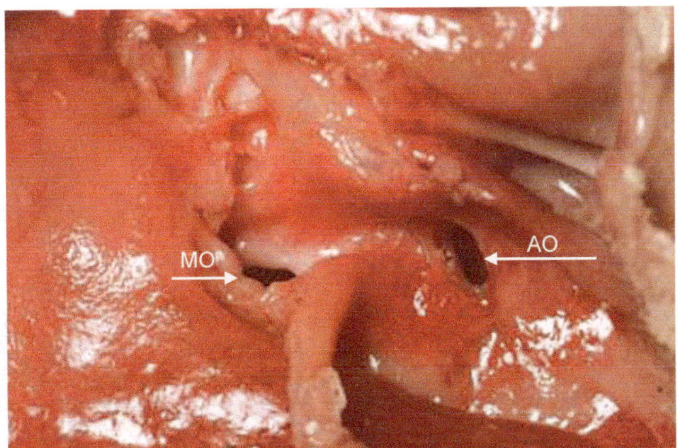

Fig. 1.3: Maxillary ostium (MO) and accessory ostium (AO)

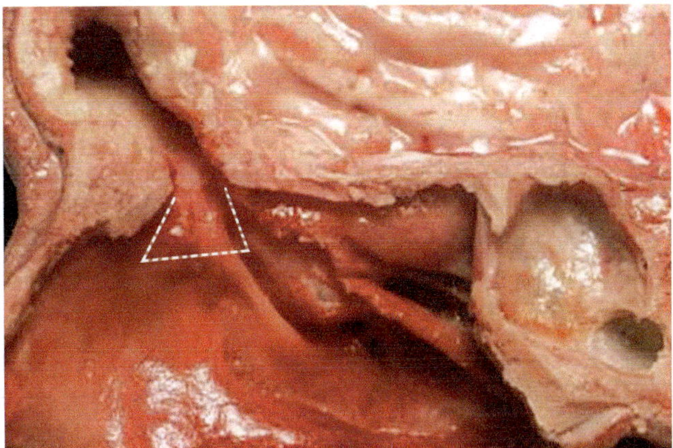

Fig. 1.4: Frontal recess area as denoted (dotted line)

mucosa may be deficient in the area of these fontanelles giving rise to accessory ostia. These ostia are usually round in shape, easily seen and do not have the tunnel like configuration of the maxillary ostium (Fig. 1.3).

FRONTAL RECESS

The infundibulum leads anterosuperiorly either directly and indirectly into the frontal recess (Fig. 1.4). The frontal recess is bounded anteriorly by the agger nasi cell, which is considered to be a part of the frontal recess. Therefore, the anterior wall of the frontal recess is formed by the anterior wall of the agger nasi cell. The posterior wall is formed by the bulla ethmoidalis. If there is a suprabullar recess it will open into the posterior wall of the frontal recess. The lateral wall of the frontal recess is formed by the lamina papyracea. The medial wall is formed by the middle turbinate. Superiorly the frontal recess opens via the frontal ostium into the frontal sinus. Seen in Figure 1.4, the frontal sinus opening is funnel shaped and is placed at the posterior and medial end of the floor of the frontal sinus. This funnel-shaped region is called the frontal infundibulum. Thus in sagittal cross section the frontal infundibulum, frontal ostium and the frontal recess together form the "hour-glass configuration" so often described.

Uncinate Process

The upper end of the uncinate process lies within the frontal recess. It shows great variation in anatomy. It can:
- Extend up to the base skull.
- Attach to the middle turbinate.
- May turn forwards to be attached to the insertion of the middle turbinate.
- Lie free in the middle meatus.
- May be pneumatized.

Most commonly (80%), it attaches to the lamina papyracea in the form of a dome. The recess, which is enclosed within this dome, is called the recessus terminalis. In this case, the frontal sinus opens medial to the uncinate process.

The frontal recess is subject to a large number of variations as each of its components themselves show variable anatomy. The anatomy of the frontal recess may be even more complex due to the presence of frontal cells. These are now classified into different types (Kuhn's classification).
- *Type 1:* a single cell above agger nasi cell
- *Type 2:* two or more cells above agger nasi cell which do not extend above the level of the frontal beak
- *Type 3:* any cell which extends above the level of the frontal beak which is less than 50% of height of frontal sinus
- *Type 4:* any cell which extends above the level of the frontal beak which is more than 50% of height of frontal sinus (given by DJ Wormald).
  - A frontal bulla is a cell which extends into the frontal sinus along the posterior wall of the frontal sinus. It pneumatizes from the area of suprabullar recess. It may appear as an isolated cell within the frontal sinus in a CT scan.

ETHMOID LABYRINTH

The ethmoidal cells are classified into anterior and posterior ethmoid cells depending, not so much on their actual locations, as on their drainage pattern. The anterior ethmoid cells drain into the middle meatus anterior to ground lamella. The posterior ethmoid cells drain into the superior meatus or the sphenoethmoidal recess posterior to ground lamella. The posterior ethmoid cells are fewer and larger than the anterior ethmoid cells. The posterior most ethmoid cell always overlies the sphenoid sinus for a variable distance.

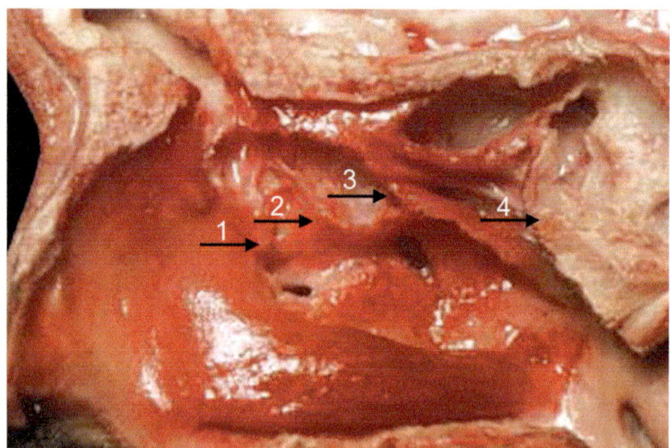

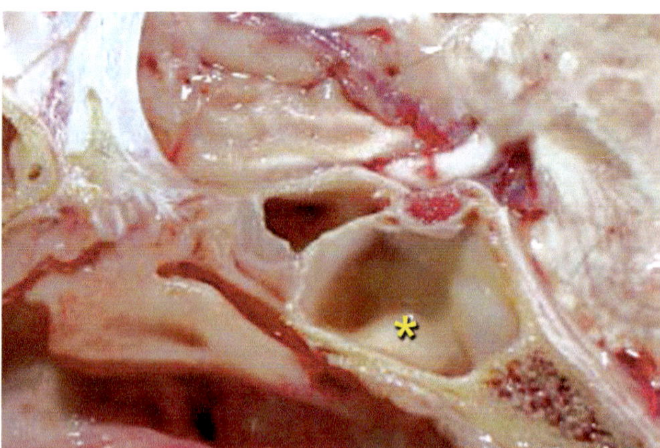

Fig. 1.5: Four lamellae (1. Uncinate process; 2. Anterior wall of bulla; 3. Ground lamella; 4. Anterior wall of sphenoid sinus)

Fig. 1.6: Sphenoid sinus shown by asterisk

Once the anterior and posterior ethmoid cells have been opened, one can appreciate the position of the four "lamellae" (Fig. 1.5). These are the uncinate process, the anterior wall of bulla, the ground lamella and the anterior wall of sphenoid sinus. Understanding the concept of these lamellae, helps the surgeons to determine the depth at which he is operating endoscopically.

SPHENOETHMOIDAL RECESS AND SPHENOID SINUS

The sphenoethmoidal recess is the region in the lateral nasal wall where the posterior ethmoid cells are related to the sphenoid sinus (Fig. 1.6). This recess contains the superior turbinate and any other supernumery turbinates, e.g. the supreme turbinate. The sphenoid ostium opens high on the anterior wall of the sphenoid into the sphenoethmoidal recess. The anterior wall of the sphenoid is relatively thinner superiorly and much thicker inferiorly at the roof of the posterior choana. The sphenoid sinus is classified into various types depending on the pneumatization (*see* Fig. 2.11).

- It may be present as a small pit in a predominantly non-pneumatized sphenoid bone, conchal type.
- It may extend up to the anterior wall of sella turcica, presellar type.
- It may pneumatize the entire sphenoid body below and behind the sella turcica, so that the pituitary forms a distinct bulge in its posterosuperior wall, sellar type.

In a highly pneumatized sphenoid sinus the lateral wall will show well-demarcated impressions of the optic nerve and the carotid artery. In 10% cases a posterior ethmoidal cell may extend posterolaterally over the sphenoid sinus for a much longer distance. This cell is then called the Onodi cell. Thus the Onodi cell when present insinuates itself between the optic nerve and the sphenoid sinus. The optic nerve therefore produces a bulge in the Onodi cell instead of in the sphenoid sinus.

Occasionally, the internal carotid artery may also present as a bulge in the lateral wall of a very large Onodi cell.

CONCLUSION

The study of the bones forming the nose and paranasal sinuses, the lateral nasal wall in a sagittal section, the endoscopic anatomy and the radiological anatomy as seen in CT scans form the four major pieces of the puzzle which completes the three-dimensional picture of nose, paranasal sinus and the skull base. Acquiring a detailed understanding of all these four components is the "rite of passage" to becoming a safe and effective endoscopic surgeon.

BIBLIOGRAPHY

1. DeLano MC, Fun FY, Zinreich SJ. Optic nerve relationship to the posterior paranasal sinuses. CT Anatomic study. Am J Neuroradiol. 1996;17:669-75. [PubMed]
2. Keros P. On the practical value of differences in the level of the lamina cribosa of the ethmoid. Z Laryngol Rhinol Otol. 1962;41:809-13.
3. Lund V. Anatomy of the nose and paranasal sinuses. In: Gleeson M, Kerr AG (Eds). Scott Brown's Otolaryngology: Basic Sciences. 6th edition. Oxford, UK: Butterworth-Heinemann. 1997;pp. 1-30.
4. Messerklinger W. Endoscopy of the nose. Baltimore, MD: Urban & Schwarzenberg; 1978.
5. Messerklinger W. On the drainage of the normal frontal sinus of man. Acta Otolaryngol. 1967;63(2):176-81.
6. Schaeffer JP. The genesis, development and adult anatomy of the nasofrontal region in man. American Journal of Anatomy. 1916;20:125-45.
7. Stammberger H. Endoscopic anatomy of lateral wall and ethmoidal sinuses. In: Stammberger H, Hawke M, (Eds). Essentials of functional endoscopic sinus surgery. St Louis: Mosby-Year Book. 1993;pp.13-42.
8. Stammberger HR, Kennedy DW. Paranasal sinuses: anatomic terminology and nomenclature. The anatomic terminology group. Ann Otol Rhinol Laryngol Suppl. 1995;167:7-16. [PubMed]

CHAPTER 2

Endoscopic Surgical Anatomy

Renuka Bradoo

"Operate on the cadaver with as much patience and meticulousness as though it were a live patient"

INTRODUCTION

The cornerstone of every safe and effective surgery is a sound knowledge of the normal anatomy and all its variations.

An exhaustive discussion of the anatomy of the lateral nasal wall as well as endoscopic anatomy of paranasal sinuses is beyond the scope of this chapter. I have therefore endeavored to present the most salient features in "bite size" capsules for ready practical references.

DIAGNOSTIC ENDOSCOPY

A thorough preoperative endoscopy not only helps to establish an overview of the area to be operated but also creates a muscle memory of the angle and trajectory in which the instruments can be easily introduced in a particular patient.

It consists of three basic passes to be carried out in a sequential manner so that no key area is missed in preoperative evaluation.

First Pass

The endoscope is passed along the floor of the nose between the inferior turbinate and the septum up to the nasopharynx (Fig. 2.1). This is usually the roomiest part of the nasal cavity. The inferior turbinate tends to have a large bulbous anterior end which tapers posteriorly to end at the posterior choana just in front of the eustachian tube orifice. The septum may show various cartilaginous and bony deviations or spurs. The roof of the posterior choana has a submucosal plexus of vessels called the Woodruff's plexus. On entering the nasopharynx one can visualize the adenoids and the opening of eustachian tube guarded by the torus tubarius, behind which lies the fossa of Rosenmüller. A 30° angled telescope can be used to visualize the opposite eustachian tube and fossa of Rosenmüller.

Second Pass

The scope is then withdrawn into the nose and tilted upwards along the roof of the posterior choana to visualize the sphenoethmoidal recess. The superior turbinate and the ostium of the sphenoid sinus can be visualized. The roof of the posterior choana, septum and the superior turbinate form an anatomical triad which help locate the sphenoid ostium. The ostium is placed close to the septum 1–1.5 cm above the roof of the posterior choana and is partially overhung by the superior turbinate (Fig. 2.2).

Third Pass

The third pass enables us to look into the structures within the middle meatus, the osteomeatal unit. The middle meatus

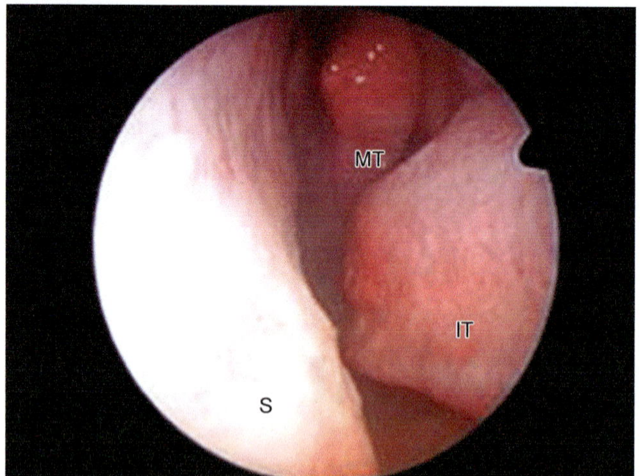

Fig. 2.1: First pass
(S-Septum, MT-Middle turbinate, IT-Inferior turbinate)

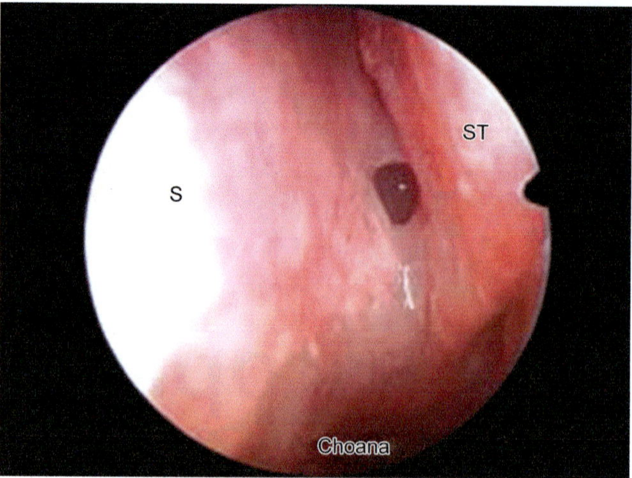

Fig. 2.2: Second pass
(S-Septum, ST-Superior turbinate)

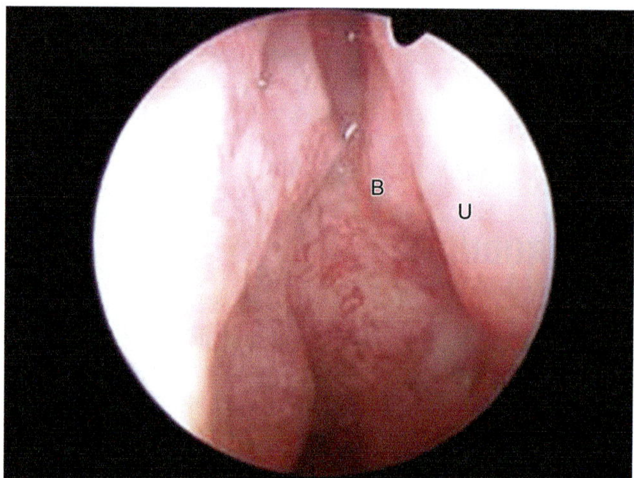

Fig. 2.3: Third pass (U-Uncinate process, B-Bulla ethmoidalis)

can be entered by retracting the middle turbinate gently. If the anterior end of the middle turbinate is bulbous and rigid, the scope can be rolled into the posterior part of the middle meatus from under the inferior edge of the middle turbinate and then withdrawn gradually to view the various structures of the middle meatus. The two main structures seen within the middle meatus are the uncinate process and the bulla ethmoidalis (Fig. 2.3). Between the two is a crescentic slit called the hiatus semilunaris inferioris. One can trace the inferior margin of the middle turbinate backward to see it turn laterally behind the bulla to attach to the lamina papyracea. This is the ground lamella.

Two other areas need to be viewed on diagnostic endoscopy. The first is the atrium, which is a relatively featureless area anterior to the middle turbinate. It shows two important anatomical landmarks. The first is the area anterior and anterosuperior to the axilla of the middle turbinate. This is the region of the lacrimal sac. If the lacrimal bone is pneumatized, then an agger nasi cell may be present which then presents as a distinct bulge in the region. The lacrimal sac extends up to at least 5–7 mm above the axilla of the middle turbinate. The second landmark is the maxillary line, which is a linear prominence extending from the bulge of the agger cell up to the peak of the attachment of the inferior turbinate to the lateral nasal wall. This line indicates the location of the nasolacrimal duct.

The second area to be examined, if possible, is the inferior meatus. The nasolacrimal duct opens in the lateral wall of the inferior meatus and is guarded by a mucosal fold, the Hasner's valve.

TURBINATES

The inferior turbinate is a separate bone unlike the superior and middle turbinate which are parts of ethmoid bone. It is

relatively straight in an anteroposterior direction. Its line of attachment to the lateral nasal wall however shows a peak or inverted "V" at the junction of anterior and middle third. This is the region at which the nasolacrimal ducts passes into the inferior meatus. The duct however does not open at the apex of the inferior meatus but runs submucosally a few mm to open in the lateral wall of the inferior meatus as stated earlier.

The anatomy of middle turbinate is easier to understand if one thinks of it as a dried-up leaf bent in various directions. The first attachment is in the sagittal plane to the cribriform plate more precisely, at the junction of the medial and lateral lamellae of the cribriform plate. It is less frequently documented that the anterior most 2–3 mm however does not attach to the cribriform plate but to the frontonasal process of the maxilla. The second attachment is in the coronal plane to the lamina papyracea, the ground lamella (the superior turbinate as well as the supreme turbinate, if present, have similar ground lamellae). The third attachment is in the horizontal plane along the perpendicular plate of the palatine bone extending up to the roof of posterior choana.

Middle Turbinate

It may show different anatomical variations:
- Quite commonly it may be ballooned out due to an air cell enclosed within it. This air cell may be pneumatized from the frontal recess, agger nasi cell or anterior ethmoids. In such a case the middle turbinate is called the concha bullosa. This balloon-like concha bullosa may block the ostiomeatal unit and the drainage of the anterior group of sinuses.
- The vertical lamella of the middle turbinate may also be pneumatized from the superior meatus to form the interlamellar cell of Grunwald.
- The middle turbinate may have a paradoxical curve bending laterally towards the middle meatus.
- Occasionally, it may be bifid.
- The ground lamella of the middle turbinate may not attach to the lamina papyracea, but may miss the lamina papyracea, pass inferiorly to it and attach to the lateral wall of the maxillary sinus instead. The maxillary sinus in this case is divided into two parts. The posterior part behaves like a posterior ethmoidal cell because it drains behind the ground lamella of the middle turbinate.
- The lower part of a normally curved middle turbinate may curve far laterally to produce a concavity within it. This concavity is called the turbinate sinus.

The superior turbinate is attached anteriorly to the middle turbinate while its posterior end partially overlies the sphenoid ostium. It overhangs a small space, the superior meatus into which open the posterior ethmoid cells. It may show variations similar to the middle turbinate like being paradoxically curved or pneumatized. The mucosa of the superior turbinate contains olfactory epithelium. However, partial resection of the turbinate during surgery does not cause any disturbance in olfaction. One or more supreme turbinate may also be occasionally found.

DISSECTION OF FRONTAL RECESS

The frontal recess is related to many critical structures like the orbit, anterior ethmoid artery and the dura. It is also subject to many anatomical variations.

When viewed from above, the frontal sinus narrows posteromedially to form a funnel-like region called the frontal infundibulum. This infundibulum leads to the frontal ostium, which in turn leads to the frontal recess in the middle

meatus. This configuration consisting of the infundibulum, the ostium, and the frontal recess has the classical "hour-glass" or "egg-cup" appearance. When viewing the opening of the frontal sinus endoscopically from within the middle meatus, one must remember that almost all of the frontal sinus lies anterior to it, as the frontal sinus ostium is in the most posterior and medial region of the frontal sinus. The thick bone of the floor frontal sinus, the frontal beak, contains no important structure.

The anterior wall of frontal recess (Fig. 2.4) is formed by the anterior wall of the agger nasi cell. The posterior wall is formed by the anterior wall of the bulla. The medial wall is formed by the middle turbinate and the lateral wall by the lamina papyracea. The uncinate process lies within the frontal recess. A variable number of frontal cells are present in the frontal recess, and these cells need to be uncapped in order to provide a wide drainage to the frontal sinus. The frontal cells are categorized depending on their number and location, with the modified Kuhn's classification being most commonly used (Refer to Chapter 1).

It is interesting to note that almost all the components of the frontal recess can show different variations. The agger cell may be absent or very large, the bulla may or may not reach up to the base of skull, the uncinate process may show variable attachments as mentioned earlier, and the number and size of the frontal cells may differ. It is therefore little wonder that the frontal recess area shows such a high interpersonal variation.

DISSECTION OF THE ETHMOID SINUS AND THE OSTIOMEATAL UNIT

Within the middle meatus lies the ostiomeatal unit (Fig. 2.5) formed mainly by the bulla ethmoidalis and the uncinate process along with the intervening space. The uncinate

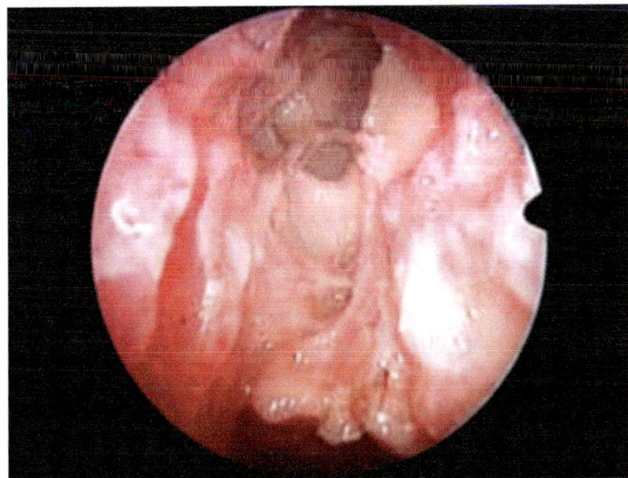

Fig. 2.4: Frontal recess

process is boomerang shaped and consists of an anterior vertical part, an intermediate part, and a posterior horizontal part. The maxillary sinus ostium most often lies lateral to the intermediate part. The uncinate process may be atrophic, flattened, and laterally rotated, in which case it is very

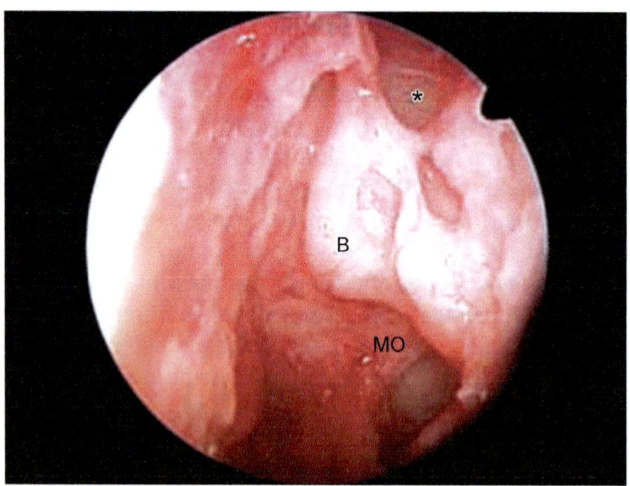

Fig. 2.5: Ostiomeatal unit (B-Bulla ethmoidalis)
* = Suprabullar recess; MO = Maxillary ostium

closely related to the lamina papyracea. On the other hand, it may be very prominent, with a distinct line indicating its attachment to the lateral nasal wall. An extremely medially rotated uncinate process may sometimes mimic a duplicated middle turbinate. The superior attachment of the uncinate process is variable, and the configuration of the frontal sinus outflow tract depends on it. In approximately 80% cases, the upper part of the uncinate process curves laterally to attach to the lamina papyracea. It encloses within it a blind recess called the recessus terminalis. When a recessus terminalis is present, the frontal sinus opens into the middle meatus, medial to this recess. It is therefore useful to remove the upper part of the uncinate process completely in order to access the frontal sinus. Occasionally, the uncinate process attaches to the base of skull or the middle turbinate, in which case the frontal sinus opens lateral to the uncinate process in the infundibulum. The uncinate process may also have multiple attachments or may itself be pneumatized (Fig. 2.6).

The bulla is the largest and most constant anterior ethmoid air cell, and although it may show variations, it is very rarely absent. It may extend all the way up to the base of skull. If the upper attachment stops short of the skull base, then the space between the skull base and the upper border of bulla is called the suprabullar recess. Posteriorly, the bulla may extend all

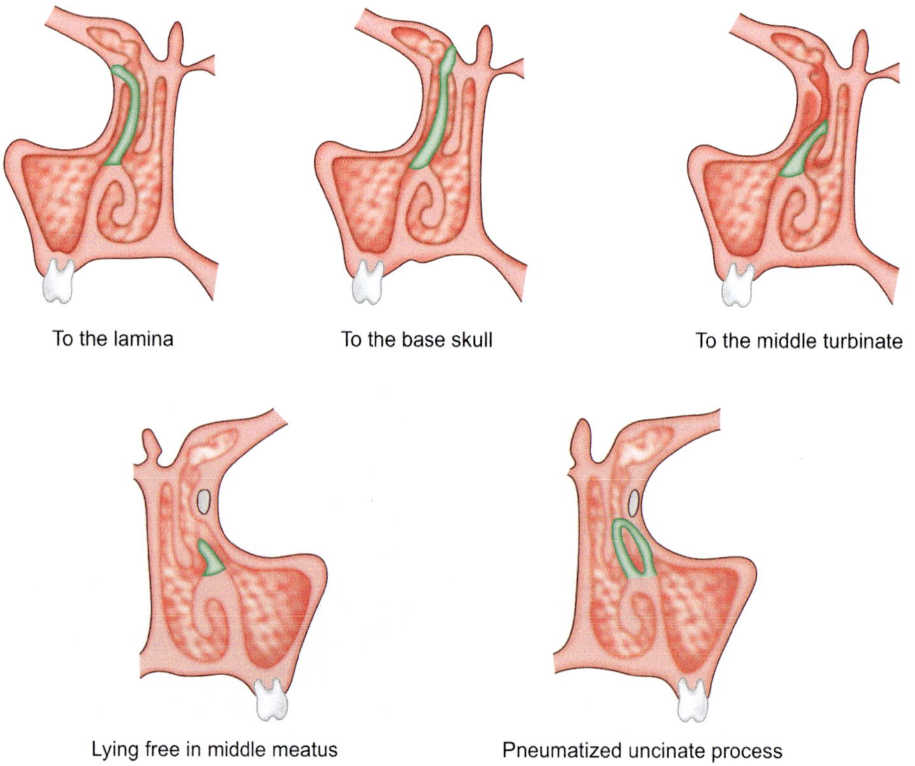

Fig. 2.6: Attachments of the uncinate

the way up to the ground lamella. If it stops short then the space between the ground lamella and the bulla is called the retrobullar recess.

The slit-like opening between the bulla and the uncinate process is the hiatus semilunaris inferioris, which leads into a tunnel-like space called the infundibulum.

The ostium of the maxillary sinus opens within the depths of this infundibulum very close to the attachment of the uncinate process. The more prominent the uncinate process, the deeper is the infundibulum, and therefore, the more relatively inaccessible is the maxillary ostium. It is therefore important to remove the entire uncinate process right up to its attachment to the lateral nasal wall in order to reveal the maxillary ostium (Fig. 2.7).

If the suprabullar and retrobullar spaces mentioned above are both present then a crescentic, slit-like opening is seen above and behind the bulla, which mirrors the hiatus semilunaris inferioris. This opening is called the hiatus semilunaris superioris, which leads to the suprabulbar and retrobulbar spaces collectively referred to as the sinus lateralis of Grunwald.

Accessory maxillary ostia may be seen in the anterior fontanelle, which lies anteroinferior to the uncinate process or in the posterior fontanelle, which is near the posterior horizontal part of the uncinate process. The accessory ostia are usually circular in shape, easily seen with a 0° endoscope, and have only two-dimensions with no depth. In contrast, the normal maxillary ostium is ovoid, tunnel like and not seen easily with a 0° endoscope as it lies in the depths of the infundibulum well hidden by the uncinate process.

The cells of the ethmoid labyrinth which open into the middle meatus are defined as the anterior ethmoid cells. For the most part they lie anterior to the ground lamella.

Occasionally, the cells may extend posteriorly to the coronal plane of the ground lamella. However, it is the pattern of their drainage rather than the actual location in relation to the ground lamella which determines their classification as the anterior ethmoid air cells.

The anterior ethmoidal artery runs obliquely in the base of the skull just behind the anterior wall of the bulla, at the point where the skull base turns from a vertical to the horizontal plane. This corresponds to the point where the vertical posterior wall of frontal sinus turns and extends backward as the cribriform plate. Since the artery lies 2–3 mm behind the anterior wall of the bulla, the intact bulla technique for the frontal recess helps to protect the anterior ethmoidal artery. However, if the anterior wall of the bulla does not reach up to the base of skull and there is a suprabullar recess, then the anterior ethmoidal artery may be damaged even in the intact bulla technique. The suprabullar recess, when present, opens into the posterior wall of the frontal recess.

Occasionally, a large cell may pneumatize the skull base along with roof of the orbit just posterior to the frontal sinus. This cell is called the supra-orbital cell and it opens into the suprabullar recess. There is usually only a thin partition between the supra-orbital cell and the frontal sinus, and very often the supra-orbital cell is mistaken for the frontal sinus in the CT scans of the paranasal sinuses. The anterior ethmoidal artery appears to lie low along the base of skull, when that region of the base of skull is pneumatized by the supra-orbital cell. In such a case, the artery usually has a bony mesentery attaching it to the base of skull or it may even be dehiscent. Dissection along the skull base in this region often shows three "openings": Those of the frontal sinus, the suprabullar recess, and the supra-orbital cells.

DISSECTION OF POSTERIOR ETHMOID CELLS

The ground lamella (Fig. 2.0) of the middle turbinate is an important landmark as it demarcates the anterior from the posterior ethmoidal cells. It is subject to many variations. It may be bowed anteriorly or posteriorly, may be pneumatized, or may be occasionally absent. It may occasionally "miss" the lamina papyracea completely and get attached to the lateral wall of the maxillary sinus. Or removing the ground lamella, one can see the posterior ethmoidal cells, which are often larger and fewer than the anterior ethmoidal cells. The posterior ethmoidal artery is sometimes seen running along the base of skull in the region of the posterior ethmoidal cells behind the ground lamella.

The most posterior ethmoid cell is easily recognized as it has a very characteristic appearance. It is pyramidal in shape and tapers to an apex away from the viewer's eye. It always

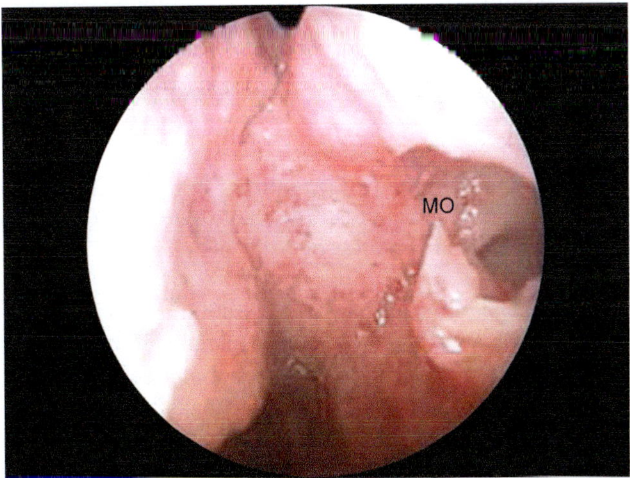

Fig. 2.7: Maxillary ostium (MO)

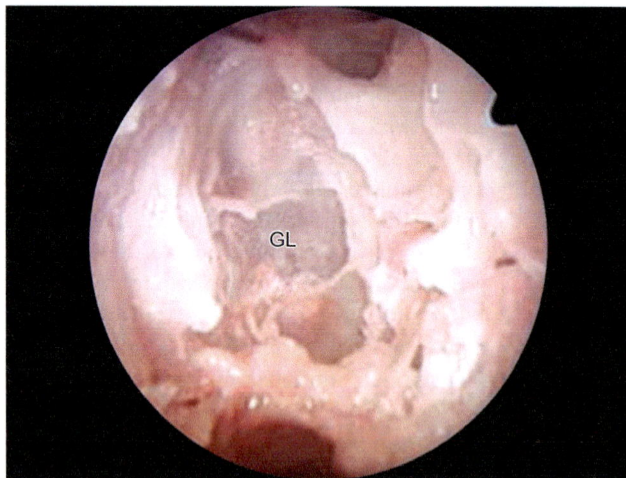

Fig. 2.8: Ground lamella (GL)

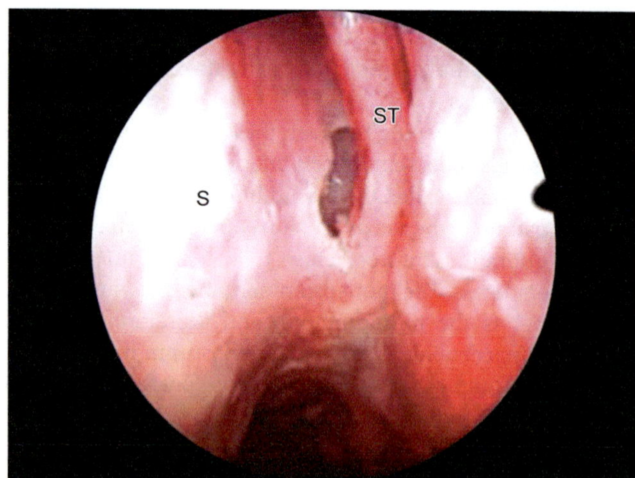

Fig. 2.9: Medial approach
(S-Septum, ST-Superior turbinate)

partially overlies the sphenoid, and hence, the sphenoid is related inferomedially to this cell. Occasionally, this cell may pneumatize over the sphenoid sinus to a greater extent. In this case, the optic nerve which routinely lies in the superolateral wall of the sphenoid, can then be related to the lateral wall of this ethmoid cell. Such a cell, which tends to "separate" the optic nerve from the sphenoid sinus, is called the Onodi cell. The optic nerve is often dehiscent in such cases. The internal carotid artery may also be seen as a bulge in the lateral wall of an extremely large Onodi cell.

"WANDERING" CELLS

The cells of the ethmoid labyrinth may "wander" and pneumatize the surrounding bones such as the lacrimal bone and sphenoid. Anterior ethmoid cells that pneumatize the lacrimal bone and the frontonasal process of maxilla anteriorly form the agger nasi cell. Similarly, if this pneumatization extends superiorly into the region of the frontal recess and the bony floor of the frontal sinus, it would form different types of frontal cells. Further pneumatization in this direction will form a pneumatized crista galli. An anterior ethmoid cell, which pneumatizes the floor of the orbit at the level of the infundibulum is the Haller cell; and one that pneumatizes the roof of the orbit behind the wall of the frontal sinus is the supra-orbital cell. A posterior ethmoid cell that pneumatizes the middle turbinate forms the concha bullosa, and one that extends backward from the posterior ethmoid cells over the sphenoid forms the Onodi cell.

Once all the posterior ethmoid cells are removed, one can delineate the entire lamina papyracea and ethmoid fovea or the skull base. Anteriorly, the lamina papyracea is related to the orbital fat, but posteriorly, the medial rectus is very often in direct contact with the lamina papyracea. The ethmoid

fovea is formed partially by the frontal bone and partially by the lateral lamella of the cribriform plate. The superolateral part, which is formed by the frontal bone, is much thicker than the medial portion formed, which is formed by the lateral lamella. The thinnest part of the base of skull is where the anterior ethmoidal artery passes through the lateral lamella of the cribriform plate into the anterior cranial fossa.

DISSECTION OF SPHENOID SINUS

The sphenoid sinus can be approached endoscopically in three ways. These are called the medial, lateral, and intermediate approaches with respect to the middle turbinate.

The medial approach (Fig. 2.9) is used to access the sphenoid sinus medial to the middle turbinate via the sphenoid ostium. The sphenoid ostium is identified as mentioned earlier, and the anterior wall of sphenoid is removed in an inferior direction. The septal branch of sphenopalatine artery runs across the anterior face of the sphenoid just above the roof of the posterior choana.

The lateral approach (Fig. 2.10) is through the posterior ethmoidal cells. The sphenoid is opened in an inferomedial direction through the posterior-most ethmoid cell. The bony partition between the two is removed to widen the opening of the sphenoid sinus. It is important to note that this bony partition is in an oblique or axial plane rather than in a coronal plane.

The sphenoid sinus is very different in appearance from the posterior-most ethmoid cell. While the ethmoidal cell is pyramidal in shape, the sphenoid is globular, like the inside of a large pot. Another landmark is the "maxillary ridge" which is a surgical landmark formed at the junction of the lamina papyracea and the floor of the orbit. If this ridge is extrapolated backward, then those cells which open above the level of this

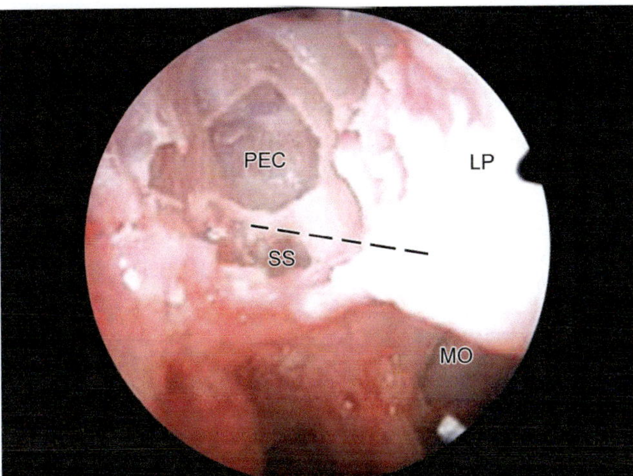

Fig. 2.10: Lateral approach (SS-Sphenoid sinus, PEC-Posterior ethmoidal cell, LP-Lamina papyracea, MO-Maxillary ostium)

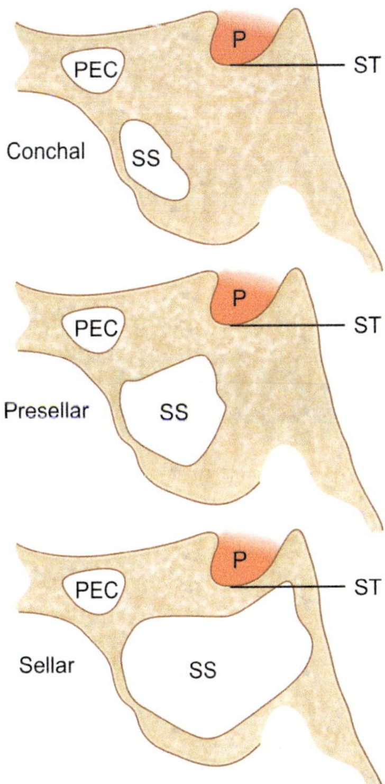

Fig. 2.11: Pneumatization of sphenoid sinus (PEC-Posterior ethmoidal cell, SS-Sphenoid sinus, P-Pituitary, ST-Sella turcica)

ridge are posterior ethmoid cells. The cell that opens below the level of this ridge is usually the sphenoid sinus.

The intermediate approach is through the middle turbinate. The turbinate is perforated a few millimeters behind the ground lamella to enter the sphenoethmoidal recess and then access the sphenoid sinus. The inferior portion of the superior turbinate very often needs to be trimmed to get access to the sphenoid sinus and to communicate the lateral sphenoid opening with the normal ostium.

The sphenoid sinus may vary in pneumatization from a small conchal sinus (Fig. 2.11) to a large sellar sinus.

The structures related to the lateral and superior wall of the sphenoid sinus can best be studied in a well pneumatized sinus. The lateral wall is related above to the optic nerve and inferoposteriorly to the internal carotid artery. A small recess is present between these two structures, which is called the opticocarotid recess. This recess is very deep if the anterior clinoid process is pneumatized. Anterior to the pituitary sella is the planum sphenoidale and it forms the lowest level of the base of the skull. If there is large lateral recess present then the vidian nerve and maxillary nerve may also be seen as ridges along the inferior and superior walls of the lateral recess, respectively.

Although the sphenoid rostrum is always in midline, the intersphenoid septum very often lies to one side, making one sphenoid much larger than the other. The larger sphenoid is called the dominant sphenoid. Intrasphenoid septae often tend to attach to important structures such as the optic nerve and carotid artery, and therefore, they should not be avulsed.

In conclusion, it is important to remember that endoscopic cadaveric dissection should always be performed in "layers". Removal of each layer will reveal different anatomical landmarks which need to be studied in detail before proceeding to the next deeper layer of cells.

BIBLIOGRAPHY

1. Bolger WE, Butzin CA, Parsons DS. Paranasal sinus bony anatomic variations and mucosal abnormalities: CT analysis for endoscopic sinus surgery. Laryngoscope. 1991;101:56-64. [PubMed]
2. Braun H, Stammberger H. Pneumatization of turbinates. Laryngoscope. 2003;113:668-72. [PubMed]
3. DeLano MC, Fun FY, Zinreich SJ. Optic nerve relationship to the posterior paranasal sinuses. CT anatomic study. Am J Neuroradiol. 1996;17:669-75. [PubMed]
4. Keros P. On the practical value of differences in the level of the lamina cribosa of the ethmoid. Z Laryngol Rhinol Otol. 1962;41:809-13.
5. Lund V. Anatomy of the nose and paranasal sinuses. In: Gleeson M, Kerr AG (Eds). Scott Brown's Otolaryngology: Basic Sciences. 6th edition. Oxford, UK: Butterworth-Heinemann. 1997;pp. 1-30.
6. Messerklinger W. On the drainage of the normal frontal sinus of man. Acta Otolaryngol. 1967;63(2):176-81.
7. Messerklinger W. Endoscopy of the nose. Baltimore, MD: Urban & Schwarzenberg; 1978.
8. Stammberger H. Endoscopic anatomy of lateral wall and ethmoidal sinuses. In: Stammberger H, Hawke M (Eds). Essentials of functional endoscopic sinus surgery. St Louis: Mosby-Year Book. 1993;pp.13-42.
9. Wormald PJ. The agger nasi cell: the key to understanding the anatomy of the frontal recess. Otolaryngology—Head and Neck Surgery. 2003;129(5):497-507. [PubMed]

CHAPTER 3

Imaging for Paranasal Sinuses

Nishit J Shah, Sunita Kanojia

INTRODUCTION

Earlier, conventional X-rays were done for all pathology of the paranasal sinuses. But with advancements in surgical techniques of sinus surgery, precise knowledge of the anatomy became essential. Structural superimposition and difficulty in differentiating the pathologies in an opacified sinus, do not permit a detailed study of the anatomy and disease pathology of the sinuses, which is important from the point of view of endoscopic sinus surgery.

Computed tomography (CT) scan helps in creating the intraoperative road maps providing precise[1] knowledge of the paranasal sinus anatomy and its anatomical variants and also helps in differentiating the sinus pathologies and their extension into the surrounding structures.

The use of CT scan combined with functional endoscopic sinus surgery has empowered the surgeon to treat patients more effectively with reduced complications and better results. As in all radiologic surveys, sinus CT scans must be read with a systematic approach.

- Ideally the scan should be at 1 mm intervals in all the three planes. In our center 1 mm cut intervals are used for cerebrospinal fluid (CSF) cases and for other cases it is 2 mm intervals in bone windows. Soft tissue cuts in coronal only are adequate to differentiate allergic fungal sinusitis (AFS) and other pathologies.
- The timing of CT scanning can have a significant impact on the correlation of CT findings and should be done once acute or reversible problems are treated to obtain maximum diagnostic yield. We usually recommend doing the scan just before the surgery.
- It is advised to blow the nose to clear out the secretions and use nasal decongestant drops to reduce the congestion due to nasal cycle just before the CT scan procedure which can be mistaken for turbinate hypertrophy.

PRE-FESS CT CHECKLIST

A systematic approach is helpful when interpreting CT scans. Reading the CT scan from anterior to posterior (on coronal views), from top to bottom (on axial sections) or from lateral to medial (sagittal sections) helps to organize one's approach in analyzing the structures to be interpreted. For initial orientation, number of important paranasal sinus structures are identified.

Coronal View

Structures Better seen on the Coronal Scan

- Nasolacrimal duct system
- Nasal septum
- *Inferior turbinate:* Hypertrophy
- *Frontal sinus:* Degree of pneumatization, interfrontal sinus septal cell and its drainage.
- Frontal recess air cells[2,3]
  - Agger nasi cells
  - *Frontal cells:* Type 1, 2, 3, 4
- Medial cells
  - Supraorbital cells
  - Frontal bullar cells

- *Middle turbinate:* Attachment/variations, horizontal ground lamella.
- *Uncinate:* Attachments, rotations
- *Maxillary sinus:* Ostiomeatal complex, degree of pneumatization, Haller cells, infraorbital nerve canal, septations in the sinus, roof of maxillary sinus, presence of foreign body in the sinus.
- *Ethmoidal cells:* Ethmoidal bulla, anterior and posterior ethmoidal cells.
- *Lamina papyracea:* Dehiscence in the lamina papyracea, shape of the medial orbital wall
- *Skull base area:* Cribriform area with Keros classification,[4] slope, thickness, and asymmetries in the height of the ethmoidal fovea and planum.
- *Anterior and posterior ethmoidal artery:* Position and dehiscence, bony mesentry.
- *Sphenoid sinus:* Intersphenoid septum attachment, sphenoid dominance, degree of pneumatization, relation to optic nerve
- Nasopharynx
- Vidian canal
- Sphenopalatine foramen
- Orbit.

Axial View

Structures Better seen on the Axial Scan

- Frontal sinus with frontal sinus drainage pathway
- Anterior and posterior walls of frontal sinus
- All walls of maxillary sinus
- Status of lamina papyracea along the entire length
- Basal lamella of the middle turbinate
- *Sphenoid sinus:* Degree of pneumatization, intersphenoid septum attachment.
- Onodi cell
- Relation of optic nerve and carotid artery to ethmoid cell and sphenoid sinus.
- Pterygopalatine fossa area, infratemporal fossa area, foramen rotundum
- Fossa of Rosenmüllar, eustachian tube area.
- Nasolacrimal duct
- Orbit.

Sagittal View

Structures Better seen on Sagittal Scan

- Frontal sinus walls and its drainage pathways
- Frontal cells and its relation to frontal sinus
- Frontal bullar cell, supraorbital cell better defined on sagittal scan

- Retro and suprabullar recesses
- Extent of Onodi cell and its content
- Sphenoid sinus ostium
- Pattern of pneumatization of sphenoid sinus
- Clival area
- Vertical segment of carotid artery.

HOW TO APPROACH CT SCAN READING?

A systematic approach is needed to start reading the scan. Let us start in a stepwise manner.

Step 1

- After placing the scan, ensure that it is of the same patient's scan, the sides are marked.
- Do the pre-FESS CT checklist as described for all the three planes identifying the important paranasal sinus structures, any anatomical variations and the disease pathology.
- Always read one side at a time.

Step 2

Plan the steps of the surgical procedures and the difficulties which can be encountered due to anatomical variations of paranasal sinuses.

Discussion of Surgical Approach with Respect to CT Scan Reading

Frontal Sinus Approach and Role of CT Scan

We will describe the left side of the patient's scans (Figs 3.1 to 3.3):

- All the three planes are required to study the frontal sinus drainage, i e. coronal, axial, sagittal scans.
- The frontal drainage pathway is studied with respect to frontal air cells. Anterior or posterior drainage is studied on coronal scans and medial or lateral drainage on axial scans.
- Type and number of frontal air cells better visualized on sagittal scan.

> Important points to be noted:
> - Degree of pneumatization of frontal sinus
> - Frontal beak
> - Degree of pneumatization of agger nasi cell
> - Types of frontal cells, presence of other frontal recess air cells and type of drainage in relation to the frontal cells
> - Interfrontal sinus septal cell and its drainage.

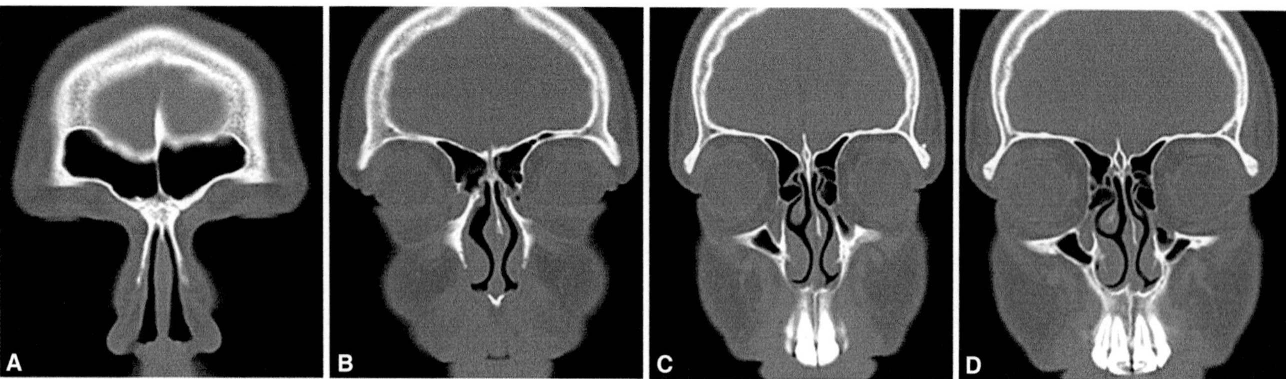

Figs 3.1A to D: *Coronal view.* (A) shows well-pneumatized left side frontal sinus with interfrontal septum attached to the midline. The frontonasal process of maxilla is seen attached to nasal bone. As we go posterior, (B) shows anterior drainage of the frontal sinus medial to the frontal cell. Lacrimal sac is seen lateral to the frontonasal process of maxilla. Further posterior (C) shows agger cell with one cell seen above it (type 1 frontal cell). (D) shows vertical attachment of the uncinate process to the lamina papyracea. Continuation of frontal cell is seen as a small medial attachment at the superior aspect of the middle turbinate

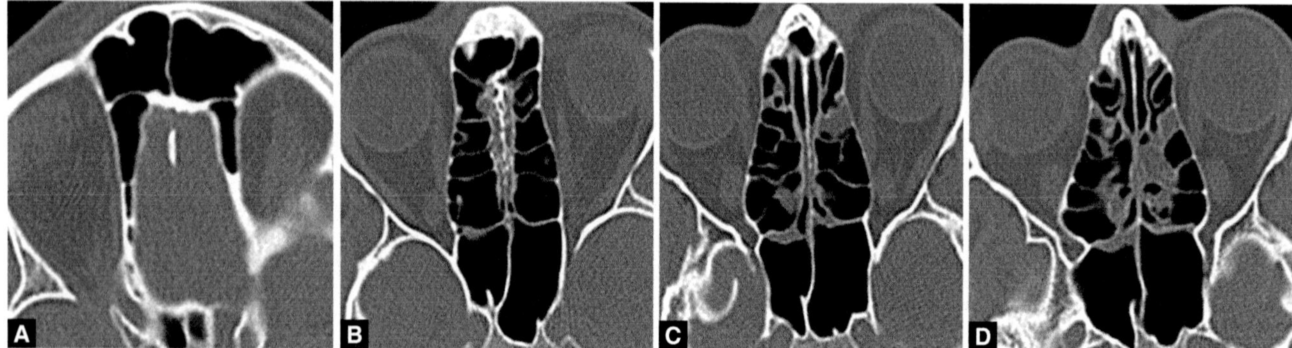

Figs 3.2A to D: *Axial view.* (A) Left side shows well-pneumatized frontal sinus with supraorbital cell. At this level, the cell appearing posterior to the frontal sinus is either suprabullar, frontal bullar or supraorbital cell. From the sagittal scan, we know the cell is suprabullar cell with pneumatization over the orbit. As we go inferiorly; (B) shows appearance of type 1 frontal cell. With more inferior scans frontal sinus drainage is seen medial to the frontal cell in (C) and agger cell in (D)

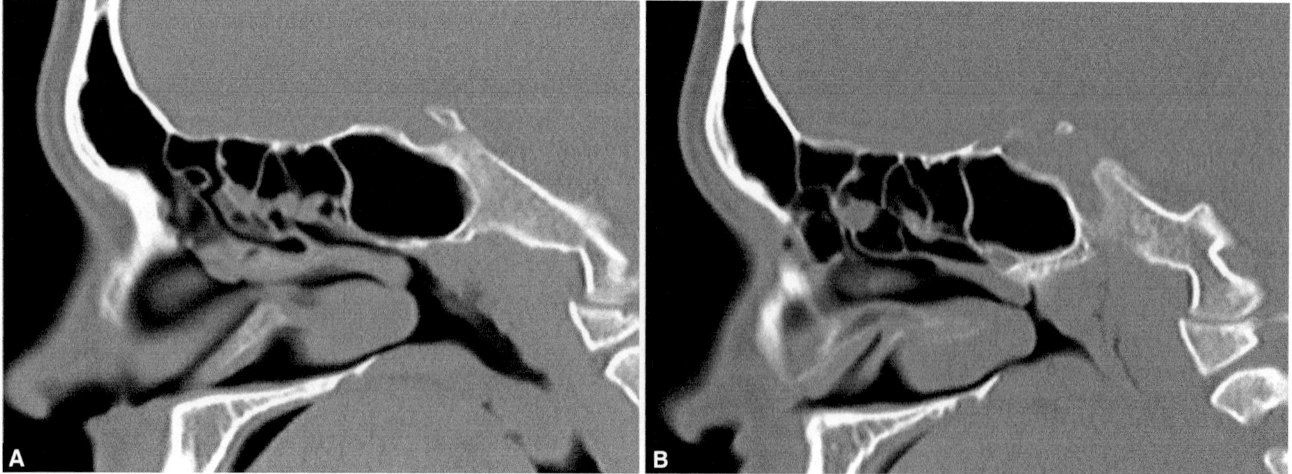

Figs 3.3A and B: *Sagittal view.* (A) medial image shows left side anterior drainage of frontal sinus to the suprabullar cell; (B) shows well-pneumatized agger cell with small type 1 frontal cell above it and suprabullar cell just superior to the frontal cell

From the Above Scans

- It is a well-pneumatized frontal sinus. Anteriorly agger cell with small type 1 frontal cell is present and posteriorly supraorbital and suprabullar cell with pneumatization till the frontal sinus ostium are seen blocking the posterior frontal sinus pathway.
- As the frontal sinus drainage pathway is followed in the coronal, axial and sagittal scans, the frontal sinus drains in the anterior and medial part of frontal recess; so the drainage of the frontal sinus is anteromedial drainage which is best seen on axial and sagittal scans.
- Sagittal scan shows good anteroposterior diameter of the frontal recess.

> **Surgical approach**
>
> - After meticulous uncinectomy, appearance of the agger nasi cell will be seen. Take Kuhn's straight curette; fracture the medial and posterior walls of the cell. With the help of debrider, agger and frontal cells are cleared, and the frontal drainage pathway identified in the anteromedial part of the frontal recess. The suprabullar cell is opened. With 45 degree scope frontal sinus opening is identified and the surrounding cells cleared; widening the frontal sinus opening.
> - In case of difficulty in instrumenting or using an angled scope, one could clear the suprabullar cell and then go back to frontal sinus surgery.

Approach to Maxillary Sinus Ostium and Role of CT Scan (Figs 3.4A and B)

- Coronal and axial scan images are best for evaluation of maxillary sinuses.
- Posterior, anterolateral and medial walls of maxillary sinus are studied on the axial scan.
- Haller cells are appreciated on coronal images.

> Important points to be noted:
> - Attachment of horizontal process of uncinate process to the inferior turbinate
> - Degree of pneumatization of maxillary sinus
> - Location of ostiomeatal unit
> - Presence of accessory ostia
> - Infraorbital nerve position and its dehiscence
> - Presence of Haller cell

From the Scans Below

- It is a well-pneumatized maxillary sinus with blocked ostiomeatal unit. There is no medial or lateral rotation of uncinate process.
- The walls of the maxillary sinus are intact.
- There is no Haller cell or accessory ostia cell present.
- The infraorbital canal is intact.

> **Surgical approach**
>
> First lateralize the inferior turbinate with the help of elevator. This will fracture the superior bent of the inferior turbinate creating more space for entry of the back bitter in the middle meatus. Since there is no lateral rotation of the uncinate process, uncinectomy can also be done with the conventional technique to open the maxillary sinus ostium.

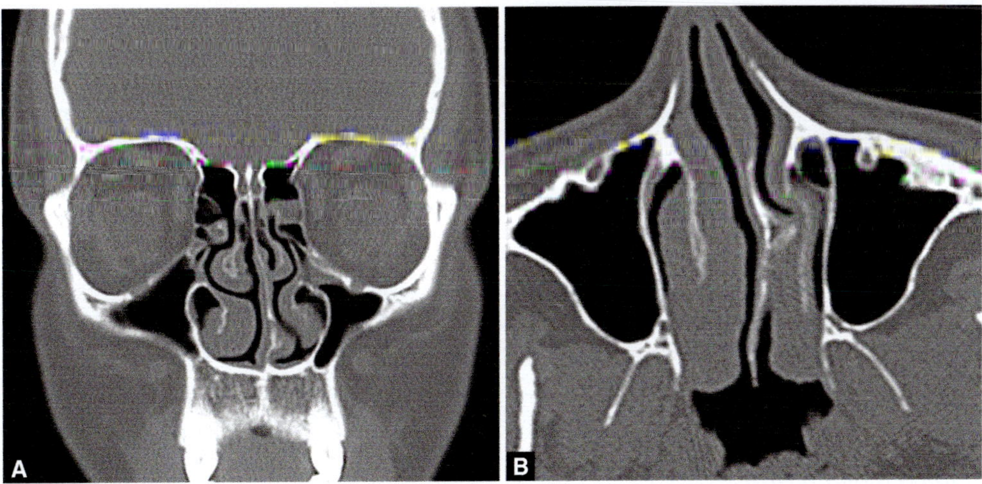

Figs 3.4A and B: *CT scans.* (A) shows pneumatized maxillary sinus with the osteomeatal unit showing the free posterior edge of uncinate process, ethmoidal bulla, infundibulum and blocked maxillary sinus ostium is seen. There is no medial or lateral rotation of the uncinate process, (B) shows well pneumatized maxillary sinus, infraorbital nerve with intact bony canal and nasolacrimal duct opening close to the inferior turbinate. The posterolateral, medial and anterior wall of the sinus is seen

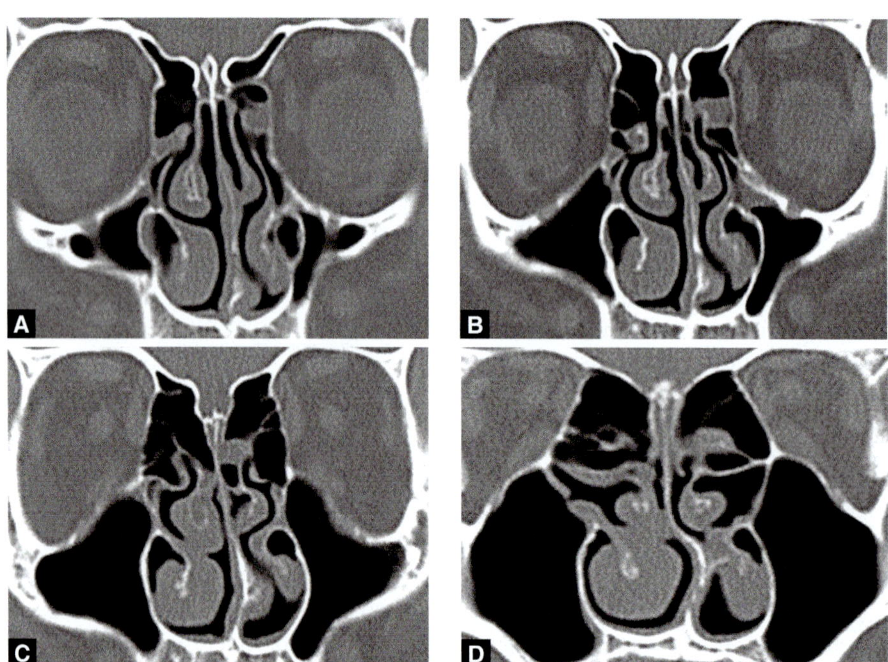

Figs 3.5A to D: *Coronal views.* (A) shows appearance of ethmoidal bulla with beaking of anterior ethmoidal artery hanging in the bony mesentry on the left side under the supraorbital cell which can be seen pneumatizing slightly over the orbit. (B) shows continuation of ethmoid bulla and suprabullar cell. (C) shows another anterior ethmoidal cell above the bulla which can be confirmed on axial and sagittal scan. (D) shows attachment of the ground lamella to lamina papyracea with septal spur indenting the inferior turbinate. Also seen, is the appearance of superior turbinate and two posterior ethmoidal cell above the ground lamella

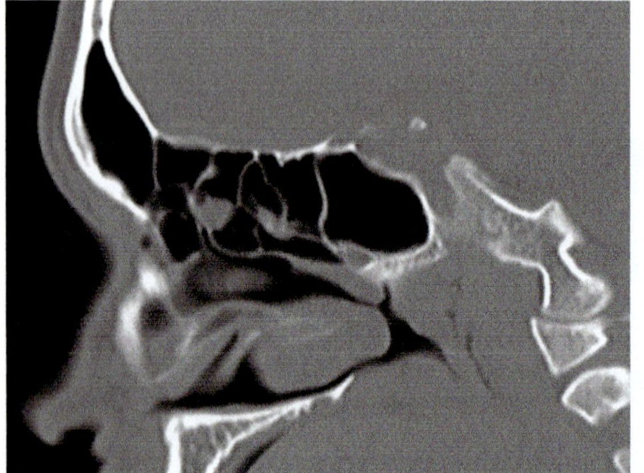

Fig. 3.6: *Sagittal view.* In this figure, bulla with two cells above it anterior to the ground lamella seen. Two posterior ethmoidal cells seen

Approach to the Ethmoid Sinus and Role of CT Scan (Figs 3.5 and 3.6)

- Scans in all the three planes required to study the ethmoidal air cells.
- However, suprabullar cells, retrobullar recess and Onodi cells are best appreciated on sagittal and axial scans, lamina papyracea best read on axial scans, Haller cells, anterior and posterior ethmoidal artey, skull base anatomy better seen on the coronal scan.

> Important points to be noted:
> - Number of anterior and posterior ethmoid air cells
> - Presence of supraorbital, Haller and Onodi cells
> - Dehiscence and bulging of lamina papyracea
> - Level of skull base and olfactory fossa
> - Position of anterior and posterior ethmoidal artery from the skull base
> - The level of the ground lamella and its pneumatization and bulging into anterior or posterior ethmoidal air cells.

From the Above Scans

- It is a well-pneumatized bulla with two cells above the bulla. Two posterior ethmoidal air cells are also seen.
- Shows anterior ethmoidal artery hanging in the bony mesentry.
- There is no dehiscence of lamina papyracea or low lying skull base with type 2 Keros olfactory fossa.

Surgical approach

With the help of straight curette or elevator, bulla is entered. Ethmoid forcep or debrider is used to remove the bulla and other ethmoidal cells. As there is no low lying skull base, ground lamella can be entered safely to open the posterior ethmoid cell. From the scan, we know there is one more cell behind this posterior cell, which is also opened. The posterior limit of this cell is the anterior face of sphenoid sinus. We use ring curette to clear the cell walls around the skull base and along the lamina papyracea. The ring curette has broader base, thus decreasing the chance of skull base penetration and with the help of sharp edges the cell walls are fractured without pulling the mucosa. As we go from posterior to anterior direction, suprabullar cells are removed and anterior ethmoidal artery identified. Since it is hanging anterior ethmoidal artery, chances of injury to the artery is high. It is safer to use ring curette or Kuhn's curette to fracture the cell walls and debrider should be used with caution in this area.

Approach to the Sphenoid Sinus and Role of CT Scan (Figs 3.7 and 3.8)

- Coronal, axial and sagittal scans are required to study the sphenoid sinus in detail.

- The degree of pneumatization, sellar area, relation of Onodi cell to sphenoid sinus and vertical part of carotid artery is best seen on axial scan.
- The optic nerve, carotid artey and intersphenoidal septum attachment are better studied on axial scan.

Important points to be noted:
- Degree of pneumatization of sphenoid sinus
- Sphenoidal dominance, inter- and intra-sphenoidal septum attachment to important structures
- Optic nerve and carotid artery and their dehiscence
- Sphenoid ostium opening
- Clival area and presence of onodi cell

From the Below Scans

- It shows left sphenoid dominance with pneumatization extending below the sella and into the pterygoid body.
- The intersphenoid septum is more or less in the midline anteriorly, but turns to the right to attach to the right internal carotid artery posteriorly.

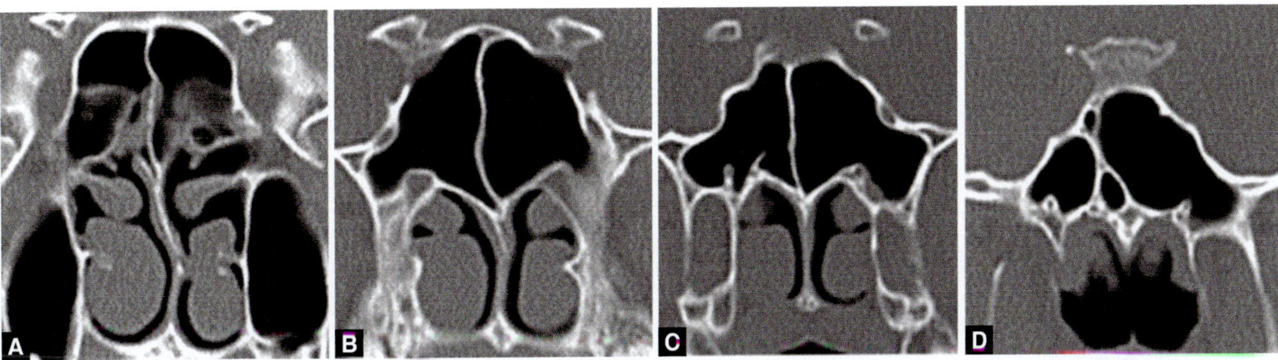

Figs 3.7A to D: *Coronal view.* (A) shows sphenopalatine foramen and start of the optic nerve. (B) shows well pneumatized sphenoid sinus with intersphenoid septum in the midline. Optic nerve and carotid artery bulge seen. (C) shows bulge of sella on the superior aspect, prominent bulge of foramen rotundum and vidian canal. Lateral pneumatization of sphenoid into pterygoids seen. (D) shows intrasphenoid septum attached on the right side, ending on the right vertical internal carotid artery

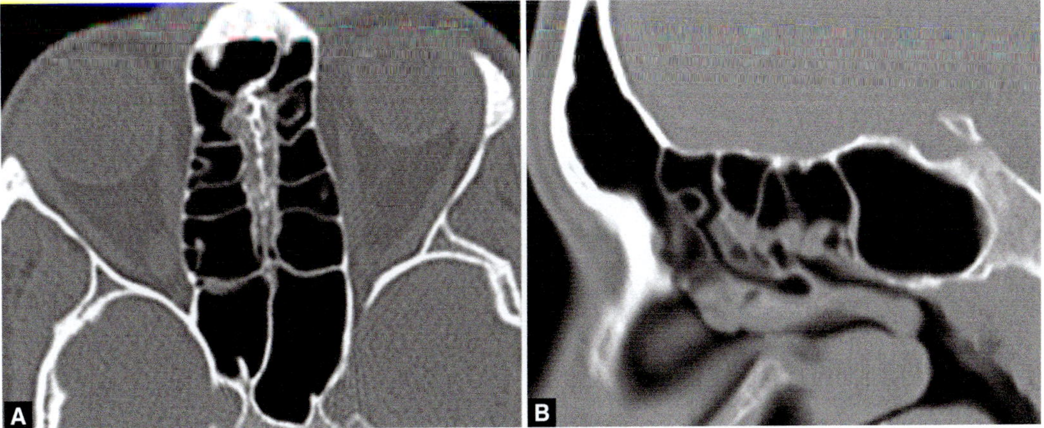

Figs 3.8A and B: (A) shows bulge of internal carotid artery. The intersphenoid septum attaches to right carotid artery. (B) shows sphenoid pneumatization extending under the sella

- There is no dehiscence of the bone over the carotid artery and optic nerve.
- There is prominent bulge of vidian canal and foramen rotundum.
- Onodi cell is not present.

> **Surgical approach**
>
> Since it is a well-pneumatized sphenoid sinus, any three approaches, i.e. lateral, medial and intermediate approach can be used to enter the sphenoid sinus and depends on the surgeon's skill and comfort. We recommend medial and intermediate approach for the beginners and lateral approach can be used by the skilled surgeon provided the landmarks are followed.

CONCLUSION

If one approaches scan reading in a systematic and thorough way, then you are more likely to have a better understanding of anatomy and pathology, enabling you to perform a complete and safer sinus surgery.

REFERENCES

1. Pinas P, Sabate J, Carmona A, Cataline-Herrera CJ, Jimenez-Castellanos. Anatomical variations in the human paranasal sinus region studied by CT. J Anal. 2000;197:221-7.
2. Lee WT, Kuhn FA, Citard MJ. 3D computed tomographic analysis of frontal recess anatomy in patients without frontal sinusitis. Otolaryngol Head Neck Surg. 2004;131:164-73.
3. Bent JP, Cuilty-Siller C, Kuhn FA. The frontal cell as a cause of frontal sinus obstruction. Am J Rhinol. 1994;8:185-91.
4. Keeros P. On the practical value of differences in the level of the lamina cribrose of the ethmoid. Z Laryngol Rhinol Otol. 1962;41:809-13.

CHAPTER 4

Preoperative Preparation of Functional Endoscopic Sinus Surgery

Arpit Sharma

INTRODUCTION

Endoscopic sinus surgery is indicated in patients of chronic rhinosinusitis who have failed to respond to maximal medical therapy. The surgery should not be performed as an alternative to medical therapy, but rather to augment the medical therapy, reduce recurrent infections, and improve overall quality of life.[1]

Functional endoscopic sinus surgery (FESS) is associated with significantly lower morbidity and higher success rates than previous open surgical approaches. Mucosal integrity is maximally preserved so that healing occurs quickly and normal mucociliary transport is restored.[2,3] However, surgery alone is rarely curative and needs to be combined with intensive medical therapy in the postoperative period. Persistent asymptomatic disease is common after surgical intervention and the goal of therapy has shifted away from short-term symptomatic improvement toward long-term disease resolution.[4] This requires continued medical therapy after surgery, endoscopic surveillance, and management of environmental and general host factors that may predispose to disease.

INDICATIONS OF SURGERY

- Chronic rhinosinusitis poorly responding to maximal medical therapy
- Nasal polyposis poorly responding to medical therapy
- Patients with chronic sinusitis and worsening asthma
- Acute sinusitis with threatened complications
- Recurrent acute sinusitis:
  - More than four times per year (adults)
  - Persistent computed tomography (CT) findings
- Allergic fungal sinusitis
- Mucoceles, tumors
- Antrochoanal polyp.

GOALS OF SURGERY

Endoscopic sinus surgery aims to reduce the disease in patients with rhinosinusitis by:
- Removal of pathological tissue from ostiomeatal complex area, which helps in restoration of mucociliary function of sinus mucosa
- Ventilation of sinuses that helps in reduction of number of mucosal glands and goblet cells population leading to decreased nasal secretions
- Clearing the pathway for better delivery and distribution of topical nasal medication in the nose and sinus mucosa
- Reduction of diseased sinus mucosa surface area by removal of polypoidal disease
- Improvement of olfaction by opening superior meatus and sphenoethmoid recess
- Relief from the nasal obstruction in cases with gross surgical anatomic variations such as concha bullosa or big spur.

PATIENT MANAGEMENT BEFORE SURGERY

Preoperative Evaluation

Key Points

- *History taking:* Chief complaints—Comorbidities, details of medical treatment received
- *Nasal examination:* Anterior rhinoscopy, endoscopy
- *Radiological investigation:* CT scan paranasal sinuses
- *Counseling:* Nature of disease, available treatment options, benefit and limitations of surgery, postoperative care, postoperative medical treatment, chances of success/failure, potential complications
- Informed consent.

Preoperative Medical Treatment

The aim is to reduce the inflammation and optimize the nasal mucosa which reduces bleeding.
- Consider oral steroids (30 mg prednisone for 3–5 days)
- Consider oral antibiotics
- Antihistamines and intranasal steroid spray are added in patients who give history of nasal allergy
- Oral steroids and steroid spray started in patients with polyposis
- Off aspirin (10–14 days)
- Off ibuprofen and other NSAIDs (5 days).

Anesthesia for Endoscopic Sinus Surgery

Generally done in general anesthesia, with mean arterial pressure between 60 mm Hg and 80 mm Hg and pulse rate below 70/minute.
- Preoperative β-blockers, clonidine and sedation can be given to allay anxiety and help in controlling blood pressure and pulse rate
- Intraoperative β-blockers and/or clonidine is given to avoid tachycardia. A pulse rate around 60/minute usually gives acceptable results
- Appropriate plane of anesthesia is recommended to avoid pain, awareness and bleeding during surgery
- It is better to avoid use of nitroprusside and nitroglycerine-like drugs to induce hypotension because they cause tachycardia and more diffuse oozing
- A head elevated position during surgery reduces venous congestion and diminishes bleeding
- Use anesthetic gases and drugs that are compatible with adrenaline
- An optimum sized endotracheal tube with good oxygenation and carbon dioxide washout is desirable.

Preparation of Nasal Cavity

Nasal packing with cotton patties soaked in 4% xylocaine with 1:1,000 adrenaline. Local infiltration with 2% xylocaine with 1:100,000 adrenaline with 24 gauge spinal needle, usual sites being above the anterior end of middle turbinate, just below and lateral to posterior end of middle turbinate and uncinate process.

Preoperative CT Scan Checklist

- Lamina papyracea dehiscence
- Kero's classification of skull base and any dehiscence in skull base
- Position of anterior ethmoidal artery and the mesentery
- Onodi cell and optic nerve.

In chronic rhinosinusitis (CRS) patients with nasal polyps, mucosal inflammatory response is more florid than in those without, and the rate of relapse after surgery for nasal polyps tends to be higher. FESS improves symptoms in nasal polyposis by removal of inflammatory tissue and reduction of the load of antigens inciting that inflammation, as well as the improvement of sinus ventilation and mucociliary clearance.

Endoscopic sinus surgery for nasal polyposis has been generally reported to be a safe and effective procedure.

POSTOPERATIVE MANAGEMENT

A significant postoperative care is required to achieve the goals of surgery and to ensure long-term results. Inflammation of CRS does not resolve immediately after surgery plus surgery itself results in scarring. So the aim of postoperative treatment is to treat the inflammation. This can be achieved by:
- Antibiotics (usually for 2 or more weeks)
- Nasal saline spray, alkaline nasal douching
- Long-term topical nasal steroids
- Slowly tapering oral steroids (in patients with diffuse polyposis)
- Possible antihistaminics
- Possible antileukotrienes
- Avoidance of allergens and environmental allergens

Also patient should be followed up with nasal endoscopy. The patients are usually seen 7 days after the surgery and then on a weekly or two weekly basis till healing is achieved. For the purpose of audit, the patients are seen at least at 3, 6, 12 and 24 months postoperatively. Any nasal crusts should be removed, scars if present should be divided, further polypoidal mucosa is removed and additional medication prescribed. The patient should be followed up till adequate healing is achieved.

These patients are prone for recurrence, and should be kept on long-term follow-up. It is recommended to continue topical nasal steroids on a regular, long-term basis to avoid recurrence.

REFERENCES

1. Kennedy DW. Endoscopic sinus surgery. In: Thaler ER, Kennedy DW. Rhinosinusitis: A guide for diagnosis and management, 1st edn. Springer 2008.pp.93-106.
2. Cohen NA, Kennedy DW. Endoscopic sinus surgery: where we are and where we're going. Curr Opin Otolaryngol Head Neck Surg. 2005;13:32-8.
3. Stammberger H, Posawetz W. Functional endoscopic sinus sugery. Concept, indications and results of the Messerklinger technique. Eur Arch Otorhinolaryngol. 1990;247: 63-76.
4. Suh JD, Kennedy DW. Treatment options for chronic rhinosinusitis. Proc Am Thorac Soc. 2011;8:132-40.

CHAPTER 5

Postoperative Management after Functional Endoscopic Sinus Surgery

Siddharth Chaudri

INTRODUCTION

The techniques of endoscopic sinus surgery aim at achieving two important goals, i.e. the functional and morphological regeneration of the nasal epithelium and improved ventilation and drainage of the paranasal sinuses. The postoperative period marks the start of the epithelial regeneration phase which is crucial for the complete healing of the mucous membrane and must therefore be accompanied by specific therapeutic procedures.

A skillful surgical technique is the primary requirement for a rapid and complete healing of the wounds. The mucous membrane should be spared as much as possible and care should be taken to avoid exposing the concha bones and lateral nasal wall in order to prevent adhesions.

Furthermore, evidence-based medicine has shown that the quality of postoperative treatment has a decisive effect on the results of endoscopic sinus surgery.[1] Postoperative nasal conditions cannot be adequately assessed by conventional mirror examinations as necessary therapeutic measures may be overlooked and thus omitted. Inadequate treatment in the postoperative phase leads to new pathological changes in the nose, and to relapses which are more difficult to treat. Such results may jeopardize the long-term results of endoscopic sinus surgery.

NEED FOR POSTOPERATIVE CARE

Unlike any other area of the body, the nasal cavity is a dynamic area where respiration continues to take place as soon as the surgery is completed. The surgical cavities are lined with mucous membrane that would normally secrete mucous that would clean and moisten the area. Postsurgery all these functions are deranged and it takes at least 4–6 weeks to return back to normal.

Postoperative treatment begins in the operation theater. Insertion of a nasal tamponade made of self-expanding oxycellulose in the dissected ethmoid bone or in the middle nasal meati helps to stop the bleeding. It also helps to separate any corresponding de-epithelialized wound surfaces, e.g. septum and inferior turbinate or middle turbinate and the lateral nasal wall. Use of splints or silicone stents may also be used for the same purpose.

Also lateralization of the middle turbinate and closure of the sinus cavity can be prevented by suturing the middle turbinate to the septum or creating raw surfaces on the medial aspect of the middle turbinate and the corresponding area of the septum leading to controlled adhesions (bolgerization).[2,3] This prevents lateralization of the middle turbinate and closure of the antrostomy.

Slight oozing postoperatively, especially after the removal of the nasal tamponade pack on the 1st or 2nd day after surgery, leads to the accumulation of blood in the nasal cavity, where it first coagulates and later dries up, forming blackish crusts. The absence of mucociliary clearance causes the mucous discharge from the opened sinus to dry out and form yellowish-brown crusts which adhere to the raw areas of mucous membrane.

Initially, these raw areas are covered with crusts, where granulations can appear on the following days and weeks. Serous and mucinous secretions tend to accumulate at the fundus of the nasal cavity and in the paranasal sinuses. Flat fibrinous exudations often form on the mucous membrane of the nasal and sinus cavities which tend to obstruct the nasal passages.

It is also important to give more than adequate washes (intraoperative douching) before nasal packing to reduce the residual blood clots and mucinous secretions which predispose to more crusting and disease recurrence.

Hence good postoperative care aims at:

- Return to normal function as quickly as possible achieving the best possible surgical outcome in a relatively short time
- To improve quality of life for patient during the mucosal healing phase
- To prevent short-term complications such as:
  - Bleeding
  - Excessive crusting
  - Infection
- To prevent long-term complications such as:
  - Synechia
  - Middle turbinate lateralization
  - Osteal stenosis

Thus, in order to achieve good results counselling of a patient about the postoperative care should be done preoperatively.

PATIENT COUNSELING AND ADVICE

As the sinuses begin to clear themselves after 2–3 weeks, one can expect to have some thick brown drainage from the nose. This is mucus and old blood and does not indicate an infection.[4] There may be some discomfort postoperatively due to manipulation and inflammation. Nausea and vomiting is expected due to the anesthesia. Some nasal and sinus pressure and pain may occur for the first 1–2 weeks after the surgery. This may feel like a sinus infection or a dull ache in the sinuses. The nasal passages and breathing should return to normal within 2–3 weeks after surgery.

Following nasal and sinus surgery patients are not allowed to blow their nose or sniff hard. Nasal irrigation is an effective method of cleaning the nasal and sinus cavities without causing any bleeding.[5]

The patients also need to be told that postoperative visits are an indispensable part of the surgery, since they help promote healing and prevent persistent or recurrent disease. During these visits, the surgical cavity is cleaned and inspected. Areas of potential adhesions may be dealt with, and the medical treatment can be adjusted.

The first postoperative visit will occur typically within the first week after surgery, and one should expect weekly postoperative visits within the first 3–4 weeks thereafter.

Continued debridement may be done at future visits. Removal of persistent inflammation or bands of scar tissue may also be done under local anesthesia, if necessary.

Patients must be instructed:[4]

- To start nasal irrigations on the day after the nasal pack removal
- Not to blow the nose for at least 2 weeks after the surgery
- Not to bend, lift or strain for two weeks after surgery as these activities may cause bleeding from the nose
- Not to suppress the need to cough or sneeze; instead, to do so with the mouth open
- To take the prescribed medicines including antibiotics as directed by the surgeon
- Not to take aspirin or aspirin-like medications for a full 7–10 days after surgery.

RESUMING ACTIVITIES[5]

- Patients are advised to maintain a vertical position and walk around as much as is comfortable beginning on the second postoperative day.
- Patients are advised to sleep with the head of the bed elevated for 7–10 days following the surgery.
- Avoid straining during elimination. Proper diet, plenty of water and walking are strongly recommended to avoid constipation
- Avoid smoking or alcohol consumption for 3 weeks after surgery as both of these activities significantly slow the healing process
- Eyeglasses may be worn immediately after surgery. Contact lenses may be used the day after surgery
- *Household activities:* From the 3rd postoperative day, patients are encouraged to be up and around the house with the usual activities. However, bending, weight lifting, and strenuous activity should be avoided for at least 2 weeks
- No swimming, athletic activity or exercises that involve straining or heavy weight lifting for at least 3 weeks following surgery
- When to return to work depends on the amount of physical activity and public contact the respective job involves and also the amount of swelling that develops
- The average person is ready to return to work or go out socially 1 week after surgery
- Not to drive while taking any sedative or prescription pain medications
- The patients must call the doctor if there is:
  - Persistent temperature above 101.5° that is not relieved by paracetamol

- Yellow or green drainage or an increase in pain, congestion with foul-smelling discharge from the nose or other evidence of infection
- Sudden swelling or skin discoloration around the eyes
- Active, persistent bleeding not resolved by decongestant spray treatment
- Any visual disturbances
- Development of any drug reaction.

NASAL IRRIGATION

Nasal irrigation is the most important instruction to be followed by patients after the surgery. This helps to clean blood clots and sticky mucous secretions, hence reducing some of the nasal obstruction and making the patients breathe easily.[6] It also helps in improving mucociliary clearance. Besides this it loosens the crusts which, makes it easier to clean for the surgeon, and less uncomfortable for the patients at the time of the postoperative visits.

Patients may irrigate their nose regularly with a saline solution which is available over the counter at the chemist. Once the saltwater solution has been instilled into the nose it will flow out again and may contain some fresh blood or blood clots.[4] This is not a matter of concern.

Sinus irrigations must be performed at least 2–3 times daily. Initially they will feel strange later they become quite soothing as they clean out the debris left behind in the sinuses after surgery making breathing easier.[5] These irrigations are critical for the success of the surgery.

Beginning the 3rd day after surgery one can begin irrigating the nose with normal saline. Otherwise, the patients may create their own dilute solution of salt water. This is done by placing a teaspoon of noniodized salt and baking soda in a cup of room temperature water. Using a nasal bulb syringe or a 20 cc disposable syringe and leaning over the sink, gently irrigate the nasal cavity one side at a time. Irrigate with as much saline as necessary until the irrigation fluid coming back is clear. After irrigating, very gently blow the nose one side at a time to clear any residual salt water.

A less effective alternative for patients who are uncomfortable with irrigation in the earlier postoperative period is to use a nasal saline spray. It is important to begin liberal use of nasal saline spray 2 days after surgery. The salt water nasal spray can dissolve any blood or mucous left in the nose after surgery and also improve the ability to breathe through the nose, while reducing swelling and speeding up the healing and recovery. Even the saline spray can shorten the duration of the swelling and improve the ability to breathe through the nose. The nasal saline spray can be used every 2–3 hours after surgery.

MEDICAL TREATMENT

The overall healing process can be further enhanced by using appropriate medications. The mucosal regeneration process cannot be separated from residual pathological findings in the nose. In particular, reactive mucosal swelling can persist for a number of weeks. The edema will eventually recede, but only through the consistent use of careful cleansing techniques and medication.

The epithelium covering the mucosal defects is very vulnerable. At first it has a thickened and undulating appearance. Secretolysis is recommended in this phase of treatment using mucolytics or enzymes. It takes weeks to months for the wound cavity to become completely re-epithelialized, as seen in the smooth mucosal surfaces of the nasal and paranasal sinus areas. Respiratory epithelium is not present at all sites, because some sites heal with multilayered scar epithelium. At this point, however, there is no longer any risk of re-stenosis of the newly created ostia or an obliteration of the ethmoid labyrinth.

Antibiotics are administered for the first 7–10 days in order to treat existing sinus infection and prevent secondary infection over the surgical wounds and raw surfaces. The choice of antibiotics may range from co-amoxyclav to cephalosporins or the newer quinolones which offer good coverage against upper respiratory pathogens.[6]

Pain killers such as paracetamol or tramadol are necessary for the first 5–7 days. It is preferable to avoid NSAIDs as they can increase the risk of bleeding. For anti-inflammatory action and in order to reduce the mucosal edema one can use anti-inflammatory enzymes such as trypsin or bromelain.

Corticosteroids offer excellent anti-inflammatory and anti-allergic action. These help to reduce edema, decrease congestion and reduce the healing time.[7]

Anti-Histamines help deal with allergy and help reduce nasal secretions. This prevents the patients from sniffing and blowing their noses.

Decongestants such as phenylephrine help to reduce nasal congestion. Local decongestants such as xylometazoline or oxymetazoline are recommended during the initial days before nasal irrigation but must be used with caution in patients with cardiovascular disease.[8]

Steroid nasal sprays[5] such as fluticasone or mometasone are used during the late postoperative phase after mucosal regeneration has started as a long-term anti allergic control.

CLEANING AND DEBRIDEMENT

So far we have discussed what the patients need to do during the postoperative period. However the surgeon also needs to play a very crucial role during the postoperative visits.

During these visits, the surgical cavity is cleaned and inspected. Unhealthy tissue may be removed, and the medical treatment strategy can be adjusted. Hence postoperative visits are an indispensable part of the surgery, since they help promote healing and prevent persistent or recurrent disease.[5,6]

The first postoperative visit will occur typically within the first 3–4 days after surgery, and then weekly postoperative visits may occur for another 3–4 weeks. Further debridement will be done at future visits which may be initially fortnightly and then monthly depending on the condition of the operated nasal and sinus cavities.[1]

Treatment in First Postoperative Week

Initially one can expect to have some thick sticky secretions from the nose. This is mucus and old blood and does not indicate an infection.

Careful suction of the nose should be performed as early as the 1st day after pack removal by the operating surgeon. Special care should be taken to remove only coagula and secretions from the nasal vestibule, the fundus of the nose, and the entrance to the middle meatus. A metallic suction tube with fingertip control is ideal for this because of its precise regulation of suction. Special care should be taken to avoid damage to the healing epithelium by not applying suction to the loose areas of mucous membrane.

Treatment in Second Postoperative Week

From the 7th postoperative day onwards, it may be necessary to remove dried-up secretions appearing as crusts or as a flat fibrinous coating. A cup crocodile forceps or nasal dressing forceps are suitable for this procedure. It is recommended that all postoperative intervention must be done by endoscopic visualization. This helps to get an accurate picture of the areas of constrictions that may require localized treatment. The use of endoscopic techniques also helps to prevent injuries to the regenerating mucous membrane.

At this time, mechanical manipulation in the ethmoidal labyrinth, in the frontal recess or in the antrostomy maxillary sinus are not necessary. Effective cleansing can usually be achieved by applying gentle suction only at their openings. Large crusts can be removed with a small cup forceps. Here special care should be taken to avoid any further damage to the epithelium. Overly-forceful removal is indicated by fresh bleeding of the mucosa.

Only a slight regeneration tendency of the epithelium can be expected in the first postoperative week. During this period fibrinous bridges that may lead to adhesions should be eliminated by suction and the selective removal of crusts.

Treatment in Third Postoperative Week

At this stage, special attention must be given to the potential adhesions between corresponding de-epithelialized mucosal areas, e.g. the middle turbinate and the lateral nasal wall where corresponding wound surfaces often adhere to each other by means of fibrinous bridges. Within 8–10 days, these fibrinous adhesions form fibrous scar bridges. In many cases, these bridges are responsible for the obstruction of the relatively large ostia of the maxillary sinus and for blocked passages to the frontal and ethmoidal sinuses. This leads to secretory congestion in these cavities.

Hence while using instruments to clean the nose, special attention should be given to removing these fibrinous bridges by suction or sectioning them. This treatment should take place in the early postoperative phase in the 1st week after surgery.

After the selective removal of crusts and suction of the secretions, the process of epithelial regeneration can be enhanced by applying low-viscosity ointments or gels containing antibiotics and corticosteroids. These methods activate wound cleansing and healing by breaking down fibrinous layers and coagulated blood. They also have an antiinflammatory effect on the swollen mucous membrane.

The cleansing of the nose with the appropriate instruments can also be enhanced by moistening the nasal region. The instillation of a physiological saline solution into the nose helps to prevent the drying up of nasal secretions and also dissolves any adhesions between mucosal surfaces.

Treatment During the Late Postoperative Phase

After the initial phase of treatment and observation, the patient must continue to remain under medical supervision. The prevailing mucosal hyperplasia starts to recede gradually. Nevertheless, flat edema beds may persist in the weeks and months that follow. These characteristic findings should not be confused with inflammatory relapses. Clearance of these is an indicator of functional regeneration not returning to its normal state until 2–6 months after surgery.

The late postoperative phase may also be accompanied by the occurrence of granulation tissue and occasional small polyps. Edematous mucosal beds may also reappear. Regular nasal endoscopy allows for a timely detection of these changes and to decide the appropriate medical treatment.

One major complication observed in this late phase is the adhesion of the middle turbinate to the lateral nasal wall; and also the inferior turbinate with the nasal septum. As long as synechia formation on the anterior section of the middle concha remains limited, cicatricotomy using scissors or a surgical scalpel is generally sufficient for correcting this situation. Re-operation is required to treat extensive adhesions with scarred occlusion of the ostia. A useful method for preventing renewed synechia formation is the insertion of small silastic splints between the corresponding wound areas for at least 8–10 days.

CONCLUSION

In conclusion, functional endoscopic sinus surgery has become a widespread tool for the treatment of chronic sinus conditions. Postoperative treatment following endoscopic paranasal sinus surgery is vital for the overall therapeutic success; and thus it is an important task for the operating surgeon.[1] As part of preoperative counseling, the patient should be informed of the various phases of wound healing and their effects on his subjective well-being. Both the patient and the surgeon must demonstrate a willingness and commitment to undergo a complex phase of postoperative treatment if they wish to achieve the common goal of improvement and healing.

During the OPD visits, under local anesthesia, aggressive postoperative care can greatly diminish the need to return to the operating room for revision surgery.

Hence effective postoperative care is crucial to obtain the best possible results.

Any and all means necessary must be taken to assure expert, detailed, and timely postoperative care.

REFERENCES

1. Gross CW, Gross WE. Postoperative care for functional endoscopic sinus surgery. Ear Nose Throat J. 1994;73(7):476-9.
2. Hanna BM, Kilty SJ. Middle turbinate suture technique: A cost-saving and effective method for middle meatal preservation after endoscopic sinus surgery. J Otolaryngol Head Neck Surg. 41(6):407-12.
3. Bolger WE, Kuhn FA, Kennedy DW. Middle turbinate stabilization after functional endoscopic sinus surgery: The controlled synechiae technique. Laryngoscope. 1999; 109(11):1852-3.
4. Cleveland Clinic, Head and Neck Institute, Section of Nasal and Sinus Disorders.https://my.clevelandclinic.org/ccf/media/files/Head_Neck/2007%20CC%20HNI%20FESS%20postop%20care.pdf.
5. Post Operative Instructions; John Hopkins, Baltimore. http://www.hopkinsmedicine.org/sinus/patient_information/post_procedure_directions.html.
6. Eugene A. Patient Guide Pre- or Postoperative instructions for Endocopic Sinus Surgery; Houston, Texas. http://texasface.com/patient-guide/pre-post-op-instructions/endoscopic-sinus-surgery.
7. Jorissen M, Bachert C. Effect of corticosteroids on wound healing after endoscopic sinus surgery. Rhinology. 2009;47(3):280-6.
8. Higgins TS, Hwang PH, Kingdom TT, et al. Systematic Review of Topical Vasoconstrictors in Endoscopic Sinus Sugery. Laryngoscope. 2011;121(2):422-32.

CHAPTER 6

Endoscopic Ethmoid Sinus Surgery

Anagha Joshi

"If the ethmoid were placed in any other part of the body, it would be an insignificant and harmless collection of bony cells; In the place where nature has put it, it has major relationships so that diseases and surgery of the labyrinth often leads to tragedy."

–Mosher 1929

The ethmoid labyrinth is truly very complex, and prior knowledge of the individual patient's anatomy is imperative before embarking on this surgery.

INDICATIONS OF ETHMOIDECTOMY

- Recurrent sinusitis
- Chronic sinusitis not responding to medical therapy
- Sinonasal polyposis
- Fungal sinusitis
- Acute sinusitis with complications
- As an approach to
  - Endoscopic orbital decompression
  - Endoscopic optic nerve decompression
  - Endoscopic repair of cerebrospinal fluid (CSF) leak
  - Endoscopic excision of nasal tumors.

PRESURGICAL CONSIDERATIONS

Review the CT scan to identify:
- Location of ethmoid variants like agger nasi cells, infraorbital ethmoid cells, and Onodi cells.
- Dehiscent or medially deviated lamina papyracea

- Lateral lamellae of the cribriform plate depth of the olfactory fossa, any asymmetry, or erosion from chronic disease.
- Anterior ethmoidal artery as it traverses the ethmoid roof. To look for bony dehiscence of the canal and its relation with the base skull.
- The attachment of the uncinate process.

STEPS OF ETHMOIDECTOMY

The basic surgical technique is based on Messerklinger's[1] anterior to posterior approach.

Uncinectomy (Infundibulotomy)

Uncinectomy or opening of the infundibulum is the first step of surgery. According to Messerklinger,[1] infundibulum is the key area for pathogenesis of sinusitis in maxillary sinus and anterior ethmoids.
- The first step in doing uncinectomy is identification of the middle part of the free border of the uncinate using a ball-tipped probe. The ball probe is inserted into the infundibulum between the anterior face of the bulla and

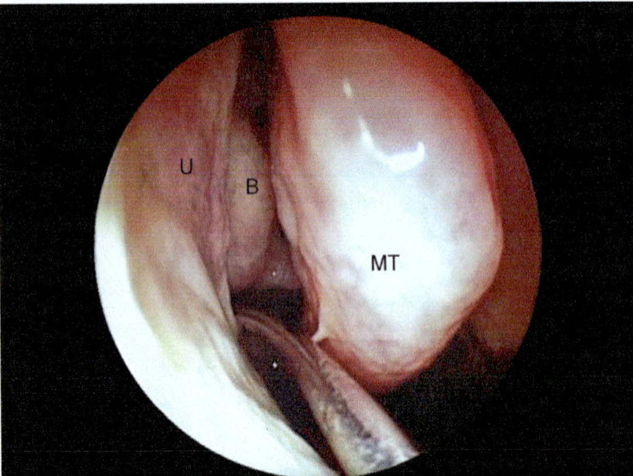

Fig. 6.1: Right nostril showing probe in the infundibulum. [MT: Middle turbinate; U: Uncinate process; B: Bulla]

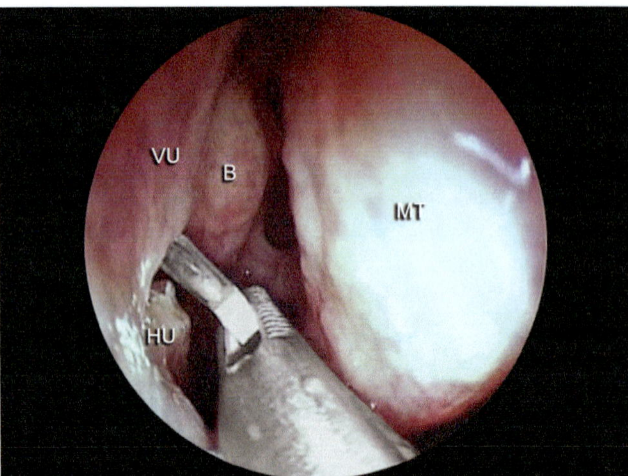

Fig. 6.2: Right nostril showing uncinectomy being done by a back-biting forceps at the junction of vertical (VU) and horizontal (HU) portion of the uncinate. [MT: Middle Turbinate; B: Bulla]

posterior border of the uncinate (Fig. 6.1). A small reverse cutting forceps is then inserted into the middle meatus and opened in the vertical plane of the meatus. The open blade is then rotated through 90° to engage the posterior edge of the uncinate process at the junction of its vertical and horizontal part (Fig. 6.2). The reverse cut should go cleanly through the entire thickness of the uncinate. One more cut is usually necessary to completely divide the horizontal part from the vertical part. The upper uncinate is then rotated medially with a ball probe and grasped with an upturned Blakesley forceps, holding it as close to the lacrimal crest attachment as possible and avulsed with a posteriorly directed force. The horizontal portion of the uncinate is then medially rotated and removed with a straight Tru-Cut forceps (Fig. 6.3).

- Another technique has been described by Wormold and McDonogh,[2] the "swing-door technique". In addition to the lower cut by the back-biter, a superior horizontal cut is made in the vertical portion of the uncinate near the axilla of the middle turbinate by a sickle knife. The whole vertical part of the uncinate is swung medially like a door and subsequently removed.
- The uncinate process can also be resected by inserting a sickle knife into the uncinate process just below the insertion of middle turbinate and then cutting along its insertion on the lateral wall in a convex arch from anterosuperior to posteroinferior. The sickle knife should not extend more than 3–4 mm through the uncinate process into the infundibulum and should always be held parallel to the lateral nasal wall to avoid injury to the lamina papyracea. The author prefers to take a horizontal mucosal incision near the axilla of the middle turbinate

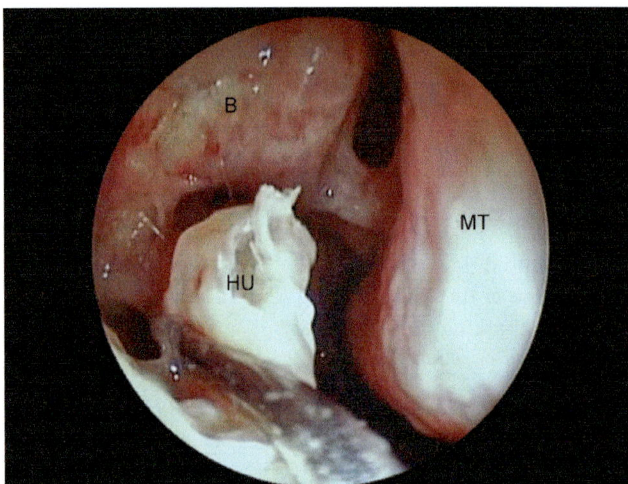

Fig. 6.3: Horizontal segment of uncinate rotated medially. [B: Bulla; HU: Horizontal segment of uncinate; MT: Middle turbinate]

before taking this incision. The uncinate process is then displaced medially, held with a Blakesley forceps and removed (Fig. 6.4).

The uppermost part of the uncinate as well as the most anterior of the ethmoid cells (agger nasi) is removed along with the clearance of the frontal recess. This is discussed elsewhere in this book.

Resection of Ethmoid Bulla (Anterior Ethmoidectomy)

After uncinectomy, middle meatal antrostomy is done. If there is a need to do frontal recess work, it is preferable to do

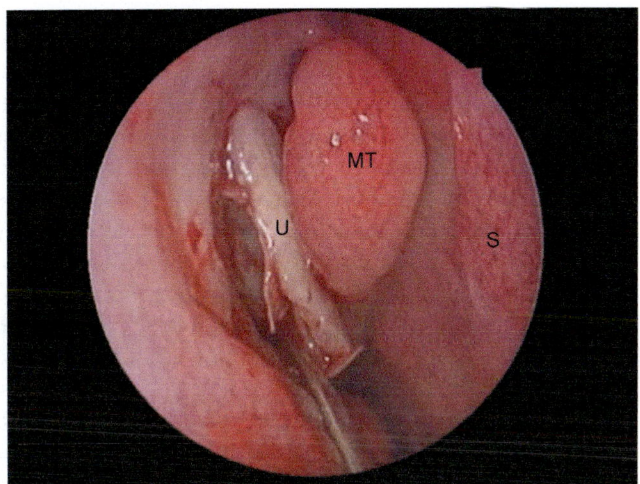

Fig. 6.4: Right nostril showing uncinectomy being done after cutting along the anterior insertion of the uncinate. A horizontal cut has been made in the vertical uncinate near the axilla of the middle turbinate. [MT: Middle turbinate; U: Uncinate process; S: Septum]

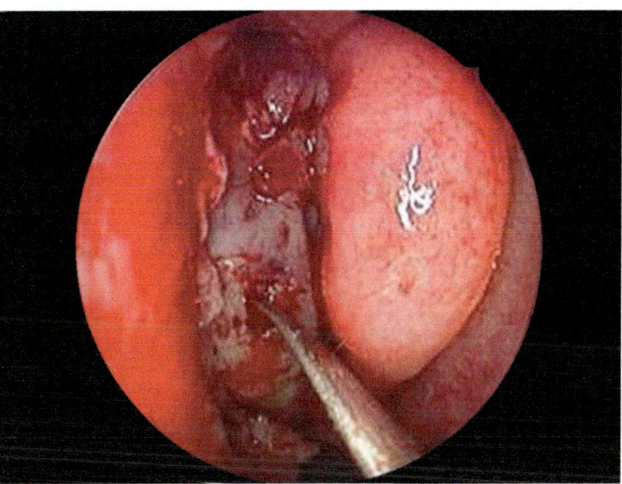

Fig. 6.5: Bulla is opened inferomedially

it with the "intact bulla technique". An intact anterior wall of the bulla provides protection to the anterior ethmoid artery during frontal recess work.

- The bulla is opened by gently inserting a Freer's elevator or a straight closed Blakesley forceps in its anterior face inferomedially (Fig. 6.5). The lumen of the bulla is identified and the anterior and medial walls are removed. This can be done with the help of either a straight Blakesley forceps or a microdebrider. The bulla is not always pneumatized. There may be only a bony ridge (called Torus Lateralis by Grunwald).[3] The bulla may be small or even absent. The suprabullar cells are then removed by using either a debrider or Tru-cut forceps to complete anterior ethmoidectomy. The lamina papyracea which marks the lateral wall of the bulla should be identified. Removal of bony septae attached to the lamina should be done with the side of the upward biting forceps to prevent accidental injury to the lamina papyracea and orbital contents. Powered instruments should never be angled directly at the lamina and it may be more judicious to use traditional instruments when skeletonizing the medial wall of the orbit.
- *Identification of the skull base:* Bony septae are removed from posterior to anterior to define the skull base. The roof of the ethmoid can be seen as a pale yellow structure.[3] As the skull base begins to curve superiorly the anterior ethmoidal artery (AEA) can be visualized as running obliquely across the skull base in its bony canal on its way from the orbit to the olfactory fossa (Fig. 6.6). As the

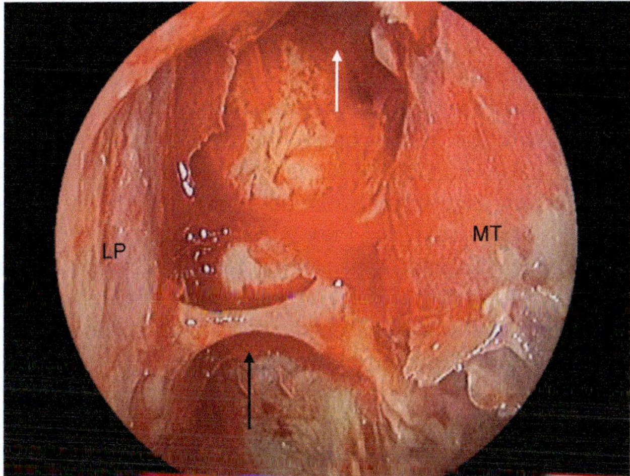

Fig. 6.6: Right ethmoid cavity showing anterior ethmoidal artery (Black arrow) running across the base skull. [LP: Lamina papyracea; MT: Middle turbinate; white arrow: Frontal sinus ostium]

AEA traverses the skull base, there can be variability in its height, as 8.5% can be suspended in a bony mesentery 2–3 mm below the skull base.[4]

- The anterior ethmoidal artery lies just posterior to the anterior face of the bulla at base skull.[5] Thus if the bulla is kept intact during dissection in the frontal recess area, the risk of bleeding from the artery is minimized.
- The point at which the artery perforates the lateral lamella of the cribriform plate is the thinnest part

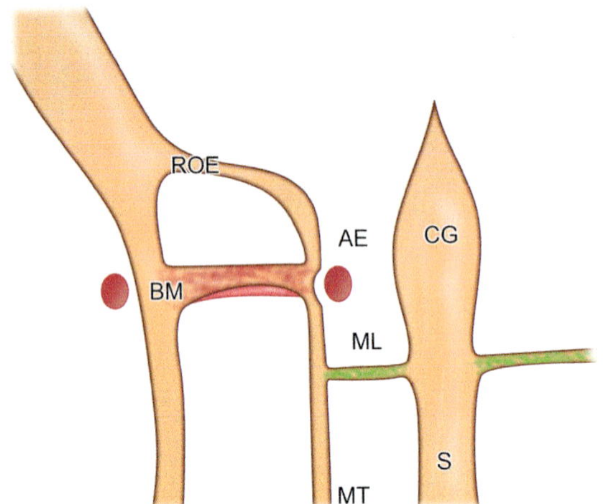

Fig. 6.7: Relative thickness of the various parts of the base skull. [ROE: Roof of ethmoid; BM: Bony mesentery of the AEA; AE: Anterior ethmoid artery, ML: Medial lamella of the cribriform plate; MT: Middle turbinate; CG: Crista galli; S: Septum]

of the anterior skull base (0.05 mm) (Fig. 6.7).[5] The underlying dura is also strongly adherent to the bone. Thus this region is vulnerable to iatrogenic CSF leaks, more so in patients with deep olfactory fossa (Keros type III).[6]

- Presence of the supraorbital ethmoid cell correlates with the AEA being at a lower level in the ethmoid cavity and hence being more at risk of damage if this anatomical variation has not been identified preoperatively on the CT scan.[7]

Ethmoid cells that extend into the maxillary sinus above the ostium are called infraorbital ethmoid cells (Haller cells). These cells can cause obstruction of the ostiomeatal complex and hence require removal.

Posterior Ethmoidectomy

If the patient has posterior ethmoid disease further dissection is indicated. At the completion of the preceding steps, at the posterior limit of the operative field, the ground lamella should be visualized. Its position is confirmed by following the middle turbinate backwards to the point where it turns laterally into the lamina papyracea.

Identification of the ground lamella may be made difficult by pathological changes or anatomic variants. If there is a prominent lateral sinus it will extend between the posterior surface of the bulla and the ground lamella. In this case, perforation of the posterior wall of the ethmoid bulla will open directly into the sinus lateralis and not into the posterior ethmoid sinus.

The lamella is not always a smooth, flat bony plate. Posterior ethmoidal cells may cause the lamella to bulge

anteriorly. Similarly, anterior ethmoidal cells particularly when associated with irregular sinus lateralis, can dent the lamella in the direction of the posterior ethmoidal sinus. If such a cell is opened during the procedure on the anterior ethmoidal sinus, identification of the ground lamella and the beginning of the posterior ethmoidal sinus may be difficult.[3] The ground lamella should be perforated medially and inferiorly. The best place is 3–4 mm above the point at which it turns upward from its posterior horizontal course.[3] If entered even just a few millimeters too superiorly, the path of the instrument will be toward the ethmoid roof, and risk of skull base injury will be much greater. Care should be taken to preserve the inferior border of the ground lamella to maintain the stability of the middle turbinate. The posterior ethmoidal cells can be recognized by their larger size as compared to the anterior ethmoidal cells. They are cleared till the lamina papyracea laterally, the skull base superiorly and the superior turbinate medially. The posterior most ethmoidal cell is pyramidal in shape. The posterior ethmoidal artery (PEA) is smaller, and therefore slightly more difficult to visualize endoscopically. A more constant relationship to look for endoscopically may be to first identify the anterior face of the sphenoid and then look approximately 8 mm anterior to that at the level of the skull base.[8] It is essential to establish the presence of an Onodi cell; a posterior ethmoid cell that pneumatizes lateral and superior to the sphenoid sinus (Fig. 6.8).[9] Identification of this cell is essential prior to endoscopic sinus and skull base surgery due to its intricate relationship with the optic nerve and carotid artery, which may lead to deleterious complications. The overall prevalence of Onodi cells in recent studies has been found to be much higher (60%[10] and 65.3%[11]) than the previous studies (8–14%).[9]

The goal of surgery is to create a marsupialized cavity, lined by healthy, intact mucosa (Fig. 6.9). After completion of ethmoidectomy, the operation then proceeds to opening and clearance of disease of the sphenoid sinus, which is described in a separate chapter.

REVISION SURGERY

The usual anatomic landmarks (uncinate process, bulla ethmoidalis, ground lamella, the middle and superior turbinates) used for performing endoscopic sinus surgery may be altered or obscured in revision surgery and in cases of severe polypoid disease.

In primary as well as revision surgery it is always prudent to clearly identify the maxillary sinus ostium as an initial landmark. In the absence of a clear free edge of the uncinate process, the insertion of the inferior turbinate can serve as guide to the position of the maxillary sinus ostium, which is located immediately superior to the midportion

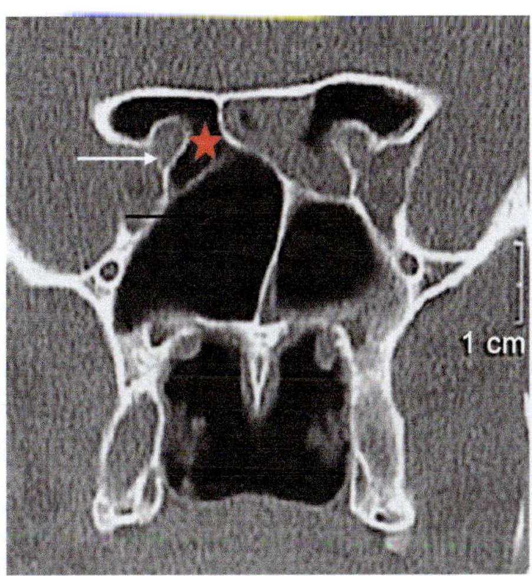
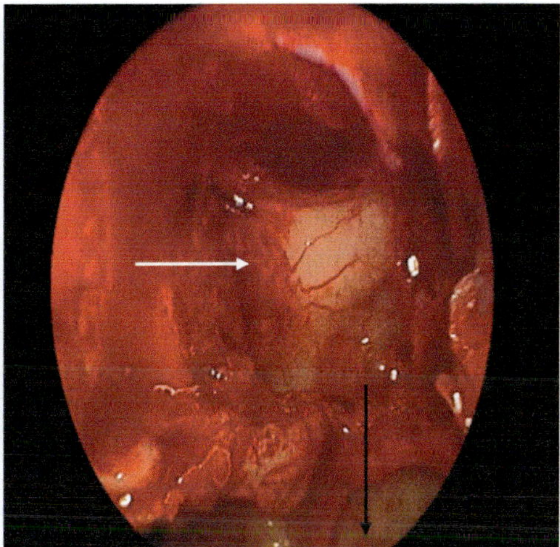

Fig. 6.8: CT scan and endoscopic picture of right nasal cavity showing optic nerve (white arrow) in an Onodi cell (red star). Sphenoid sinus is shown by black arrow

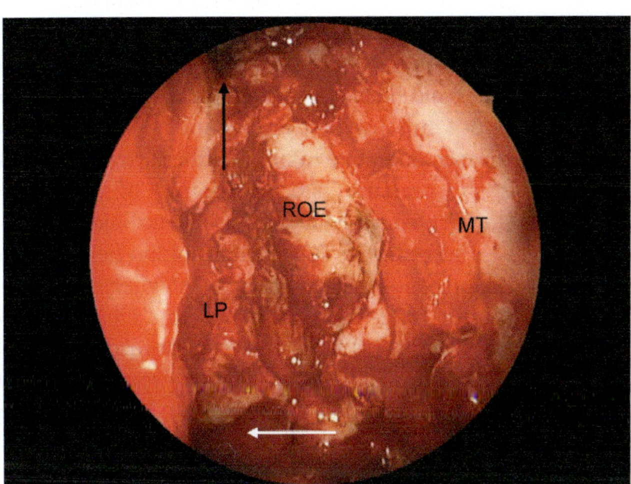

Fig. 6.9: Operated right ethmoidal cavity. The cavity is lined by mucosa. [LP: Lamina papyracea; MT: Middle turbinate; ROE: Roof of ethmoid; black arrow: pointing towards frontal sinus; white arrow: maxillary sinus ostium]

of this turbinate. A curved probe can be inserted just above the insertion of the inferior turbinate and advanced in an inferolateral direction to palpate for the position of the ostium. The ostium is then enlarged posteriorly and anteriorly. The position of this ostium can now be used as a landmark; the superior border of the maxillary antrostomy depicts the junction of the medial orbital floor and the lamina papyracea. Hence by identifying this, the lamina papyracea can be identified.

The skull base provides the second critical landmark after identification of the lamina papyracea and must be identified

carefully. (This identification is achieved more easily and more safely in the posterior ethmoid or sphenoid sinus.) The skull thus identified can then be followed and delineated anteriorly.

More common findings within the ethmoid cavity during revision surgery are a lateralized middle turbinate, retained uncinate process, and residual agger nasi cells. Removal of bony lamellar remnants, the use of Tru-Cut forceps, and judicious use of the microdebrider help achieve resection of disease as well as a mucosal-lined cavity.

CLEANING AND PACKING

Any loose bony fragments, exposed bony chips, blood clots, discharge, etc. should be removed. It should be ensured that there is no active bleeding. The cavity is irrigated with saline and packed with non-absorbable pack, preferably polyvinyl alcohol (PVA) sponge to control any postoperative bleeding. Additional theoretical benefits of nasal packing include preventing adhesion formation, middle turbinate lateralization, and restenosis after surgery. These packs can be kept for upto 4 days.

MUCOSAL PRESERVATION AND PREVENTION OF ADHESIONS

- Mucosa should be preserved meticulously to enhance quicker recovery and to prevent adhesions. Use of micro-debrider or through-cutting instruments is recommended.
- All bony spicules without mucosal covering should be removed completely.
- Prevention of lateralization of middle turbinate

- Preservation of mucosa of the arch of middle turbinate
- *Bolgerization:* This is performed by denuding the medial surface of the middle turbinate and the opposing nasal septum to create raw surfaces that are in contact with each other. This leads to the formation of favorable adhesions that medialize the middle turbinate.[12] Although originally performed with a sickle knife, this technique can easily be performed with a microdebrider and is successful in 93% patients.[13]
- Medialization can also be achieved by trans-septal suturing of both middle turbinates[14] or by use of trans-septal metallic clips.[15]
- Placement of middle meatal spacers or packing for 3–4 days after surgery not only serves to laterise the middle turbinate but also prevents bleeding and synechie.[16]

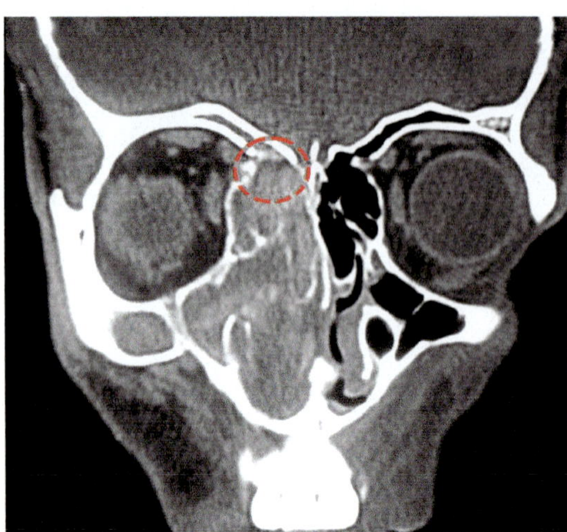

Fig. 6.10: Dehiscent orbitocranial canal of anterior ethmoidal artery

OPTIMIZING THE SURGICAL FIELD

It is essential to reduce the amount of blood obscuring the visual field during surgery. This will allow proper visualization of the landmarks that are critically important for a safe and successful surgery. Measures taken intraoperatively to reduce bleeding include reverse Trendelenburg positioning, the application of topical and local vasoconstrictors,[17,18] maintaining the mean arterial pressure at around 75 mm Hg and the heart rate less than 60 beats/min.[19,20] This is best achieved with total intravenous anesthesia.[21] All preventable causes of excessive surgical bleeding should be addressed preoperatively and is dealt with elsewhere in this book. Care should be taken not to suction blood away from raw mucosal edges, because this will promote further bleeding. Instead, saline irrigation is preferable to wash away excessive blood. Most of the bleeding that clouds the end of the endoscope occurs proximal to the position of the endoscope. The surgeon should actively seek such bleeding sites and coagulate these to ensure that when the scope touches the side wall, accumulated blood does not run down the scope and contaminate the end. Suction instruments can be used to ensure optimal visualization of the dissection in the bloody surgical field.

MANAGEMENT OF COMPLICATIONS

Anterior or Posterior Ethmoid Artery Transection

As the AEA traverses the skull base, there can be variability in its height, as 8.5% can be suspended in a bony mesentery 2–3 mm below the skull base.[4] AEA is at risk during surgery in these cases if attention has not been paid to it when reading the

CT scan (Fig. 6.10). The PEA is smaller, more posterosuperior in location, entering the bony roof of the posterior ethmoid cells at the junction between the lamina papyracea and the frontal bone 2–8 mm anterior to the optic nerve, hence at a lesser risk for intraoperative injury. If either artery is injured during surgery, pressure and application of hemostatic material within a pledget should be applied immediately.

Bipolar cauterization is used to control the hemorrhage. Unipolar suction cautery should be avoided when controlling bleeding at the skull base to avoid the creation of a cerebrospinal fluid (CSF) leak. The retraction of a bleeding artery into the orbit will lead to a rapidly expanding orbital hematoma (Fig. 6.11). This can quickly lead to orbital compartment syndrome, which can result in vision loss from compression of the optic nerve.[22] An emergency ophthalmologic consultation should be sought for, and temporary medical measures such as orbital massage and administration of mannitol and acetazolamide should be instituted. Absolute indication for lateral canthotomy in the anesthetized patient is an intraocular pressure greater than 40 mm Hg. This can lower the intraocular pressures by approximately 33 mm Hg.[23]

Management of Damage to the Lamina Papyracea

Intermittent palpation of the eye while dissecting in this region is essential in being able to identify the lamina without penetrating it. Examining the CT scan preoperatively will allow the surgeon to assess for any dehiscences or anatomic variability in the structure of this bone. There have been several case reports suggesting the rapidity and severity of orbital injury following powered instrumentation use.[24]

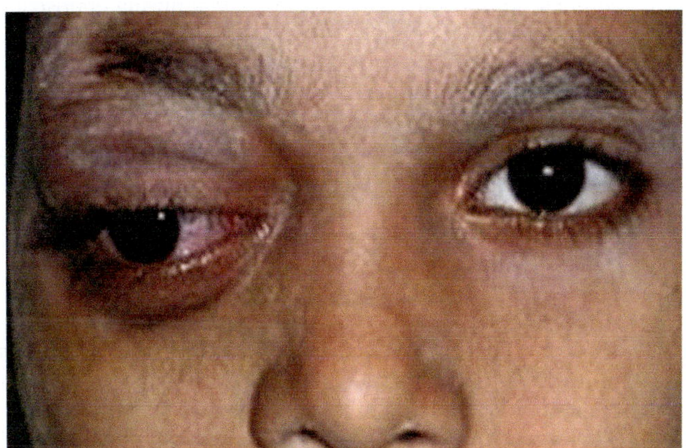

Fig. 6.11: Right eye proptosis due to orbital hematoma

Powered instruments never should be angled directly at the lamina, and it may be more judicious to use traditional instruments when skeletonizing the medial wall of the orbit. If lamina papyracea is entered during ethmoidectomy further dissection should be terminated in the immediate region, and the fat should not be removed or resected. The surgeon should immediately check the eye for edema, ecchymosis, and proptosis. If the eye remains within normal limits, then the lamina papyracea should be positively identified and skeletonized in the region adjacent to the dehiscence. Thereafter, surgery may be continued provided that the lamina can be clearly visualized and respected throughout the remainder of the surgery. If a piece of fat obscures an area of dissection cavity, bipolar cautery can be carefully applied to reduce the fat. At the end of the case, even if no sign of orbital injury is evident, nasal packing within the middle meatus should be avoided.

If there are any clinical signs of an orbital hematoma, sinus surgery should be terminated and treatment for orbital hematoma instituted without delay. An ophthalmology consultation may be required for measurement of intraocular pressures. Medical measures include orbital massage administration of mannitol or acetazolamide. Eye massage helps to redistribute intraocular and extraocular fluid.

Intraoperative CSF Leak

When a leak occurs, the surgeon should stop and review the anatomy. Landmarks (e.g., posterior wall of the maxillary sinus, attachments of the middle turbinate, anterior face of the sphenoid sinus, skull base) should be identified to re-orient oneself, and then the preoperative imaging should be used to help localize the probable site of the leak. The most likely sites of injury are the lateral and medial lamellae of the cribriform plate; therefore, surgeons should review these areas for any dehiscences, asymmetries, thinness/thickness, or any bony abnormalities on the preoperative imaging. On coronal images, the height of the maxillary sinus should be compared with the height of the ethmoid sinuses. The ratio of maxillary-to-ethmoid height can vary from 1:1 to 2:1. Meyers has shown how a higher ratio can lead to inadvertent injury to the anterior skull base during surgery.[25] If a CSF leak is suspected, an attempt should be made to correlate the radiographic site with the region endoscopically. Proper site preparation, graft selection, and preservation of outflow tracts are essential for success of the repair. If the site cannot be completely identified or if the operating surgeon does not feel equipped to repair the defect, then adequate hemostasis should be obtained and the nasal cavity lightly packed to help apply gentle pressure to the defect. The patient should then be referred to an experienced endoscopic sinus surgeon. It is prudent to administer perioperative parenteral antibiotics (e.g., ceftriaxone) that effectively cross the blood–brain barrier.[26]

POSTOPERATIVE CARE

This has been discussed in detail elsewhere in this book.

SUMMARY

For successful endoscopic sinus surgery, a clear understanding of the anatomy is vital.

By applying anatomic knowledge with careful surgical technique, one can maximize success whilst minimizing the risks involved in endoscopic ethmoid surgery.

REFERENCES

1. Kennedy DW. Endoscopic Sinus Surgery. In: Thaler ER, Kennedy DW (Eds). Rhinosinusitis: A Guide for Diagnosis and Management, 1st edn. Springer 2008.pp.93-106.
2. Wormold PJ, McDonough M, The "swing- door" technique for uncinectomy in endoscopic sinus surgery J Laryngol Otol, 1998;112(6):547-51.
3. Stammberger H, Michael Hawke. Essentials of Endoscopic Sinus Surgery. St. Louis: Mosby–Year Book 1993.pp.164-8.
4. Moon HJ, Kim HU, Lee JG, et al. Surgical anatomy of the anterior ethmoid canal in the ethmoid roof. Laryngoscope. 2001;111: 900-4.
5. Stammberger H. Functional Endoscopic Sinus Surgery: The Messerklinger Technique. St. Louis: Mosby-Year Book; 1991. pp. 70-6.
6. Kuhn FA. Chronic frontal sinusitis: The endoscopic frontal recess approach. Operative Tech Otolaryngol Head Neck Surg. 1996;7:222.
7. Anagha AJ, Kshitij DS, Renuka AB. Radiological correlation between the anterior ethmoidal artery and the supraorbital ethmoid cell. Indian J Otolaryngol Head Neck Surg. 2010;62(3):299-303.

8. Han JK, Becker SS, Bomeli SR, et al. Endoscopic localization of the anterior and posterior ethmoid arteries. Ann Otol Rhinol Laryngol. 2008;117(12):931-5.

9. Stammberger HR, Kennedy DW. Paranasal sinuses: anatomic terminology and nomenclature. The Anatomic Terminology Group. Ann Otol Rhinol Laryngol Suppl. 1995;167:7-16.

10. Thanaviratananich S, Chaisiwamongkol K, Kraitrakul S, et al. The prevalence of an Onodi cell in adult Thai cadavers. Ear Nose Throat J. 2003;82(3):200-4.

11. Senja T, Azadeh E, Norman J, et al. High-resolution computed tomography analysis of the prevalence of Onodi cells. Laryngoscope. 2012;122(7):1470-3.

12. Bolger WE, Kuhn FA, Kennedy DW. Middle turbinate stabilisation after functional endoscopic sinus surgery: the controlled synechiae technique. Laryngoscope. 1999;109: 1852-3.

13. Friedman M, Landsberg R, Tanyeri H. Middle turbinate medialisation and preservation in endoscopic sinus surgery. Otolaryngol Head Neck Surg. 2000;123(1 Pt 1):76-80.

14. Thornton RS. Middle turbinate stabilisation technique in endoscopic sinus surgery. Arch Otolaryngol Head Neck Surg. 1996;122(8):869-72.

15. Moukarzel N, Nehme A, Mansour S, et al. Middle turbinate medialisation technique in functional endoscopic sinus surgery. J Otolaryngol. 2000;29(3):144-7.

16. Kuhn FA, Citardi MJ. Advances in postoperative care following functional endoscopic sinus surgery. Otolaryngol Clin North Am. 1997;30(3):479-90.

17. Wormald PJ, Athanasiadis T, Rees G, et al. An evaluation of effect of pterygopalatine fossa injection with local anesthetic and adrenalin in the control of nasal bleeding during endoscopic sinus surgery. Am J Rhinol. 2005;19(3):288-92.

18. Cohen-Kerem R, Brown S, Villaseñor LV, et al. Epinephrine/Lidocaine injection vs. saline during endoscopic sinus surgery. Laryngoscope. 2008;118(7):1275-81.

19. Wormald PJ, van Renen G, Perks J, et al. The effect of the total intravenous anesthesia compared with inhalational anesthesia on the surgical field during endoscopic sinus surgery. Am J Rhinol. 2005;19(5):514-20.

20. Nair S, Collins M, Hung P, et al. The effect of beta-blocker premedication on the surgical field during endoscopic sinus surgery. Laryngoscope. 2004;114(6):1042-6.

21. Eberhart LH, Folz BJ, Wulf H, et al. Intravenous anesthesia provides optimal surgical conditions during microscopic and endoscopic sinus surgery. Laryngoscope. 2003;113 (8):1369-73.

22. Stankiewicz JA, Chow JM. Two faces of orbital hematoma in intranasal (endoscopic) sinus surgery. Otolaryngol Head Neck Surg. 1999;120:841-7.

23. Yung CW, Moorthy RS, Lindley D, et al. Efficacy of lateral canthotomy and cantholysis in orbital hemorrhage. Opthal Plast Reconstr Surg. 1994;10:137-41.

24. Bhatti MT, Giannoni CM, Raynor E, et al. Ocular motility complications after endoscopic sinus surgery with powered cutting instruments. Otolaryngol Head Neck Surg. 2001;125: 501-9.

25. Meyers RM, Valvassori G. Interpretation of anatomic variations of computed tomography scans of the sinuses: a surgeon's perspective. Laryngoscope. 1998;108:422-5.

26. Welch KC, Palmer JN. Intraoperative emergencies during endoscopic sinus surgery: CSF leak and orbital hematoma. Otolaryngol Clin North Am. 2008;41(3):581-96.

CHAPTER 7

Endoscopic Surgery for the Frontal Sinus

Abhineet Lall, Milind V Kirtane

INTRODUCTION

Even after 100 years of frontal sinus surgery[1] and over three decades of evolution of endoscopic sinus surgery, frontal sinus surgery still remains an enigma.

Why is it so Difficult?

- Complex anatomy
- Narrow space
- Surrounding vital structures
- Awkward approach
- Multiple cells
- Difficult landmarks, unlike maxillary and sphenoid
- Blood trickles on the scope, unlike maxillary and sphenoid
- High failure rate
- High chances of iatrogenic stenosis

EMBRYOLOGY

The frontal sinus should be considered as an extension of the ethmoid sinus. The nasofrontal region is located antero superior to the middle meatus. In the embryo this region is a smooth mucosal surface. With development, it sees the appearance of conchae, thereby creating multiple furrows or pits. The frontal sinus is believed to develop from these furrows.[2-6] Mucosa lined air cells keep on advancing, absorbing the cancellous bone. Frontal sinus may also develop as a direct extension of the frontal recess, or may develop as an anterosuperior pouch of the ethmoid infundibulum. Davis[7] published his study based on the dissection of 101 cadavers in various stages of development, wherein he showed that 41%

develop from the frontal recess furrow, 18.4% develop directly from frontal recess, 15.6% as a direct extension of the ethmoidal infundibulum, 24% as an extension of infundibular cell, and 1% from the suprabullar cell.

ENDOSCOPIC ANATOMY

The frontal recess often inappropriately called the fronto-nasal duct, is actually a narrow space surrounded by the ethmoidal cells. These ethmoidal cells develop by extramural migration from the ethmoid sinus.[8] Getting into the frontal sinus essentially means removing these anterior ethmoidal air cells, and the key lies in reading these cells well on the imaging scans. Of them the most prominent is the agger nasi cell[9,10] (Fig. 7.1). Kuhn[11,12] has given a classification to describe the frontoethmoidal cells. A modification to type 4 cell has been suggested by PJ Wormald (Table 7.1).

TABLE 7.1: Modified Kuhn classification for the frontoethmoidal cells
• Agger nasi cell
• Supraorbital ethmoid cell
• Frontoethmoid cells: *Type 1:* Single frontal recess cell above the agger nasi cell (Fig. 7.2) *Type 2:* Tier of cells in the frontal recess above the agger nasi cell (Fig. 7.3) Type 3: Single massive cell pneumatization cephalad into the frontal sinus *Type 4:* A cell pneumatizing through into the frontal sinus and extending greater than 50% of the vertical height of the frontal sinus (Fig. 7.4)
• Frontal bullar cell
• Suprabullar cell
• Interfrontal sinus septal cell

Supraorbital Cell (Figs 7.5A and B)

It is an ethmoidal cell that extends over the orbit from the frontal recess.[13] During endoscopic sinus surgery, it may occasionally be confused with the frontal sinus, but it is pertinent to remember that the frontal sinus opening will be anterior and medial to the supraorbital cell.

Frontal Bullar Cell (Fig. 7.6)

It is a an ethmoidal cell above the ethmoidal bulla. It pneumatizes along the skull base into the frontal sinus from the posterior frontal recess. Its posterior wall is the anterior cranial fossa skull base and anterior border must extend into the frontal sinus. It may be misinterpreted as a type III cell, but the difference is that the frontal bullar cell is located behind the true frontal sinus pneumatization tract.

Interfrontal Sinus Septal Cell (Fig. 7.7)

It is the pneumatization of the interfrontal sinus septum.[14] Som and Lawson[15] have shown that unlike conventional thinking that these cells may be ectopic ethmoidal cells, they are actually diverticula from the frontal sinus.

Recessus Terminalis

Equally important here is to understand the concept of recessus terminalis. The uncinate process has a variable superior attachment and accordingly affects the drainage pathway of the frontal recess. The uncinate process may be:

a. *Directly attached to the lamina papyracea:* In this case it forms a recessus terminalis. The frontal recess here drains medial to the attachment, into the middle meatus (Fig. 7.8A).

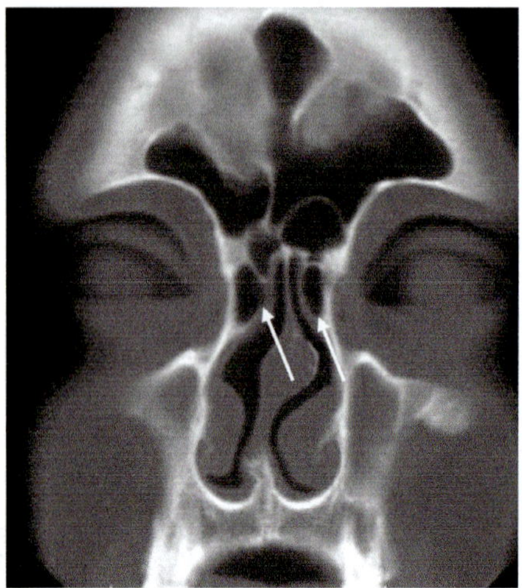

Fig. 7.1: Agger nasi cell: The most anterior ethmoidal cell (white arrows)

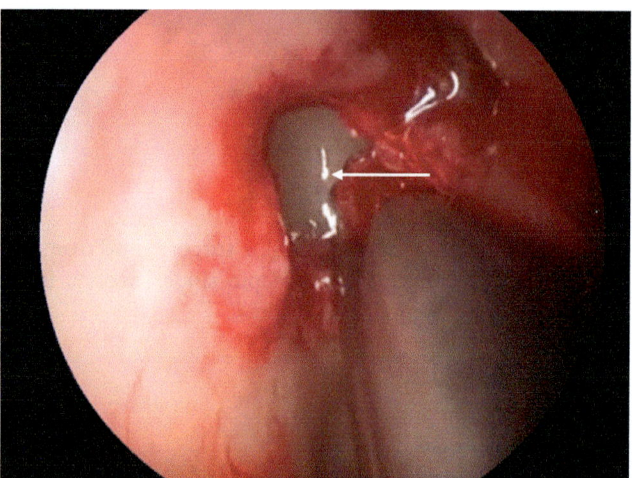

Fig. 7.2: Endoscopic view of a type 1 cell (white arrow)

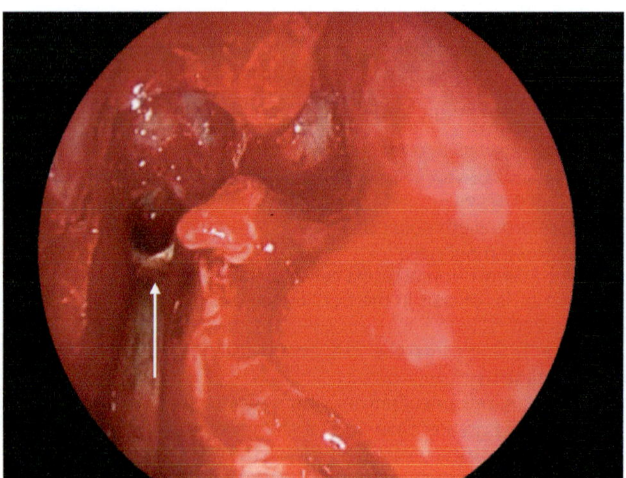

Fig. 7.3: Type 2 cells: Two or more cells above and behind the agger nasi cell

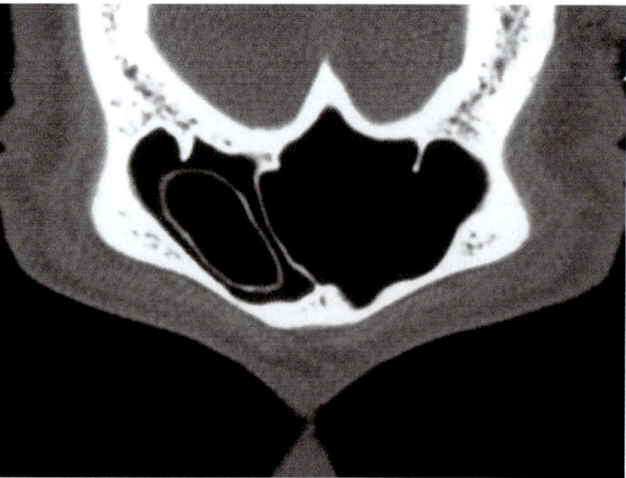

Fig. 7.4: Type 4 cell: Single large cell above the agger nasi, pneumatized into the frontal sinus (> 50% the height of the frontal sinus)

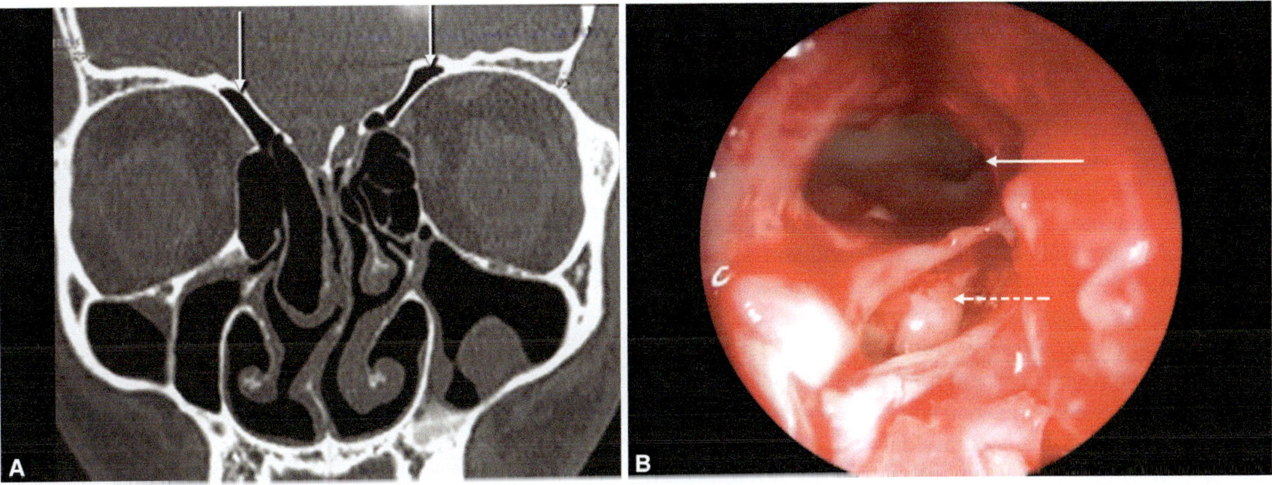

Figs 7.5A and B: (A) CT image showing supraorbital cells (white arrows); (B) Endoscopic view of an opened frontal sinus (white arrow) anterior and medial to a supraorbital cell (dotted arrow)

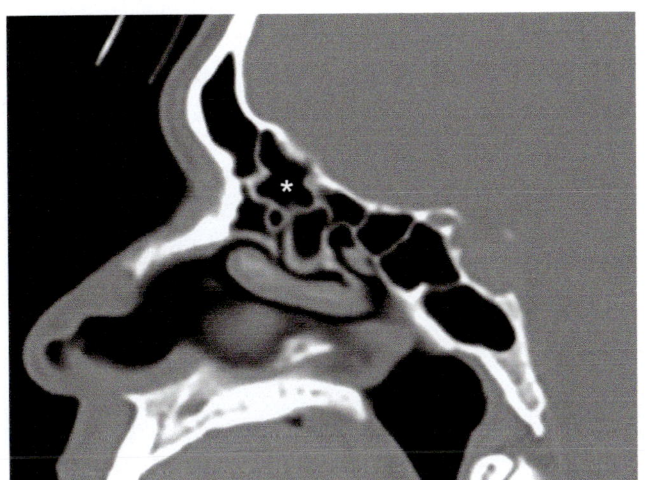

Fig. 7.6: CT scan image showing a frontal bullar cell (asterisk)

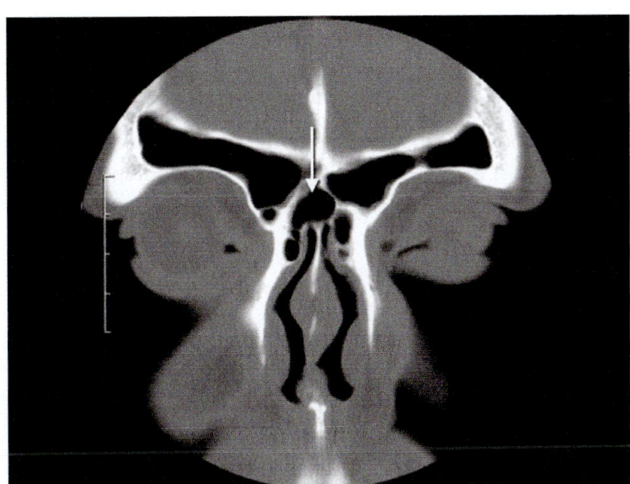

Fig. 7.7: CT image showing an interfrontal sinus septal cell (white arrow)

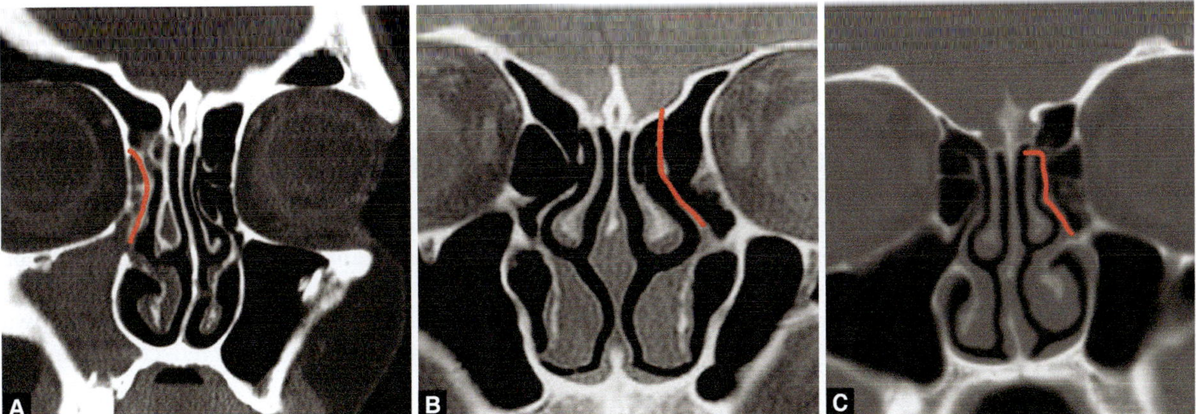

Figs 7.8A to C: CT images showing variable attachment of the uncinate process (red line)

b. *Attached to the skull base:* The frontal recess here drains into the ethmoidal infundibulum (Fig. 7.8B).

c. *Attached to the middle turbinate:* Here again, the frontal recess drains into the ethmoidal infundibulum (Fig. 7.8C).

Lien et al[16] evaluated the role of various cells in causing frontal sinusitis. They evaluated a total of 384 sides, of which 51 sides were diagnosed as having frontal sinusitis. On comparing the frontal recess cells in patients with and without frontal sinusitis, they found suprabullar cell and recessus terminalis to have an increased association with frontal sinusitis on univariate analysis. However on a multivariate analysis, supraorbital ethmoidal cell and frontal bullar cell were found to have an increased association with frontal sinusitis.

Agger nasi cell, frontoethmoidal cell type 1, 2, 3 and interfrontal sinus septal cell did not show an increased association.

OTHER FACTORS AFFECTING THE FRONTAL SINUS OUTFLOW TRACT[17]

Thickness of the Frontal Beak

Measurement of the thickness of the frontal beak is shown in Figure 7.9. It is measured in the parasagittal image at a point where the frontal beak is most prominent.

Anteroposterior Diameter of the Frontal Isthmus

It is the shortest length between the most prominent point of the frontal beak and the posterior wall of the frontal sinus (Fig. 7.10).

Anteroposterior Diameter of the Frontal Recess

It is the length between the most prominent portion of the frontal beak and the attachment of the ethmoidal lamella on the skull base (Fig. 7.10).

Park et al[17] have shown that the volume of the agger nasi cell has a positive co-relation with the AP length of the frontal isthmus and a weak positive co-relation with the AP length of the frontal recess. This would actually mean that greater the pneumatization of the agger nasi cell, more is the surgical space available, thereby leading to a larger frontal sinus opening.

Apart from the above measurements, an AP diameter of the frontal sinus should also be measured on axial scan, especially when a median drainage procedure is being considered. An ostium diameter of at least 5 mm is desirable.[18]

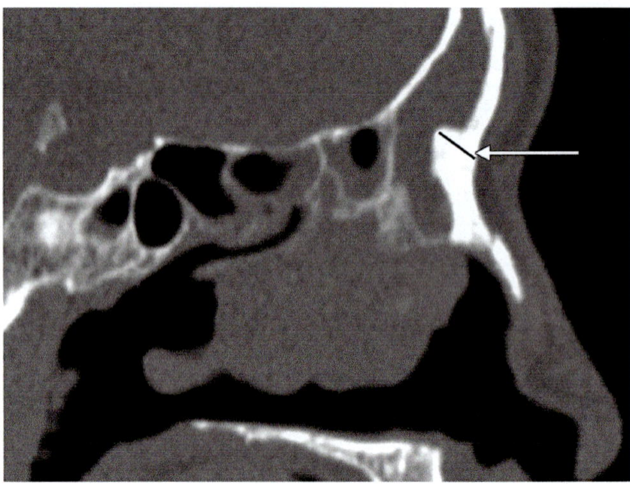

Fig. 7.9: The arrow in the parasagittal CT scan shows the thickness of the frontal beak.

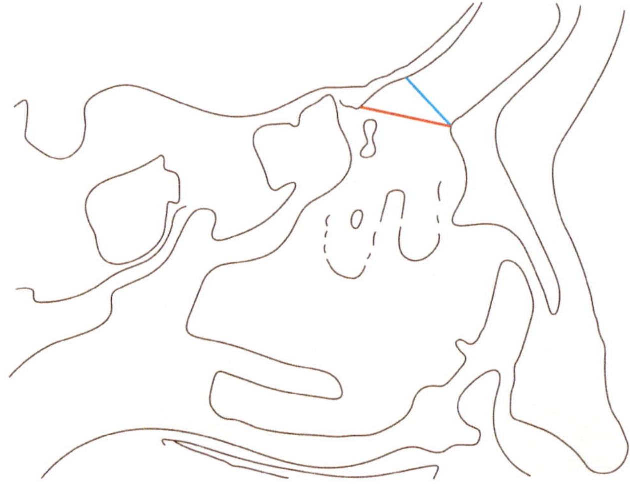

Fig. 7.10: Anteroposterior (AP) diameter of the frontal isthmus (shown by the blue line) and the frontal recess (shown by the red line)

PATHOLOGIES AFFECTING THE FRONTAL SINUS

Rhinosinusitis

Rhinosinusitis in adults has been defined[19] as inflammation of the nose and paranasal sinus characterized by 2 or more symptoms, one of which should be either nasal blockage/obstruction/congestion or nasal discharge, along with the presence of facial pain/pressure or reduction/loss of smell.

It can also be defined on the basis of endoscopic evaluation wherein the presence of nasal polyps and/or mucopurulent discharge primarily from the middle meatus and/or edema/mucosal obstruction primarily in the middle meatus is looked for.

The above symptoms and endoscopic findings may/may not be coupled with CT scan changes.

Acute Rhinosinusitis

An acute episode of rhinosinusitis is one which has been of a duration of <12 weeks, and if the problem is recurrent, there should be complete resolution of symptoms between the episodes.[19]

Pathogens
- *Streptococcus pneumoniae*
- *Haemophilus influenzae*
- *Moraxella catarrhalis*
- Other streptococcal species
- Anaerobic bacteria
- *Staphylococcus.*

Management[20]
See Flow chart 7.1.

Chronic Sinusitis[19,20]

- Duration >12 weeks
- Chronic rhinosinusitis with nasal polyps is rhinosinusitis as defined above, along with endoscopically visualized polyp in the middle meatus.
- Chronic rhinosinusitis without nasal polyps is rhinosinusitis as defined as above with no visible polyp in the middle meatus.

Flow charts 7.2 and 7.3 describe the management of chronic rhinosinusitis without and with nasal polyposis respectively.

IMAGING FOR THE FRONTAL SINUS

Computed Tomography (CT)

The conventional practice of asking for coronal computed tomography sections of the paranasal sinus may not be sufficient in frontal sinus surgery. We need to supplement them with axial sections and sagittal sections.

Coronal CT sections: These are the most basic sections required for endoscopic sinus surgery, as we are essentially operating in a coronal plane.

Axial CT sections: These sections give us an idea of the AP diameter for the frontal sinus and a better perspective on the frontal sinus outflow tract.

Sagittal sections: These sections are useful to delineate the anterior ethmoidal cells in the frontal recess.

Leunig et al[22] have shown that there is a definite advantage in obtaining multiplanar CT reconstructions for agger nasi cell, Kuhn's frontoethmoid cells, frontal bullar and suprabullar cell. However, the same was not true for interfrontal septum pneumatization.

Flow chart 7.1: Management of acute rhinosinusitis[19]

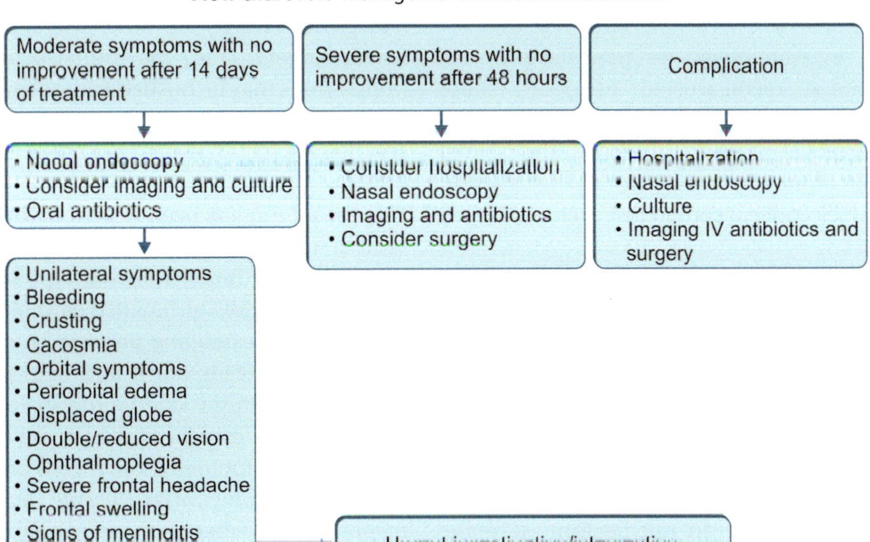

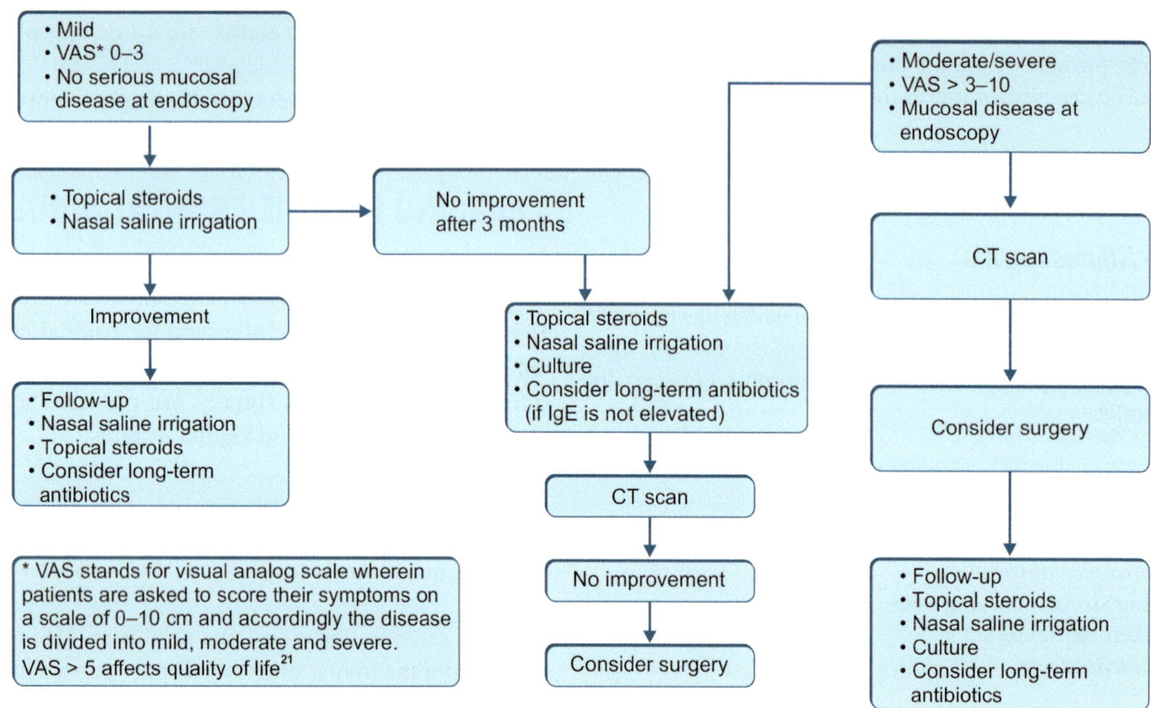

Flow chart 7.2: Management of chronic rhinosinusitis without nasal polyposis[19]

MAGNETIC RESONANCE IMAGING

There is no added advantage of magnetic resonance imaging (MRI) over CT scan for the frontal sinus in inflammatory lesions of the paranasal sinus.[23] MRI has a role in expansile lesions of the frontal sinus and neoplasms, mainly to rule out any dural involvement. MR cisternography is useful to see the site of CSF leak.[24]

Three-dimensional Reconstructed Images

With improvement in technology, we now have at our disposal 3-dimensional reconstructed images.[25] These reformatted images help improve our understanding of the frontal sinus drainage pathway, anatomy, and spatial relationship between ethmoidal cells. Wormald[26] suggested that a 3D building block concept should be developed based on two dimensional CT.

APPROACHES TO THE FRONTAL SINUS

Endoscopic Frontal Sinusotomy

This is the most routinely practised approach for frontal sinusitis needing surgery. The aim of the surgery is to open the frontal ostium and achieve a patent drainage channel. Using a 0° endoscope, initially an uncinectomy is done. One then encounters the ethmoidal bulla. The author's preference is an intact bulla technique. This helps in preventing exposure of the supraorbital cell and anterior ethmoidal artery. However, one can also remove the bulla to create greater space.

The first cell encountered is the agger nasi cell, and this is removed using a curette. The other Kuhn's frontoethmoidal cells are removed as they are seen on the CT scans. Here, Wormald's concept of developing a 3D building block prior to surgery is especially useful.[26] An angled scope, 45° or 70°, is used when dissecting the frontal recess. Angulated curette and giraffe forceps are other useful instruments in frontal recess surgery. Once the frontal ostium is visualized, the frontal sinus may be flushed with saline.

Axillary Flap Technique (Fig. 7.11)

This technique has been described by PJ Wormald[26] and is used in surgery for frontal sinus disease. Using a 0° endoscope uncinectomy is done. A mucosal flap based posteriorly over the axilla of the middle turbinate is elevated, starting 8 mm above the axilla and extending posteriorly for 6 mm. The incision then runs vertically down and then posteriorly to become continuous with the middle turbinate. A part of the frontal process of the maxilla is then removed using a Kerrison's bone punch. Frontoethmoidal cells are then cleared as in a frontal sinusotomy. After clearing the recess and achieving patency of the ostium, the axillary flap is reposited to enable epithelialization and to prevent adhesions.

Flow chart 7.3 : Management of chronic rhinosinusitis with nasal polyposis

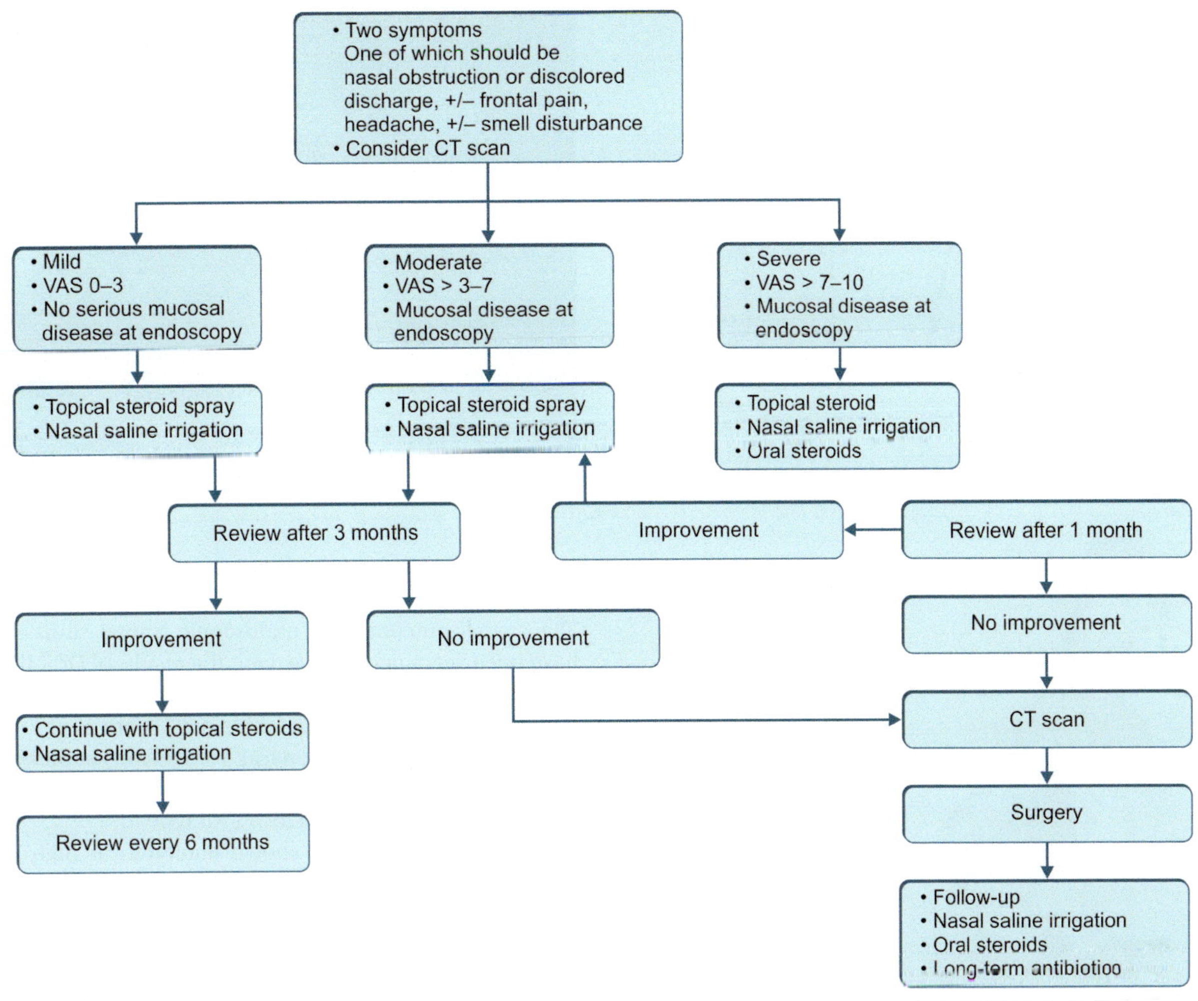

ENDONASAL FRONTAL SINUS SURGERY TYPE I–III

Professor Draf has described frontal sinus surgery taking into consideration the extent of surgery required for the disease.[27]

Type I

Type I is indicated in conditions exhibiting minor pathology of the frontal sinus and involves only ethmoidectomy. It is based on the premise that clearing the frontal recess should provide adequate aeration to the frontal sinus.

Type II

Draf IIa involves drilling and removing the frontal sinus floor from the lamina papyracea to the middle turbinate.

Draf IIb involves drilling and removing the frontal sinus floor from the lamina papyracea to the nasal septum.

The average diameter of the neo-ostium created by a Draf IIa is 5.6 mm.[28] Draf IIb is indicated when there is a need to create a larger opening and when the resultant opening after a IIa is smaller than 5 × 7 mm.

Indications for a Draf Type II

- Revision surgery
- Acute sinusitis with complication
- Benign tumor removal.

Type III/Median Drainage

Type III or median drainage is the same as endoscopic modified Lopthrop as described by Gross et al.[29] It is a type

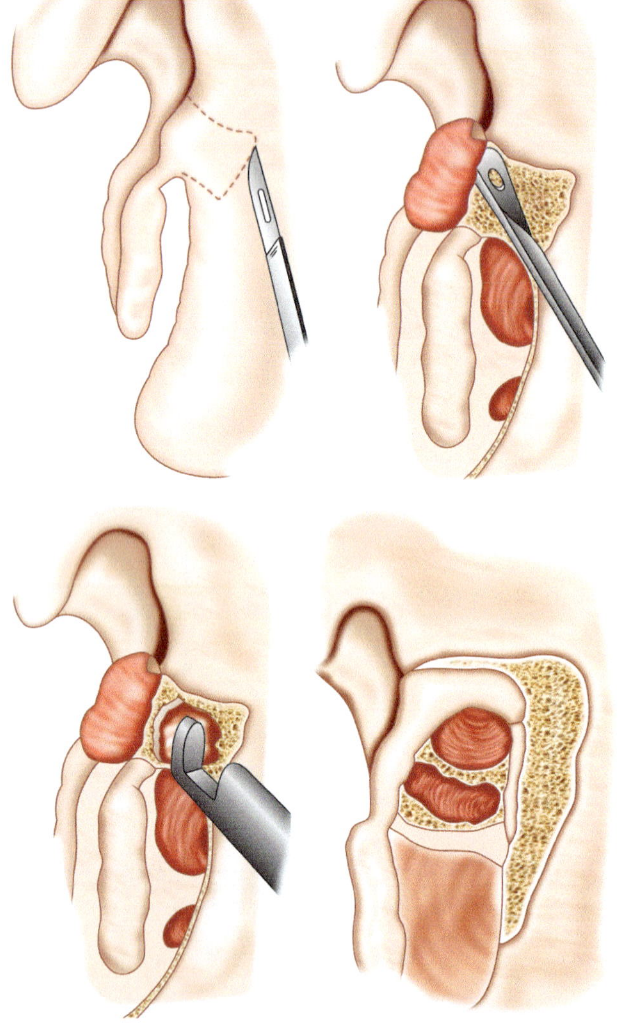

Fig. 7.11: Various steps of an axillary flap technique

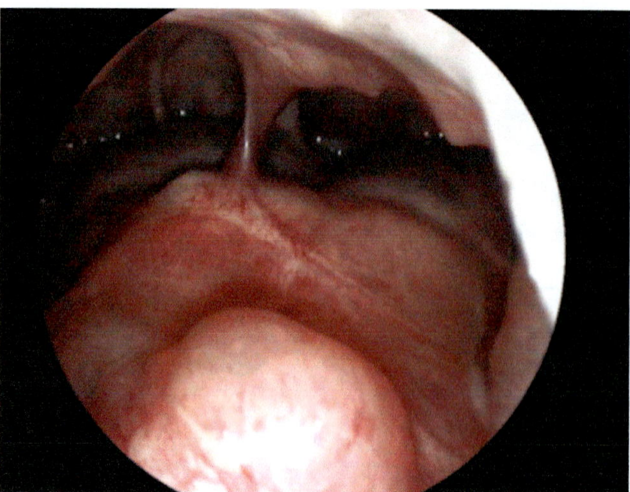

Fig. 7.12: Outcome of a Draf III procedure as seen endoscopically

IIb drainage on both sides with removal of the upper nasal septum and frontal sinus septum or septa. Identifying the first olfactory fiber and creating a "frontal T" are the key points so as to achieve maximum opening. The "frontal T" is where the long crus is represented by the posterior border of the perpendicular ethmoid lamina and the shorter wings on both sides are provided by the margins of the frontal sinus floor resection. The middle turbinate is trimmed from anterior to posterior. Figure 7.12 shows the postoperative result following a Draf type III procedure.

Indications for Draf Type III

- Revision surgery
- In patients of Samter's triad, it can be a primary modality
- Frontal sinus tumors.

Outcomes of Frontal Sinus Drilling

The overall outcomes for endoscopic frontal sinus surgery have been very encouraging, with the results of Draf III being as high as 90% inspite of the fact the cases selected for a Draf III have adverse prognostic features.[30] Weber et al[31] studied the outcomes of Draf endonasal frontal sinus surgery over a median of 5 years and showed a success outcome of 85.7% for type 1, 83.8% for type 2 and 91.5% for type III.

Metson et al[32,33] have shown outcomes as high as 80% after frontal sinus drill out procedure.

The olfactory outcomes have also been encouraging after an endoscopic Lothrop/Draf III.[34,35]

FRONTAL SINUS TREPHINATION

Alexander Ogston[1] in 1884 possibly gave the first insight into a trephination procedure. He placed a vertical incision in the midline of the forehead and raised a subperiosteal flap to expose the anterior table. He then made a "six penny piece" size trephine through the anterior table to clear the sinus. Trephination is still as relevant today in this endoscopic era.[36] Frontal ostium may occasionally be difficult to identify endoscopically, and dissection in such cases can be done by instilling fluorescein stained saline into the sinus through a trephine.

Causes of Failure

1. *Retained frontal recess cells:* This is perhaps the most important cause of failure in frontal sinus surgery.[37]

   Ability to develop a 'building block' concept in the preoperative planning as advocated by PJ Wormald[26] would help us overcome this problem.

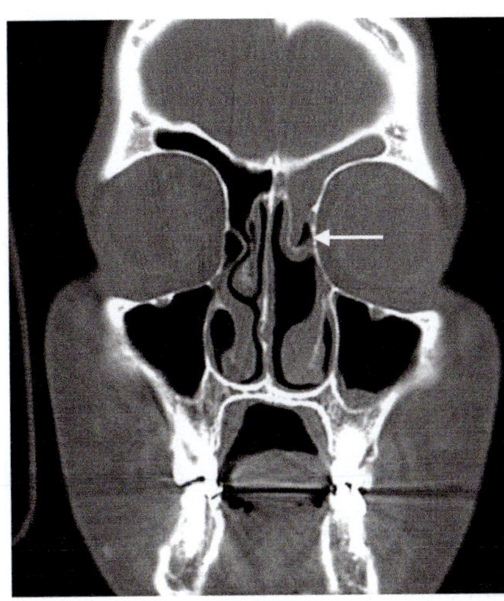

Fig. 7.13: CT scan showing a lateralized middle turbinate remnant (arrow)

2. *Retained uncinate process:* As described earlier, the manner in which the uncinate has its superior attachment, determines the drainage of the frontal sinus.

   An incompletely performed uncinectomy becomes a problem especially when its superior attachment forms a recessus terminalis.

3. *Lateralized middle turbinate:* A floppy middle turbinate can lateralize post-surgically and block the frontal recess (Fig. 7.13). Care should therefore be taken to keep the middle turbinate medialized by using techniques described in chapter 25.

Frontal sinus rescue procedure[38] *(Fig. 7.14):* This procedure has been described in patients with a lateralized middle turbinate remnant.

The initial step involves a parasagittal incision so as to separate the scarred tissue from the frontal sinus outflow tract (Figs 7.14A and B). The medial and lateral mucosa over the remnant middle turbinate is gently

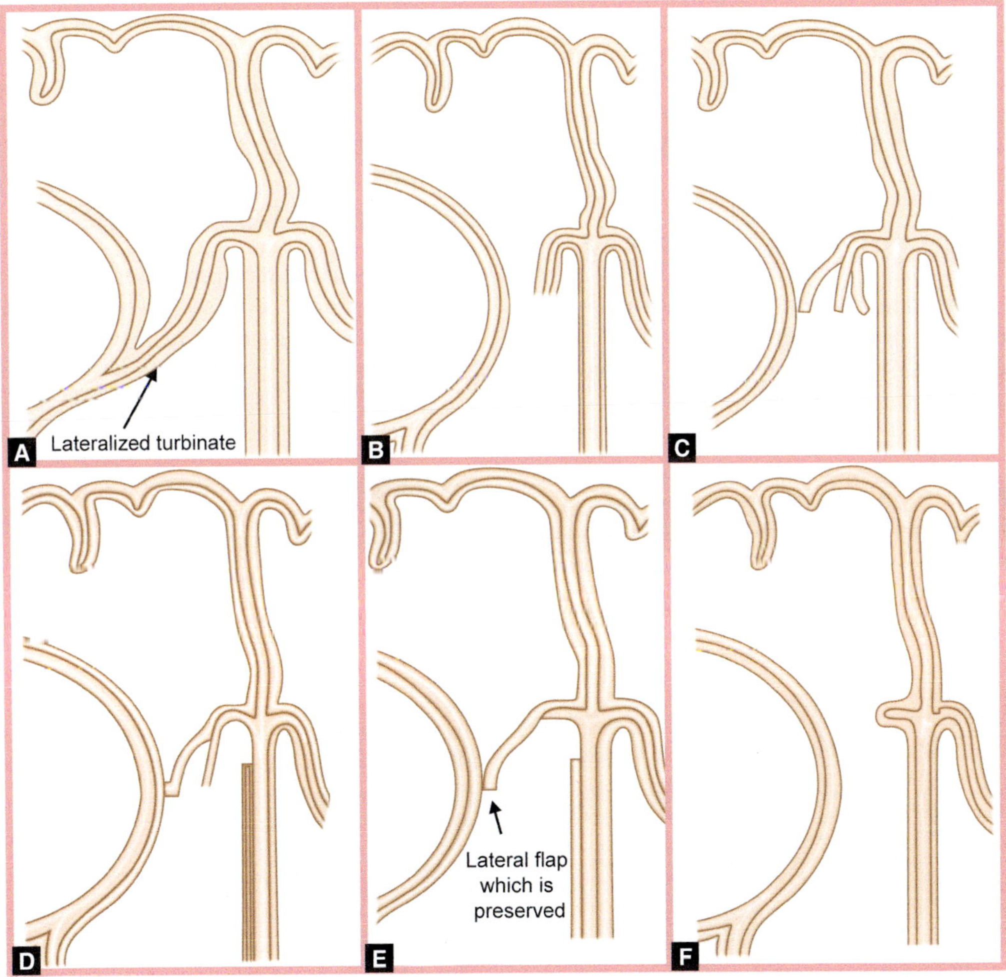

Figs 7.14A to F: Various steps of a frontal sinus rescue procedure

separated (Fig. 7.14C). The medially elevated mucosa is discarded (Fig. 7.14D). The lateral mucosal flap is preserved (Fig. 7.14D) and forms the mucoperiosteal flap. The bony middle turbinate is then removed gently (Fig. 7.14E). The mucoperiosteal flap is reposited on the raw area initially occupied by the middle turbinate (Fig. 7.14F).

4. *Osteoneogenesis:* Osteitis and osteoneogenesis occurs due to a combination of factors, which include surgical trauma, persistent inflammation, and chronic refractory infection. It is more likely to occur if mucosa in the frontal recess has been denuded during previous endoscopic surgery. Figures 7.15 and 7.16 show iatrogenic frontal stenosis.

5. *Inflammatory mucosal thickening:* Scarring and inflammatory mucosal thickening is seen frequently in the frontal recess in the postoperative setting. It has been reported up to 15%[39] in patients not requiring revision, and up to 50%[40,41] in those requiring revision surgery.

6. *Recurrent polyposis:* Recurrent polyposis has been reported in 29.9% to 40%[41,42] of patients undergoing revision surgery.

Saline irrigation during surgery helps flush out all the allergic mucin and goes a long way in preventing recurrent polyposis.

STENTING IN THE FRONTAL RECESS

The concept of stenting is as old as frontal sinus surgery. Lynch[43] in his original description of external fronto-ethmoidectomy has described postoperative stenting. The same principle has been applied in the endoscopic era.

Material for Stenting

A number of materials such as rubber tube[43], gold[44], pliable silastic sheet/tube[45] have been used as stents. Commercially available silastic stents may also be used.

Indication for Stenting

Stenting is a prerogative of the operating surgeon and depends on the underlying mucosal destruction and pathology. Hosemann et al[46] showed the need for stenting if the neo-ostium created was less than 5 mm.

Duration of Stenting

There are no current guidelines to determine the duration of stenting. Literature is divided between a shorter period[47] (6–8 weeks) of stenting as against Weber et al[48] who advocated a longer period (6 months) of stenting. Freeman[49] advocated a shorter period (up to 6 weeks of stenting) to prevent postoperative stenosis and a longer period (up to 6 months) to correct the frontal recess stenosis.

Postoperative Care of the Stent

The postoperative management of the stent involves regular saline irrigation, endoscopic cleaning and intranasal corticosteroids. The stents can be removed in the office using an endoscope.

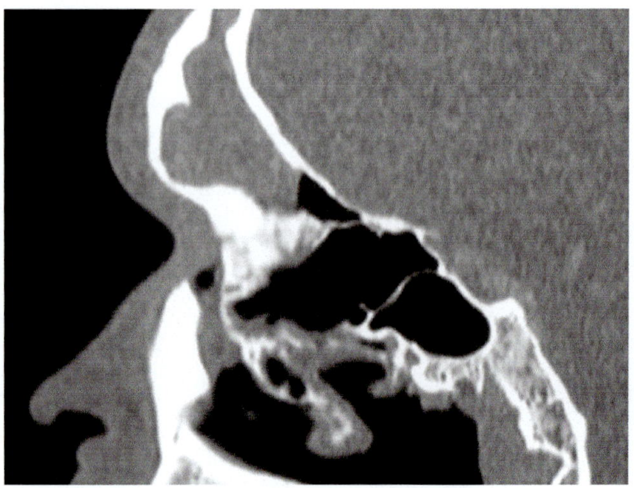

Fig. 7.15: CT scan showing extensive osteoneogenesis in the frontal recess area

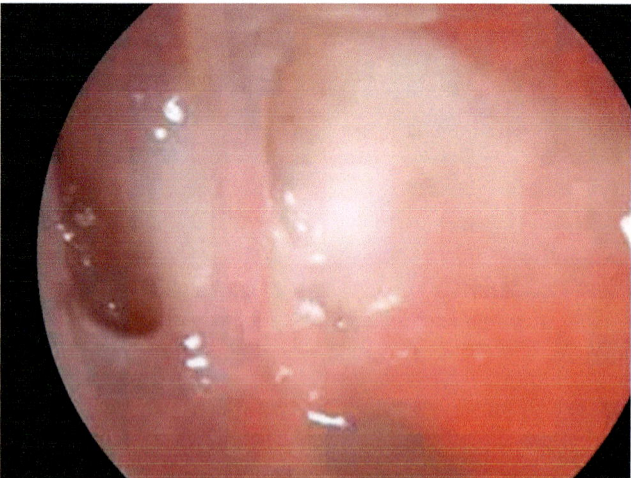

Fig. 7.16: Endoscopic view corresponding to the CT image (shown in Figure 7.15) showing extensive fibrosis and scarring

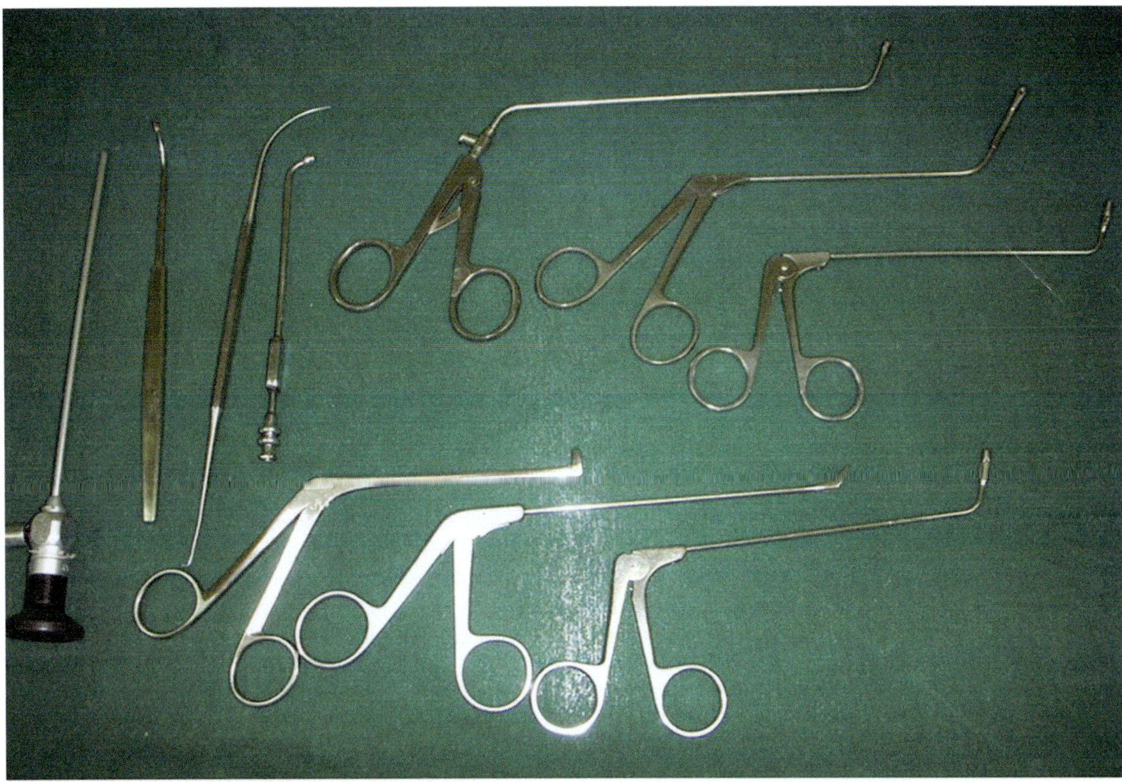

Fig. 7.17: Instruments which are used for a mucosa preserving frontal sinus surgery

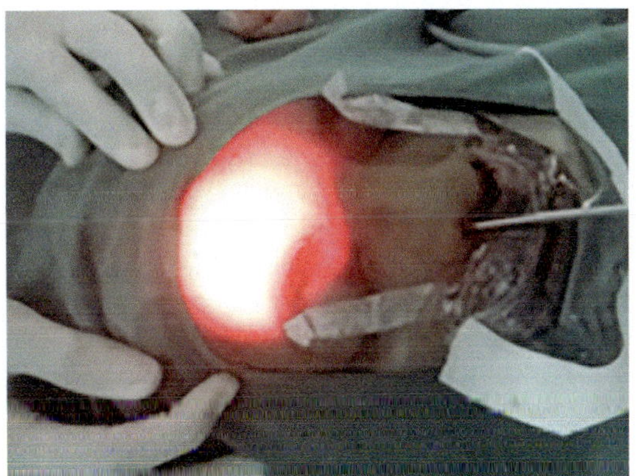

Fig. 7.18: Frontal glow indicating patency
of frontal ostium and recess

CONCLUSION

Endoscopic surgery for frontal sinus disease is more challenging than that for the other sinuses because of various factors mentioned earlier.

To achieve a successful outcome, the surgeon should:
- Be able to read CT scans well to understand the complex anatomy and pathology.
- Use the specially designed instruments (Fig. 7.17) to ensure adequate exenteration of disease.
- Be careful to preserve mucosa during exenteration of cells, so as to avoid scarring, adhesions and osteoneogenesis.
- Use frontal sinus stents when indicated.
- Ensure diligent postoperative care and nasal toilet.

REFERENCES

1. Jacob JB. 100 years of frontal sinus surgery. Laryngoscope. 1997;107:1-36
2. Kuhn F. Surgery of the frontal sinus (David Kennedy's book).
3. Kasper NA. Nasofrontal connections: a study based on one hundred consecutive dissections. Arch Otolaryngology Head Neck Surgery. 1936;23:322-43.
4. Van Alyea OE. Ethmoid Labyrinth: Anatomic study with consideration of the clinical significance of its structural characteristics. Arch Otolaryngol Head Neck Surgery. 1939;29:881-901.
5. Van Alyea OE. Frontal cells. Arch Otolaryngol. 1941;34:11-23.
6. Van Alyea OE. Frontal sinus drainage. Ann Otol Rhinol Laryngol. 1946;55:267-78.
7. Davis WB. Development and anatomy of nasal accessory sinuses in man. Philadelphia WB Saunders; 1914.
8. Marquez S, Tessema B, Clement PA, Schaefer SD. Development and extramural migration: the anatomical basis of paranasal sinus. The Anatomical Records, 2008;291;1535-53.

9. Kuhn FA, Bolger WE, Tisdall RG. The agger nasi cell in the frontal recess obstruction: an anatomical, radiological and clinical correlation. Oper Tech Otolaryngol Head Neck Surgery. 1991;2:226-31.

10. Wormald PJ. The Agger Nasi Cell. The Key to understanding the anatomy of the frontal recess. Otolaryngol Head Neck Surgery. 2003;129:497-507.

11. Kuhn FA. Chronic frontal sinusitis: the endoscopic frontal recess approach. Operative Techniques Otolaryngol Head Neck Surgery. 1996;7:222-9.

12. Bent J, Kuhn FA, Cuilty C. The Frontal cell in the frontal recess obstruction. Am J Rhinol. 1994;116:185-91.

13. Owen G, Kuhn FA. The Supraorbital ethmoid cell. Otolaryngol Head Neck Surgery. 1997;116:254-61.

14. Merritt R, Kuhn FA. The interfrontal Sinus Septal cell. Am J Rhinol. 1996;10:299-301.

15. Som PM, Lawson W. The frontal intersinus septal air cell: a new hypothesis of its origin. Am J Neuroradiology. 2008;29:1215-7.

16. Lien CF, Weng HH, Chang Y, Lin YC, et al. Computed tomographic analysis of frontal recess anatomy and its effect on the development of frontal sinusitis. Laryngoscope 2010;120:2521-7.

17. Park SS, Yoon BN, Cho KS, Poh HJ. Pneumatization pattern of the frontal recess: relationship of the anterior to posterior length of the frontal isthmus and/or frontal recess with the volume of agger nasi cell. Clinical and Experimental Otorhinolaryngology. 2010;3:76-83.

18. Draf W, Hosemann W, Keerl R, Weber RK. Modern Frontal Sinus Surgery. Karl Storz Media 05/2007.

19. Fokken W, Lund V, Mullol J, et al. European position paper on rhinosinusitis and nasal polyps 2012.

20. Fokken W, Lund V, Mullol J, et al. European position paper on rhinosinusitis and nasal polyps 2007.

21. Lim M, Lew-Gor S, Darby Y, et al. The relationship between subjective assessment instrument in chronic rhinosinusitis. Rhinology. 2007;45:144-7.

22. Leunig A, Sommer B, Betz CS, Sommer F. Surgical anatomy of the frontal recess—Is there a benefit in multiplanar CT reconstruction. Rhinology. 2008;46:188-94.

23. Haehnel S, Ert Wagner B, Tasman Abel Jan, Forsting M, Jansen O, et al. Relative value of MR imaging as compared with CT in the diagnosis of inflammatory paranasal sinus disease. Radiology. 1999;210:171-6.

24. Selcuk H, Albayam S, Ozer H, et al. Intrathecal gadolinium enhanced MR cisternography in the evaluation of CSF leakage. Am J Neuroradiol. 2010;31:71-5.

25. Reitzen SD, Wang EY, Butros SR, et al. Three dimensional reconstruction based on computed tomography images of the frontal sinus drainage pathway. Journal of Otology and Laryngology. 2010;124:291-6.

26. Wormald PJ. Surgery of the frontal recess and frontal sinus. Rhinology. 2005;43:82-5.

27. Draf W. Endonasal micro-endoscopic frontal sinus surgery the fulda concept. Operative Techniques in Otolaryngology Head Neck Surgery. 1991;2:234-40.

28. Samaha M, Cosenza DO, Metson R. Endoscopic frontal sinus drill out in 100 patients. Arch Otolaryngol Head Neck. 2003;129:854-8.

29. Gross WE, Gross CW, Becker D, et al. Modified Lopthrop procedure as an alternative to frontal sinus obliteration. Otolaryngology Head Neck Surgery. 1995;113:427-34.

30. Georgalas C, Hansen F, Videler WNJ, et al. Long term results of Draf III (modified endoscopic Lothrop) frontal sinus drainage procedure in 122 patients: a single centre experience. Rhinology. 2011;49:195-201.

31. Weber R, Draf W, Keerl R, et al. Micro-endoscopic pansinus-operation in chronic sinusitis—results and complication. Am J Otolaryngol. 1997;18:247-53.

32. Metson R, Gliklich RE. Clinical outcome of endoscopic surgery for frontal sinusitis. Arch Otolaryngol Head Neck Surgery. 1998;124:1090-6.

33. Philphott CM, Mckierman DC, Javer AR. Selecting the best approach to the frontal sinus. Indian Journal of Otolaryngology Head Neck Surgery. 2011;63(1):79-84.

34. Minovi A, Hummer T, Vral A, et al. Predictors of the outcome of nasal surgery in terms of olfactory function. Eur Arch Otorhinolaryngol. 2008;265(1):57-61.

35. Yip JM, Seiberling KA, Wormald PJ. Patient reporting olfactory function following endoscopic sinus surgery with modified endoscopic Lothrop procedure/draf3. Rhinology. 2011;49:217-20.

36. Seibering K, Jardeleza C, Wormald PJ. Minitrephination of the frontal sinus: Indication and uses in today's era of sinus surgery. Am J Rhinol Allergy. 2009;23(2):229-31.

37. Huang BY, Lloyd KM, DelGaudio JM, et al. Failed endoscopic sinus surgery: spectrum of CT findings in the frontal recess. Radiographics. 2009;29:177-95.

38. Citardi MJ, Batra PS, Kuhn FA. Frontal sinus rescue. The Frontal Sinus (editors Stillianos Kountakis, Brent Senior and Wolfgang Draf) Springer publication 2005.

39. Friedman M, Bliznikas D, Vidyasagar R, et al. Long term results after endoscopic sinus surgery involving frontal recess dissection. Laryngoscope. 2006;116(4):573-9.

40. Musy PY, Kountakis SE. Anatomic findings in patients under-going revision endoscopic sinus surgery. Am J Otolaryngol. 2004;25:418-22.

41. Schaitkin B, May M, Shapiro A, et al. Endoscopic sinus surgery: 4 year follow up on the first 100 patients. Laryngoscope. 1993; 103(10):1117-20.

42. Chiu AG, Vaughan WC. Revision endoscopic frontal sinus surgery with surgical navigation. Otolaryngol Head Neck Surg. 2004;130(3): 312-8.

43. Lynch RC. The technique of radical frontal sinus stenting which has given me the best results. Laryngoscope. 1921;31:1-5.

44. Kanowtiz SJ, Jacobs JB, Lebowitz RA. Frontal sinus stenting The Frontal Sinus (editors Stillianos Kountakis, Brent Senior and Wolfgang Draf) Springer publication 2005.

45. Neel HB, Whicker JH, Lake CF. Thin rubber sheeting in frontal sinus surgery. Animal and clinical studies. Laryngoscope 1976; 86:524-36.

46. Hosemann W, Kuhnel TH, Heed P, et al. Endonasal frontal sinusotomy in surgical management of chronic sinusitis. A critical evaluation. Am J Rhinol. 1997;11:1-19.

47. Rains BM. Frontal sinus stenting. Otolaryngol Clinics of North America 2001;34:101-10.

48. Weber R, Mai R, Hosemann W, et al. The success of 6 months stenting in endonasal frontal sinus surgery. Ear Nose Throat J. 2000;79:930-32.

49. Freeman SB, Blom ED. Frontal Sinus stents. Laryngoscope. 2000;110:1179-82.

CHAPTER 8

Endoscopic Maxillary Sinus Surgery

Milind Navalakhe

HISTORY

- The treatment of maxillary sinusitis by opening and irrigation of sinus via a variety of routes has a long and varied history.
- Highmore advocated decompression by thrusting silver bodkin through an empty tooth socket. Cowper in 1707 and Meibomius in 1718 recommended irrigation through alveolar tooth margin after molar tooth extraction. Lamorier in 1743 and Desault in 1798 preferred the canine fossa approach. In 1835, John Hunter and in 1893, Zuckerkandl advocated perforation of middle meatus, but later abandoned the technique because of potential orbital damage.
- Inferior meatal antrostomy was first described by Gooch in 1770, but routine puncture of inferior meatus was not common until advocated by Krause in 1887 using needle, Mikulicz in 1887 using trocar, and Lichtwitz in 1890 using stylette.
- Shortly after its introduction, it was largely superseded by more radical canine fossa approach described by Caldwell in 1893, Spicer in 1894, Luc in 1897. Caldwell-Luc approach was the primary operation during the first part of the 20th century, but there was increasing trend toward lavage, followed by inferior meatal antrostomy with Caldwell-Luc reserved for any failures.[1]
- In the UK, in 1980s endoscopic surgery was first introduced. In 1903, Killian proposed removal of anterior and inferior walls but with preservation of

supraorbital rims. The primary objective of Messerklinger approach, championed by Stammberger is the removal of pathology in the osteomeatal complex sufficient to achieve ventilation and drainage, thereby addressing the underlying pathology by a conservative approach technique, hence term "Functional" endorsed by Kennedy.[2]
- The title, FESS (functional endoscopic sinus surgery) is therefore only appropriate when performing limited surgery with preservation of existing structures.

ANATOMY

The maxillary sinus is the largest paranasal sinus and lies lateral to middle meatus in which it drains. It is commonly referred as antrum and first described in detail by Nathaniel Highmore in 1651.[3] A consensus is lacking regarding shape of this structure due to high variability in its development. Cullen and Vidic attempted to describe it as elliptical, triangular, irregular, and the spherical shape in 1972. Then in 1996, Anon described it as a pyramidal shaped in three-dimensional views.

It is large, pyramidal shaped chamber, with its limit being:
- Superiorly, orbital floor
- Inferiorly, hard palate and alveolar process of maxilla
- Laterally, zygomatic process
- Posteriorly, a thin plate of bone separating the cavity from infratemporal and pterygopalatine fossa where maxillary artery and vein run

- Medially, uncinate process, fontaneles and inferior turbinate.

The apex of sinus points laterally and extends into zygomatic process, sometimes into the zygomatic bone. The base of sinus faces medially and forms the lateral wall of nasal cavity. It is located within the maxillary bone which is the second largest of facial bones.

PNEUMATIZATION AND GROWTH

The degree of pneumatization varies with age. The shape of sinus changes with age. At birth, the maxillary sinus has rounded or elongated shape and gradually becomes pyramidal. It appears at 65th day of gestation and by 13th years of age maxillary sinus reaches its definitive shape.

CLINICAL ANATOMY

In adults, maxillary sinus is roughly described as triangular in shape, measuring 25 mm along the anterior limb of its base, 34 mm in depth, and 33 mm in height. The primary or natural ostium of this sinus is located in the superior aspect of the medial wall of the sinus and drains via its infundibulum into the ethmoid infundibulum, and thus the hiatus semilunaris. The ostium is located 1.3–11.5 mm from nasolacrimal duct and this proximity of duct to natural ostium makes it vulnerable to injury during middle meatus antrostomy.

The natural ostium tends to be elliptical, measuring from 1 mm to 20 mm in length. In addition, accessory maxillary sinus ostia are found in 15–40% of subjects. These ostia may be located in the ethmoid infundibulum or the membranous region of medial sinus wall, i.e. membranous meatus or fontanel. This region is located inferior to uncinate process and superior to the insertion of the inferior turbinate.

PHYSIOLOGY OF SINUS DRAINAGE

Normal drainage of paranasal sinuses is a complex function of both the secretion and transport mechanisms, and to large extent dependent upon the amount of mucus produced, its composition, the effectiveness of cilliary beating movement, mucosal resorption and condition of ostium.

In maxillary sinus, secretion transport starts from the floor of sinus. The mucus is transported along the anterior, medial, posterior and lateral wall of the sinuses as well as along the roof. All these secretion routes converge at the natural ostium of the maxillary sinus. When the secretion has passed through the maxillary sinus ostium, it is not yet in the free middle meatus, and must pass through a very narrow and complicated system of clefts in the lateral nasal wall. Secretion from the sinus is always transported via the natural ostium, even when there is one or more accessory ostium in the area of the fontanel. While an inferior meatal nasoantral window may provide good ventilation to the diseased maxillary sinus, but this window does not achieve considerable active outwardly directed transportation of secretion.[4]

PATHOLOGY

Rhinosinusitis is a common pathology seen in all paranasal sinuses. It is defined as a condition manifested by an inflammatory response involving the mucus membrane of the nasal cavity and paranasal sinuses.

The most common site for mucosal thickening in decreasing order is as follows (Fig. 8.1):

Anatomical obstruction of maxillary sinus ostium in chronic rhinosinusitis can be because of:

- Mucosal hypertrophy
- Deviated nasal septum
- Ipsilateral concha bullosa
- Contralateral concha bullosa producing septal deviation
- Extensive nasal polyposis
- Prominent Haller cell.

CLINICAL FEATURES OF RHINOSINUSITIS

Major symptoms	Minor symptoms
Facial pain/pressure	Headache
Facial congestion/fullness	Fever
Nasal obstruction/blockage	Halitosis
Nasal discharge/ posterior discolored drainage	Fatigue
Hyposmia/anosmia	Dental pain
Purulence on nasal examination	Ear pain/fullness/pressure
Fever	Cough

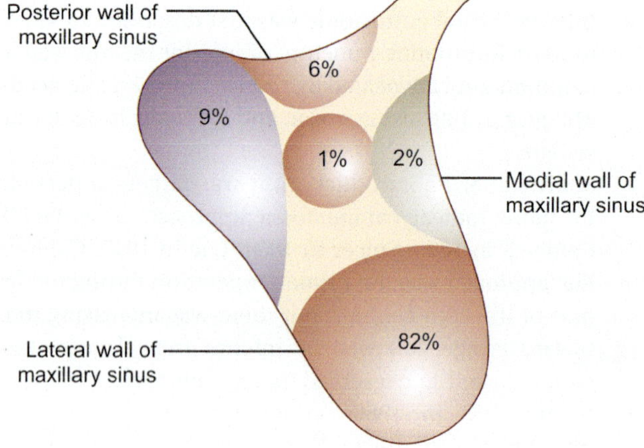

Fig. 8.1: Mucosal thickening in decreasing order

MEDICAL MANAGEMENT OF RHINOSINUSITIS

- In case of acute sinusitis antibiotics for 7–10 days is effective in controlling infection. Often a course of 3 or 4 weeks may be necessary for chronic forms; change in antibiotic may be needed.
- Antihistamines and topical decongentants like oxymetazoline and phenylephrines produce vasoconstriction and therefore shrinkage of congested nasal mucosa.
- Topical corticosteroids help in reducing edema. And hence it provides added relief in treatment of acute recurrent sinusitis.
- Oral steroids are also given in cases of polyposis for 2 weeks, as it helps in reducing the size of the polyp by its anti-inflammatory action.
- Nasal irrigation is also helpful in chronic sinusitis in removing crusts with soda bicarbonate and salt solution.
- In case of invasive fungal infection for example, mucormycosis, antifungals like injection amphotericin given intravenous (IV) with a total dose of 4 gm in divided doses and oral antifungal like itraconazole or voriconazole 200 mg BD is given for 2–3 months.

PREOPERATIVE EVALUATION OF PATIENT

- A complete history and thorough ENT examination are required before planning any surgery. Contrast-enhanced computed tomography (CT) scan of the paranasal sinuses and diagnostic nasal examinations (DNE) are important tools before surgery.
- Imaging of paranasal sinuses plays a larger role in functional endoscopic sinus surgery by not only defining the extent of inflammatory sinus disease, but also to help in determining the course of treatment and a successful surgical outcome. Anatomical variants in the paranasal sinuses and nasal fossa may be recognized on CT scan. In case of polyposis oral steroid is given for 2 weeks prior to CT scan. A contrast-enhanced CT scan will be useful in vascular lesions like an angiofibroma.
- The diagnostic nasal examination is important both for medical and surgical treatment of sinonasal disease.
- It is directed toward confirming the history and documenting the evidence of sinonasal disease, in particular, obstruction of ostia of sinuses.[5]

INDICATIONS OF MAXILLARY SINUS SURGERY

- Chronic rhinosinusitis
- Acute recurrent rhinosinusitis
- Nasal polyposis

- Mucoceles
- Allergic fungal sinusitis and mycetoma
- Management of epistaxis.

PREOPERATIVE PREPARATION OF PATIENT

- The patient is explained about the procedure and complication of both surgery and anesthesia in detail and written informed consent is taken.
- The patient is given preoperative antibiotics, nasal and systemic steroids, such as prednisolone or methylprednisolone. Steroid is useful in reducing inflammation and hemorrhage in patient with extensive nasal polyposis.
- The procedure can be performed under either general or local anesthesia. The patients to be operated under general anesthesia include:
  - Pediatric patients
  - The adult patients who are anxious and uncooperative.
  - In patients with more advanced pathology such as nasal polyposis or cases where a chance of bleeding is more.
- In both cases vasoconstriction is must. Patient's nose should be packed with 4% xylocaine with adrenaline soaked cottonoid prior to surgery for decongestion and better visualization.
- Local anesthesia is carried out by infiltrating with 2% lignocaine (1:80,000 adrenalin) into uncinate process, around the sphenopalatine foramen and middle turbinate.

STEPS OF SURGERY

- Once thorough vasoconstriction of nasal mucosa is accomplished, a complete examination should be performed. This is best done with 0° or 30° telescope. The nasal cavity should be examined with particular attention being paid to middle meatus and any other abnormality on CT scan.
- If a deviated nasal septum is present, then septoplasty is indicated to correct nasal obstruction independent of sinus disease, or to remove a septal deviation at the level of middle turbinate which prevents adequate access for the instruments to perform the procedure.
- Mucosa over the uncinate process is infiltrated with 2% lignocaine with 1:200,000 adrenalin. The blanching of mucosa is seen due to ischemia.
- *Uncinate process is removed in a variety of ways:*
  - The base of uncinate is incised with a sickle knife and then elevated with a Freer's elevator, superior attachment is twisted inside and inferior attachment twisted outside with straight Blakesley forceps. The uncinate bone is then removed. Any remnants of the uncinate process can be removed secondarily with

Ostrum's forceps and inferior uncinectomy can be performed with the same forceps.

- Uncinectomy can also be performed with microdebrider.
- The next step is removal of the bulla ethmoidalis. This is accomplished either with the straight Blakesley forceps or a microdebrider.
- A middle meatal antrostomy is performed. If maxillary ostium is visualized easily and is adequate in size, a middle meatal antrostomy is probably not necessary. On the other hand if the ostium cannot be visualized or seems to be small, it should be enlarged with a reverse biting forceps anteriorly or with a straight tru-cut forceps posteriorly until it is 1.5–2.0 cm in diameter. Any disease present in the maxillary sinus should be cleared.
- Nasal packing is done to achieve hemostasis.

TIPS FOR COMPLETE CLEARANCE OF ANTROCHOANAL POLYP

- Use of angled scope
- Use of angled instruments
- Use of long bladed instruments
- If the stalk still cannot be approached, then inferior meatal antrostomy can be done for better access.

POSTOPERATIVE CARE

- Proper postoperative care is essential. The objective is to keep the sinuses open and draining and to prevent scarring, which might subsequently occlude ostia.
- Pack is removed after 48 hours of surgery.
- In early postoperative period, the cavity should be inspected, and any clots or crusts should be removed.
- The patient is explained about nasal irrigation to keep the nasal cavity clear.
- The patient is given antibiotic for 2 weeks along with antihistaminic and steroidal nasal sprays to aid in healing.

COMPLICATIONS

- Bleeding
- Injury to orbit
- Injury to the nasolacrimal duct
- Cerebrospinal fluid (CSF) leak
- Synechiae.

DIFFICULTIES ARISING IN ENDOSCOPIC MAXILLARY SINUS SURGERY

- Maxillary sinus ostium is difficult to identify in some cases, probably due to edematous mucosa or more commonly due to posteroinferior remnants of the uncinate process. These uncinate remnants should be identified and removed. When palpating for the ostium of the maxillary sinus, it is best to palpate along the bony insertion of the inferior turbinate.
- Anterior wall, floor, lateral wall of the maxillary sinus are difficult to approach. To overcome these difficulties long bladed and angled instruments like 45°, 90° or 120° forceps along with 45° or 70° endoscopes may have to be used.

REFERENCES

1. Tange RA. Some historical aspects of the surgical treatment of the infected maxillary sinus. Rhinology. 1991;29(2):155-62.
2. Stammberger H, Posawetz W. Functional endoscopic sinus surgery. Concept, indications and results of the Messerklinger technique. Eur Arch Otorhinolaryngol. 1990;247(2):63-76.
3. Wendler D. Nathanael Highmore (1613-1685) and the maxillary sinus. Anat Anz. 1986;162(5):375-80.
4. Mann WJ, Tóth M, Gouveris H, Amedee RG. The drainage system of the paranasal sinuses: a review with possible implications for balloon catheter dilation. Am J Rhinol Allergy. 2011 Jul-Aug;25(4):245-8. doi: 10.2500/ajra.2011.25.3647.
5. Nouraei SA, Elisay AR, Dimarco A, Abdi R, Majidi H, Madani SA, Andrews PJ. Variations in paranasal sinus anatomy: implications for the pathophysiology of chronic rhinosinusitis and safety of endoscopic sinus surgery. J Otolaryngol Head Neck Surg. 2009;38(1):32-7.

CHAPTER 9

Approach to the Sphenoid Sinus

Nishit J Shah, Rahul P Tejankar

INTRODUCTION

The sphenoid sinus is located at the skull base and is related to all the three cranial fossae, i.e. anterior, middle and the posterior.

The sphenoid sinus was assumed to be a dangerous sinus in the pre-endoscopic era as it is surrounded by several neurovascular structures, including the optic nerve, the internal carotid artery (ICA), the maxillary nerve, and the vidian nerve.

But it is one of the easiest sinuses to deal with as this is the only sinus whose ostium is visible even without surgery and lies straight ahead behind and medial to the superior turbinate.

ANATOMY

The central portion of the body of the sphenoid is pneumatized by the two sphenoid sinuses. The sphenoid sinuses are variably pneumatized. They are often asymmetrical showing right or left side "dominance".

Depending on the extent of pneumatization, the sphenoid sinus can be classified into three types:

1. *Sellar:* The most common type (75–86%), where pneumatization extends into the body of the sphenoid beyond the floor of the sella, reaching sometimes the clivus.
2. *Conchal:* The area below the sella is a bone with very little pneumatization (<2%).

3. *Presellar:* The sphenoid is pneumatized to the level of the frontal plane of the sella and not beyond (10–25%).

The superior wall of the sinus is in continuity with the roof of the ethmoid sinus and it is part of the anterior and middle floors of the skull base, being in direct contact to the olfactory nerves, optic nerves and hypophysis.

The anterior wall is connected to the perpendicular plate of the ethmoid and vomer in the midline, as well as the lateral masses of the ethmoid on each side. The anterior wall harbors the sphenoid ostium.

The floor of the sinus forms the dome of the choanae and of the nasopharynx.

The lateral wall of the sphenoid sinus can show various prominences, the most important being the carotid canal and the optic canal: the internal carotid artery is the most medial structure in the cavernous sinus, and rests against the lateral surface of the sphenoid bone. The optic canal is found in the posterosuperior angle between the lateral, posterior and superior walls of the sinus, horizontally crossing the carotid canal from lateral to medial. Pneumatization of the sphenoid above and below the optic canal can result, respectively, in a supra optic recess and an infraoptic recess (the optico carotid recess). The infraoptic recess lies between the optic nerve superiorly and the carotid canal inferiorly, and can sometimes pneumatize the anterior clinoid process. The canals of two other nerves can be encountered in the lateral wall of the sphenoid sinus if there is extensive pneumatization of the sphenoid till or beyond the pterygoids, below the level of the carotid canal; the second branch of the trigeminal nerve superiorly through the foramen roduntum and the vidian nerve in the pterygoid canal inferiorly.

The sphenoid sinus drains through a single ostium into the sphenoethmoid recess: this ostium is classically situated 7 cm from the base of the columella at an angle of 30° with the floor of the nose in a parasagittal plane, and this usually corresponds to a location halfway up the anterior wall of the sinus. Endoscopically, the posteroinferior end of the superior turbinate points superiorly and medially toward the ostium and thus represents a very important landmark to identify it.

The average volume of the sinus is about 6–7.5 mL, with average size of presellar sinus is 2.5 mL and that of the postsellar sinus is 8.5 mL. The average dimensions of the sinus: anteroposterior: 2.5 cm, transverse: 2.8 cm and vertical: 2.2 cm.

Congenital bony defect in the lateral wall of sphenoid sinus (the lateral craniopharyngeal canal) is called Sternberg's canal and is usually associated with spontaneous CSF leak and encephalocele. This canal extends from the junction of the body of the sphenoid bone and the posterior root of the lesser sphenoid wing, just medial to the superior orbital fissure inferiorly to connect with either the pharynx at the processus vaginalis, or when sufficient pneumatization has occurred into the lateral wall of the sphenoid sinus.

SURGICAL APPROACHES

Trans-septal Sphenoidotomy

It is the traditional and oldest of the approaches; "follow the septum, enter the sphenoid." Various incisions and approaches were popular earlier. Example:

Sublabial Trans-septal Approach

The operation is begun by a transfixation incision along the left nasal septum. A mucoperichondrial tunnel is elevated along the left septum from anterior to posterior. Inferior tunnels are then elevated bilaterally in a submucoperiosteal plane lateral to the nasal spine. The mucosa is left intact and not elevated along the right side of the quadrangular cartilage. A vertical incision is then made in the posterior quadrangular cartilage near the perpendicular plate of the ethmoid. The mucoperiosteum along the right nasal septum is then elevated posteriorly over the perpendicular plate and vomer. The cartilaginous septum is then separated from the nasal spine and maxillary crest and translocated to the right. The bony septum is taken down to the sphenoid rostrum. A sublabial incision is made between the canine fossae

bilaterally and the sublabial and transnasal exposures are connected. The hypophysectomy speculum is then inserted through the sublabial incision between the mucosal flaps to the sphenoid rostrum. The anterior wall of the sphenoid and intersinus septum is removed and the sellar bone exposed.

External Rhinoplasty Approach

Popularized by Parnes and Koltai among others, the external rhinoplasty technique has the advantages of enhanced exposure while limiting the problems with sublabial dissection (gingival numbness, denture problems, contamination of the field with oral flora). A standard external rhinoplasty incision employing the inverted "V" is made and columellar flaps are raised to the midportion of the lower lateral cartilages. Complete exposure of the lateral crura and the upper lateral cartilages is unnecessary. The caudal edge of the quadrilateral cartilage is exposed by dividing the intercrural ligaments between the medial crura. A mucoperichondrial flap on one side of the quadrilateral cartilage is developed and continued over the perpendicular plate of the ethmoid and vomer. Dissection proceeds onto the maxillary crest and the floor of the nose, connecting the medial and inferior tunnels. The quadrilateral cartilage is detached posteriorly at the bony cartilaginous junction and the mucoperiosteum on the opposite side of the ethmoid and vomer is elevated. The cartilage is then disarticulated from the maxillary crest. The mucoperiosteal elevation is continued on the maxillary crest and the floor of the nose on the opposite side. The nasal speculum is inserted, displacing the septal leaflets laterally. The perpendicular plate of the ethmoid is resected, taking care to preserve the vomer, which serves as a midline guide to the anterior face of the sphenoid. The anterior sinus wall is opened, the intersinus septum is removed, and the sinus mucosa is exenterated.

Columellar Flap Modification

It is a modification of external rhinoplasty approach. A complete transfixation incision is made at the caudal septum and an incision is made at the base of the columella. The quadrangular cartilage is accessed via this incision and it requires no separation of the medial crura. The operation then proceeds in the previous manner.

Advantage: These are midline approach and safer and provided equal access to both sides of the sphenoid sinus and sella.

Disadvantage: These trans-septal approaches are usually not preferred because of the associated nasal morbidity usually secondary to improper handling of septum during surgery.

Transantral Sphenoidotomy

This approach was used when Caldwell-Lucs approach was the standard for chronic maxillary, ethmoid and sphenoid sinusitis.

This procedure begins with sublabial maxillary sinusotomy, followed by posterior ethmoidectomy through superomedial aspect of maxillary antrum and then the anterior sphenoid wall is exposed and entered.

Advantage: This approach gives access to extreme lateral extension of sphenoid sinus, e.g. pterygoid recess.

Disadvantage: It is the oblique angle taken toward the sphenoid which does not allow for easy orientation with midline structures. Because of the potential complications due to this, the transantral approach is seldom used.

External Transorbital Transethmoidal Sphenoidotomy

First described by Chiari in 1912, this procedure includes a Lynch type incision for external ethmoidectomy and is followed by sphenoidotomy.

Advantage: Lack of oral communications of trans-septal, no nasal complication like septal perforation and it gives excellent control of the orbit.

Disadvantage: The midline is not followed and loss of orientation could be disastrous if the lateral wall of the sphenoid sinus is mistaken for the intersinus septum. Other disadvantages include the external scar and inaccessibility of the suprasellar region.

Transpalatal Sphenoidotomy

The surgery starts with dividing the palate. Many incisions are proposed to do so, a midline palatal split through the medial raphe is the quickest and easiest procedure to perform and allows good exposure. Once the hard palate is reached, it is removed as necessary for exposure along with the posterior vomer. This allows direct access to the rostrum of the sphenoid and nasopharynx.

Advantage: Good exposure to nasopharynx and pterygopalatine space.

Disadvantage: It may lead to palatal shortening and velopharyngeal insufficiency.

Endoscopic Endonasal Sphenoidotomy

This is the preferred surgical approach for sphenoid sinus surgery.

This approach is the least invasive, direct and safe. It is safe as it deals with the medial part of the anterior sphenoid wall thus avoiding the injury of optic nerve and carotid artery in the lateral sphenoid wall.

Paraseptal Approach

The access to sphenoid sinus can be gained directly by lateralizing middle and superior turbinate and identifying the sphenoid os (direct/bulls eye) (Fig. 9.1). After ensuring correct identification of the sphenoid sinus, it is entered medially adjacent to the septum approximately 1.5 cm above the choana, approximately one-third of the way up the anterior sphenoid wall, 7 cm and 30° from the anterior nasal spine. Precaution taken during this maneuver is to stay in the inferior half of the turbinates as the space between nasal septum and lateral nasal wall tapers superiorly like tip of pyramid, and pushing the scope and instruments superiorly may damage the olfactory fibers, traumatize the cribriform area and also because of this narrow space the blood trickles down over the scope and obscures the surgical field view. Sometimes the inferior half of the middle turbinate may be removed if necessary for making space to negotiate the scope and instruments together.

This approach is more physiological as it deals directly with the sinus ostium with minimum disruption of ostiomeatal complex (Fig. 9.1).

Intermediate Approach

After opening of the anterior ethmoidal air cells, one has to go through the posterior end of middle turbinate, identify the horizontal lamella of superior turbinate and create a superior meatal window to gain access to the sphenoethmoidal recess

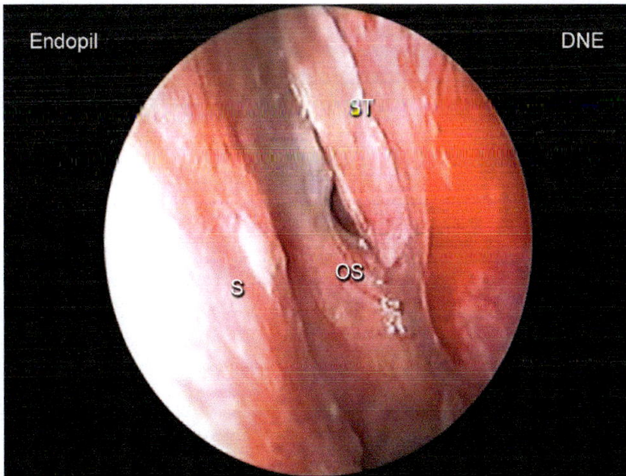

Fig. 9.1: Left nasal cavity showing paraseptal approach exposing sphenoid ostium (OS) just behind superior turbinate (ST) and lateral to septum (S)

and the natural sphenoid ostium, and is widened. Sometimes resection of the inferior one-third of superior turbinate may be required (Figs 9.2 to 9.4).

Lateral Approach

This involves prior clearance of the anterior and posterior ethmoid air cells before gaining access to sphenoid sinus. The posterior ethmoid sinuses are entered through the ground lamella which will then expose the anterior wall of the sphenoid sinus. The sinus can then be opened inferiorly, medially. Care should be taken opening the sinus superiorly, because a CSF leak can result if the thin roof of the sinus is entered.

The various landmarks which can help a surgeon identify sphenoid sinus correctly during the lateral approach are; superior turbinate (sphenoid sinus ostium lies just posterior and medial), imaginary line along the medial orbital floor and the bony ridge of middle meatus antrostomy (the cells above this line are the posterior ethmoidal cells and sphenoid sinus lies below this line), color of bone (color of skull base is white as opposed to sphenoid which has a bluish hue), lie of bone (ethmoids cells give a feel of going away while the bone of sphenoid is more perpendicular) (Figs 9.5 to 9.7).

Endoscopic Transnasal with Posterior Septectomy

This technique is mainly used for lesion/diseases of the lateral recess of sphenoid, sellar, parasellar and clivus and nasopharynx region or extensive sphenoid lesions and revision surgery (Fig. 9.8).

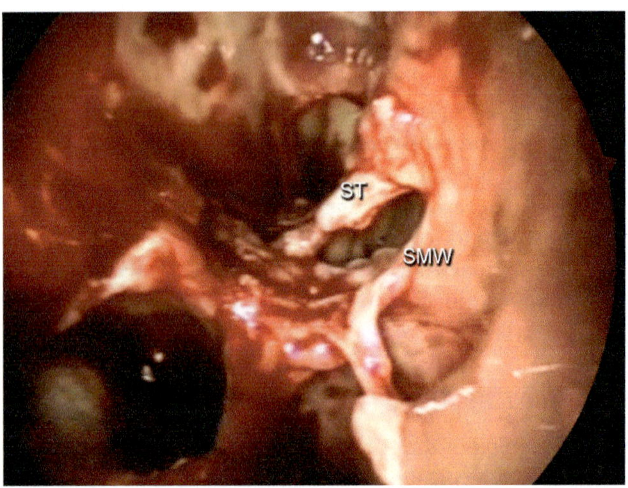

Fig. 9.2: Right nasal cavity showing anterior edge of superior turbinate (ST) for an intermediate approach via superior meatal window (SMW)

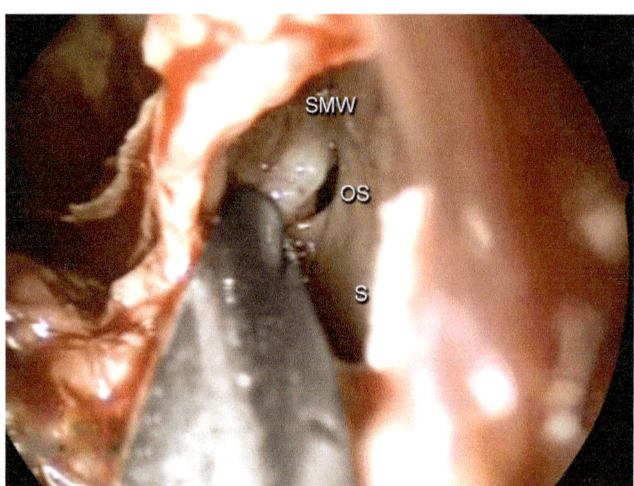

Fig. 9.3: View through the intermediate approach localizing the sphenoid ostium (OS)

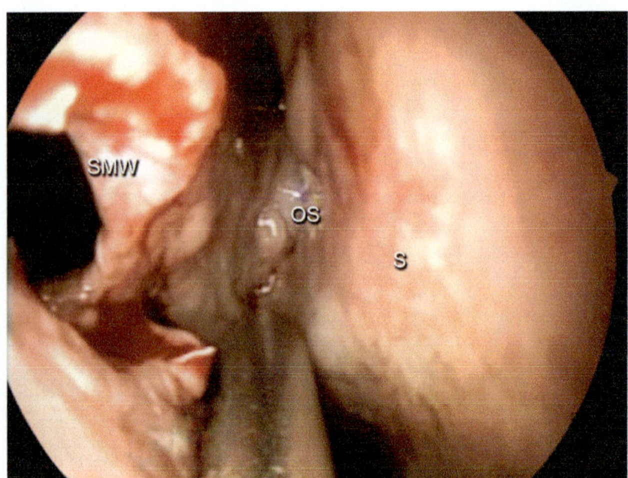

Fig. 9.4: Same view of the right sphenoid ostium via a paraseptal approach

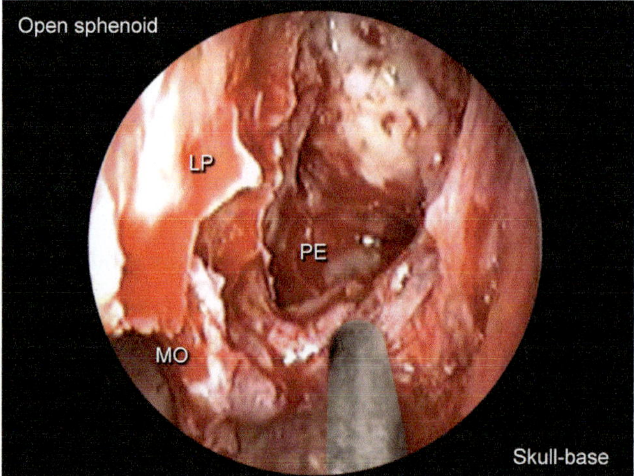

Fig. 9.5: Right nasal cavity showing maxillary ostium (MO) laterally, superior turbinate ground lamella (suction tip) and posterior ethmoid (PE) opened

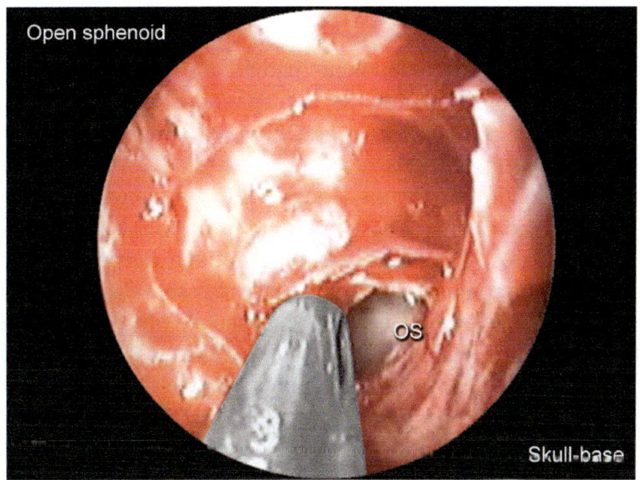

Fig. 9.6: Same patient with the sphenoid sinus opened inferolateral to the orbital apex via a lateral approach

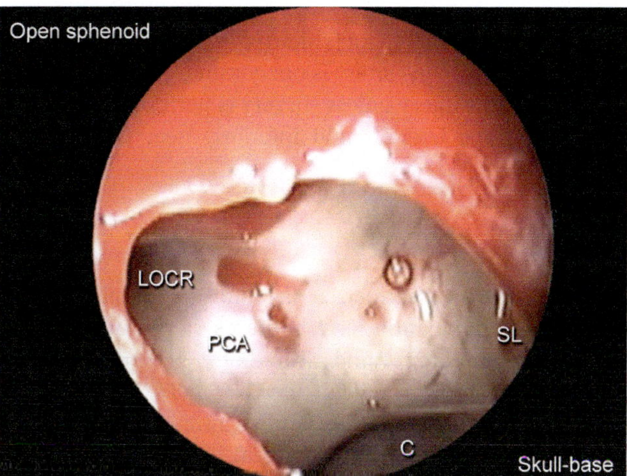

Fig. 9.7: View of paraclinoid carotid artery (PCA), lateral opticocarotid recess (LOCR), clivus (C) and sella (SL) in widened right sphenoid

Advantage: The main advantage of this technique lies in revision surgery where all the essential landmarks are lost; here by following the septum the surgeon easily can identify the sphenoid. The septum is attached to the sphenoid rostrum in the midline.

PATHOLOGIES

Usually sphenoid sinus diseases are mostly inflammatory in nature and a primary sphenoid sinus tumor is a rare occurrence.

Infections and inflammation of the sphenoid sinus (bacterial sinusitis, fungal sinusitis, polyps, mucocele) are mostly accompanied by involvement of the other sinuses. Isolated sphenoid sinus disease is uncommon. The diagnosis in such cases is generally delayed, as the sphenoid sinus is located in the deep apex of the nasal cavity and is dependent on imaging.

Tumor of the sphenoid sinus is a rare entity, though tumors of skull base and pituitary do regularly present through the sphenoid sinus.

COMPLICATIONS OF SPHENOID SURGERY

Epistaxis

Epistaxis usually occurs from the artery of the pterygoid canal, artery of palatovaginal canal, or the septal branch of sphenopalatine (SP) artery.

The most prominent artery encountered during sphenoidotomy is the septal branch of the sphenopalatine (posterior nasal artery), which is a distal branch of the internal maxillary artery (IMA). This branch arises directly

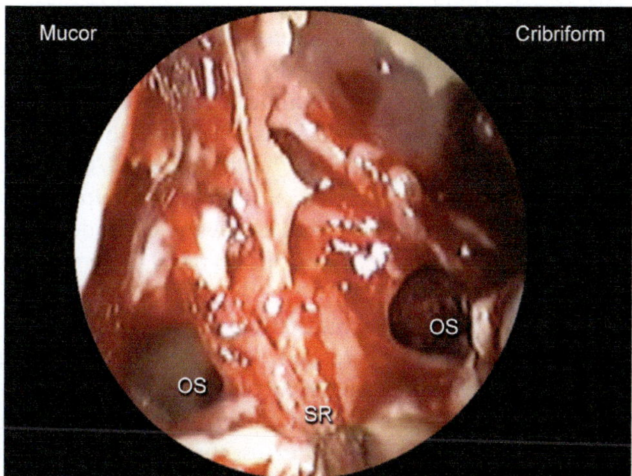

Fig. 9.8: Endoscopic septectomy for trans-septal approach to the sphenoid. Both sphenoid ostia seen on either side of the rostrum (SR)

from sphenopalatine artery in the sphenopalatine foramen and traverses across the anterior face of sphenoid near the insertion of superior turbinate posteriorly, and superior-to-posterior lateral nasal arterial branch which supplies the middle turbinate. This artery is typically encountered when opening the sphenoid sinus too inferiorly near the horizontal portion of the superior turbinate. This can be easily cauterized (monopolar/bipolar) and rarely requires SP artery ligation.

The artery of palatovaginal canal (pharyngeal branch of internal maxillary artery) traverses through palatovaginal canal. This canal is related laterally to medial pterygoid plate and medially to sphenoid rostrum. This vessel gets injured during opening of sphenoid ostium more laterally and inferiorly.

The artery of pterygoid (vidian) canal arises from internal maxillary artery. This artery is not commonly encountered in routine sinus surgery unless surgery is performed to remove sphenoid bone laterally and inferiorly near the pterygoid plate.

Carotid Artery Damage

Carotid may be lacerated at the time of surgery and is a dreaded complication and requires a multidisciplinary effort with a calm mind. The bony wall covering the carotid may be thin or dehiscent in 5–8% of population. This vascular injury during endoscopic surgery is a high pressure and high volume type in a small surgical field contaminating the endoscope easily leaving the surgeon without view. The first and foremost thing for a surgeon is to keep calm and ask his ENT/neurosurgery colleague's help. Two surgeon four hand technique allows one surgeon to keep surgical field clean and this enables the other surgeon to obtain a sufficient view to perform maneuvers necessary for hemostasis. Also, one must ask the anesthetist to stabilize the patient hemodynamically. After localizing the site of bleed, the surgeon can use variety of methods to stop the bleeding. Muscle piece/Surgicel/Floseal/Gelfoam/endoscopic vascular clamps with self-knotting clips can be used to plug and stop small tears in ICA and larger defects in ICA may need endovascular occlusion by an interventional radiologist.

Usually muscle is harvested from thigh or from sternocleidomastoid and is crushed and used for patching. Hemostasis can be achieved by this in almost all cases.

SURGIFLO (J&J) is porcein gelatin with thrombin and hemostasis is achieved almost in less than 1 minute; Floseal (Baxter) is porcein gelatin and gives hemostasis within 2 minutes. The drawback of using these agents is that they cause postoperative granulations and adhesion formation, high rate of antibody formation and are mainly useful for microvascular control.

Neck exploration with ligation of internal carotid artery (ICA) followed by clipping the carotid artery below the anterior cerebral artery through craniotomy may rarely be requied if facilities of intervention radiology is not available.

Venous hemorrhage from cavernous sinuses and intercavernous sinus may occur in cases of transsphenoidal surgery and usually stops after bipolar cauterization of the small bleeders or with help of packing with Gelfoam/Surgicel/Floseal.

Maxillary and vidian nerve injury are related to the lateral recess of sphenoid; so in an over pneumatized sphenoid sinus they are at a risk injury leading to facial numbness and eye dryness.

Optic nerve injury can occur in sphenoid sinus surgery if the operating surgeon is not careful about the optic nerve course and its relation to the sphenoid sinus, its bony dehiscence and presence of an Onodi cell, pneumatization of anterior clinoids.

The optic nerve runs along the superolateral aspect of the sphenoid sinus and sometimes produces a prominent lateral bulge (8%) which can be identified intraoperatively and radiographically. The optic nerve may sometimes be only covered with mucosa, i.e. Bony dehiscence (4%) or the bone over the optic nerve may be as thin as less than 0.5 mm (78%). An Onodi cell is a sphenoethmoidal cell, which pneumatizes the superolateral aspect of sphenoid sinus and its presence places the optic nerve at risk especially while dealing with posterior ethmoids or assuming that the sphenoid sinus can be entered directly posteriorly to the ethmoids following the lamina papyracea. An Onodi cell is best detected if there is a horizontal septation within the sphenoid sinus as seen on the first coronal CT cut in which complete posterior bony choana can be identified. Excessive pneumatization of anterior clinoids cause the optic nerve to run exposed in the roof of sphenoid along its mesentery.

Intravenous corticosteroids and optic nerve decompression is usually undertaken in cases of traumatic optic neuropathy.

Iatrogenic cerebrospinal fluid (CSF) leaks are usually seen in revision surgery cases. During routine sinus surgery, the regions most at risk for CSF leak are lateral lamella of cribriform, cribrifom plate. Posteriorly these structures abut the planum sphenoidale (roof of sphenoid sinus). Skull base injury is best avoided by the entering sphenoid through its ostium and then identifying the roof of sphenoid sinus by removing the anterior wall with a sphenoid punch. More sturdy instruments like Hajek Kofler punch, Kerrisons punch should be used with caution near the skull base as they have a potential to fracture the bone in an unpredictable manner.

If CSF leak occurs, the first step is to identify its exact location and depending on the size of defect; different methods for closure can be used.

Stenosis and synechie are late complications of sphenoidotomy. Stenosis usually occurs if the ostium is not widened enough or if the ostium is widened circumferentially (circumferential defects lead to cicatrical stenosis). In early postoperative period this scarring can be removed with balloon dilatation or with Stammberger punch. Revision surgery is required for late and complete stenosis.

Meningitis and postoperative infective hydrocephalous are rare complications.

Rhinologic complications happen due to improper manipulation of the septum and rarely due to improper handling of the septum per se.

These complications include septal perforation, synechiae, anosmia, and cosmetic deformity.

LANDMARKS AND PRECAUTIONS DURING SPHENOID SURGERY

Sphenoid surgery becomes relatively easy and uncomplicated if we remember all our "anatomical friends" and the "things not to do."

- The superior turbinate is a reliable and consistent anatomic marker for localization of the sphenoid sinus, especially, in revision surgeries where middle turbinate has been already removed. The average distance of anterior end of superior turbinate to sphenoid ostium is around 2 cm.
- Sphenoid ostia lies 1–1.5 cm above choana medially against nasal septum.
- After identification of the ostium the first step of any sphenoid surgery is widening of the sphenoid ostium. The safest direction of widening of sphenoid ostium is inferomedially. After widening, the disease (infection) can be dissected out bluntly or with microdebrider (instruments should not point superolaterally during polyps removal as the thin stalk of polyp may be attached to optic nerve or carotids and always towards floor and medially). The optimum widening of the ostium is usually around 10–15 mm.
- In revision surgeries, the usual landmarks like middle and the superior turbinates are absent, in these cases the reference plane of sphenoid sinus is usually approximated with help of a line along the medial orbital floor (MOF) and bony ridge of antrostomy and the cells above this line are the posterior ethmoidal cells and sphenoid sinus lies below this line; also the reference plane of the sphenoid lies 20–30° above superior part of inferior turbinate.

  In skull base surgeries, after posterior septectomy, the best way to identify and enter the sphenoid is by identifying the "bow sign" and the "bird beak" After excising the perpendicular plate of the ethmoid and vomer, the peculiar bowing of the anterior sphenoid wall (bow sign) is identified. Also, the medial anterior wall of sphenoid sinus along with rostrum of sphenoid bulges anteriorly similar to bird beak with bilateral bony apertures of sphenoid sinus laterally. This position of the bird beak between the 2 apertures is the best place to enter the sphenoid sinus.

- Wider exposure of the sphenoid sinus is required in trans-sphenoidal approaches enabling "binostril 2-surgeons 4-hand technique" without crowding of the instrument, enabling sharp dissection and improved ability to control bleeding. For this the inferior one-third of the superior turbinate is usually sacrificed along with exenteration of Onodi cells along with posterior septectomy. A panoramic view should be obtained exposing bilateral optico-carotid recess, ICA, cavernous sinus, optic nerve in one endoscopic view. The sella, clivus, planum are identified in midline.
- For widening during these approaches a plethora of instruments can be used like punches (up/down), Stammberger mushroom punch, drill, Tru cut forceps, microdebrider. Sharp instruments and microdebrider are usually avoided (Refer Chapter 19 on pituitary surgery).
- Patterns of septation in the sphenoid sinus are highly variable making it an unreliable guide to the midline. Moreover, the septa may be attached to the bony bulges over the optic nerve or the internal carotid artery, which have to be trimmed with precision with help of Tru cut forceps or drill but never be pulled. For determining the midline of sphenoid we again rely on the sphenoid keel and rostrum, and never the sphenoid sinus septations.
- During surgical procedures, the surgeon must always remember that the optic canal and the bulge of the internal carotid artery may only be covered by a very thin and occasionally fragmented bony layer in the area of the sphenoid and that these two vital structures may not be well protected and thus this warrants a careful dissection and careful entry into the sphenoid sinus. If a small or narrow instrument is pushed hard onto the face of sphenoid to enter the sphenoid, the bone may give way and the instrument introduced into the sinus with force and may injure the carotid/optic nerve/cavernous sinus region leading to injury to these structures. Therefore an instrument with large blunt surface (e.g Freer's elevator) is used and the penetration point should be medial and inferior.
- The most posterior point of an Onodi cell of the posterior ethmoid may extend up to 1.5 cm beyond the most anterior point of the anterior wall of the sphenoid sinus. This is particularly important if the sphenoid sinus is to be opened endoscopically via the ethmoid. The anterior wall of the sphenoid sinus must never be sought behind the furthermost point of posterior ethmoid. This is the precise point where the risk of injury to the optic nerve is the greatest.
- In cases of extensive lateral pneumatization of the sphenoid sinus, the maxillary nerve and vidian nerve (forming the superior and inferior boundaries of lateral recess respectively) may bulge into the lateral wall of the sinus or may be entirely surrounded by pneumatization and, thus, liable to iatrogenic injury.

SPHENOID AS A ROUTE

Endoscopic transsphenoidal route is gaining more and more value to treat skull base pathologies like pituitary tumors, sphenoid mucocele, meningiomas, petrous apex granulomas, optic nerve decompression, craniocervical junction abnormalities, cavernous sinus diseases, craniopharyngiomas, clival chordomas, Sternberg canal CSF leaks. The advantages of the extended transsphenoidal approach over a traditional craniotomy are the avoidance of frontal or temporal lobe retraction or sylvian fissure dissection and the potential associated brain injury.

BIBLIOGRAPHY

1. Moeller CW, Welch KC. Prevention and management of complication in sphenoidotomy. Otolaryngol Clin North Am. 2010;43(4):839-54.
2. Peter-John Wormald. Endoscopic Sinus Surgery: Anatomy, Three-dimensional Reconstruction and Surgical Technique. Thieme Medical Publishers, 3rd edition, 2012.
3. Sareen D, Agrawal AK, Kaul JM. Study of sphenoid sinus anatomy in relation to endoscopic surgery. Int J Morphol. 2005;23(3): 261-6.
4. Solares CA, Ong YK, Carrau RL. Prevention and management of vascular injuries in endoscopic surgery of the sinonasal tract and skull base. Otolaryngol Clin North Am. 2010;43(4):817-25.

CHAPTER 10

Sinonasal Polyposis

Sujata Muranjan

INTRODUCTION

The term Polyp is derived from the Greek word "polypous" which means "multifooted". This is a misnomer since a polyp has only a single stalk. By definition, polyps are soft, yellowish, boggy structures usually insensitive to touch arising from the lining mucosa of the nose and the paranasal sinuses. The ideal nomenclature for this condition would therefore be "Sinonasal polyposis".

Nasal polyps were first described in India and by 1000 BC curettes had been devised to remove them.[1] The condition occurs in approximately 2% of the population[2] and is seen in almost all ethnic races in the world. The male:female ratio is 2:1. From the standard classification and differentiation between ethmoidal and antrochoanal polyps, the concept and understanding of nasal polyps has undergone a considerable change. Numerous complex mechanisms have now been postulated to describe the etiology. Understanding the pathogenesis is challenging, the treatment difficult and a "complete cure" at times impossible. A systematic approach is therefore essential for establishing a rational therapy.

PATHOPHYSIOLOGY AND THEORIES

Though several etiologies have been proposed to describe sinonasal polyposis a lot of lacunae still remain in the understanding of the disease process.

Allergy was initially proposed as the causative etiology. Following an antigen-antibody reaction in the target organ there was resultant release of various pharmacologically active chemical mediators, histamine being the chief one. This was thought to cause diffusion of fluid from capillaries into the tissue. Prolonged tissue edema was conducive to the development of hydrophilic colloids with changes in the ground substance of the nasal mucosa. Much of the edema fluid, high in protein content, became thicker as the disease progressed especially in presence of infection.[3] The prolapsed edematous and thickened tissue finally led to formation of polyps which could grow to an extent to cause significant mechanical nasal obstruction. This allergy theory however is now refuted by the fact that there is no clear evidence that H1 antihistamines are effective in nasal polyposis. Recent studies also show that IgE mediated allergy does not play a role in the development of nasal polyps. This is supported by the fact that nasal polyps are rare in children with perennial allergic rhinitis. They are also seen more commonly in non-allergic adults and the incidence of nasal polyps in allergic patients is usually under 5%, which is similar to that of the general population.

Over the years the understanding of the disease has changed and recent research now states that nasal polyps are thought to be a part of an "inflammatory reaction" involving the lining mucous membrane of the nose and paranasal sinuses. The disease is now regarded as part of a spectrum of chronic rhinosinusitis.[4] In fact some otolaryngologists consider that most polyps are due to infective sinusitis or other diseases of the upper respiratory tract and that only a few are the result of allergy.[5,6] A more consistent theory explains nasal polyps to result from a self-propagating inflammatory cascade. Viral, bacterial or fungal infections lead to an inflammatory response in the host. Contact areas and narrow clefts in the ostiomeatal region create turbulence of air flow in the lateral wall of the nose. This is supported by the fact that early nasal polyps are consistently related to sinus ostia and the ostiomeatal region in the middle meatus (Fig. 10.1).

Recurrent inflammation leads to ulceration of lining mucosa and prolapse of the submucosa with re-epithelialization and new gland formation. A polyp thus forms as an inflammatory process from epithelial cells, vascular endothelial cells and fibroblasts. The bioelectric integrity of Na^+ and Cl^- channels is affected which in turn results in an increased movement of water into the cell and the interstitial fluid. This causes growth and enlargement of the nasal polyp.

Polyps are also devoid of sensory, autonomic, vasomotor or secretomotor nerves. A few nerve fibers may be present in the stalk of some polyps. This status of denervation causes a decrease in secretory activity of the glands and induces an abnormal vascular permeability, leading to an irreversible tissue edema.[7] Release of chemical mediators also causes widespread mast cell degranulation and release of histamine. This in turn leads to microvascular plasma exudation.

Various "chemical mediators" play a pivotal role in the pathophysiology of this disease. Cytokines are secreted proteins which mediate and regulate immunity, inflammation, and hematopoiesis. Granulocyte monocyte colony stimulating factors (GM-CSF) are up regulated in various tissue compartments viz. epithelium and stroma of nasal polyps. Pro-inflammatory cytokines like interleukin (IL) 1, IL-3, IL-4, IL-5, IL-6, IL-8, and IL-10 are responsible for the chemical reactions in polyps. Immunoglobulins like IgG,

IgA, IgM and IgE have also been detected along with adhesion molecules like vascular adhesion molecule 1 (VCAM-1) and growth factors such as tumor necrosis factor (TNF), platelet derived growth factor, vascular permeable factors (VPFs), vascular endothelial growth factors (VEGFs), insulin like growth factor (I) and stem cell factor. Both interleukin IL-3 and IL-4, as well as IL-1 and tumor necrosis factor (TNF) can induce VCAM-1 expression in microvascular endothelium from the polyps. The interaction between adhesion molecules VLA-4 and VCAM-1 play an important role in the extravasation of eosinophil's into nasal polyps.[7] Thus whatever be the causative factor, nasal polyps represent a common clinical end point for a myriad of inflammatory disease processes involving the nose and paranasal sinuses (Flow chart 10.1).

OTHER DISEASES ASSOCIATED WITH NASAL POLYPOSIS

There are other diseases with differing etiologies associated with nasal polyps (Table 10.1). Despite having similar macroscopic findings, each of these disorders represents a complex pathology and varying treatment strategy.

"Allergic fungal sinusitis" is a disease seen in an atopic host in which there is a Type I hypersensitivity reaction to fungal specific antigens. Inhalation of fungi by such a host triggers off an intense inflammatory response leading to mucosal edema and exudate. This exudate comprises of allergic mucin and fungus and is associated with formation of nasal polyps (Fig. 10.2). Accumulation of this exudate in the sinus cavities can lead to considerable expansion of the sinuses and distortion of normal sinus anatomy. Though *Aspergillus* is a

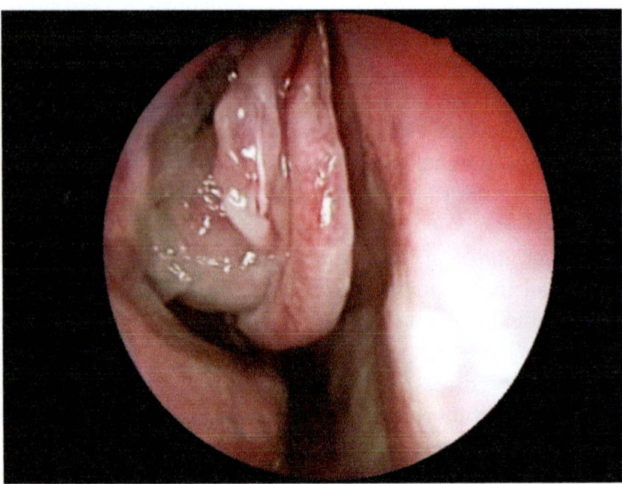

Fig. 10.1: Early polyps in the middle meatus

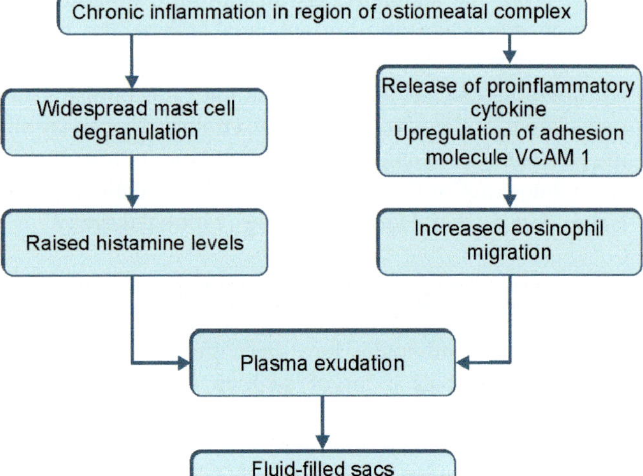

Flow chart 10.1: Inflammatory pathways causing nasal polyp formation

TABLE 10.1: Other diseases causing nasal polyps
• Allergic fungal sinusitis (AFS)
• Samter's disease
• Kartagener's syndrome
• Young's syndrome
• Cystic fibrosis

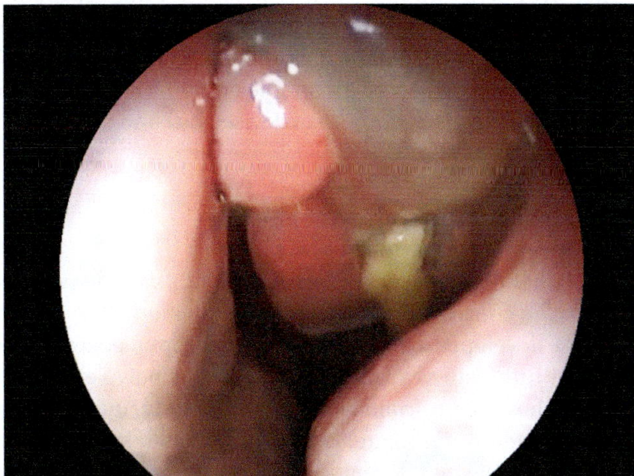

Fig. 10.2: Polyps with allergic fungus

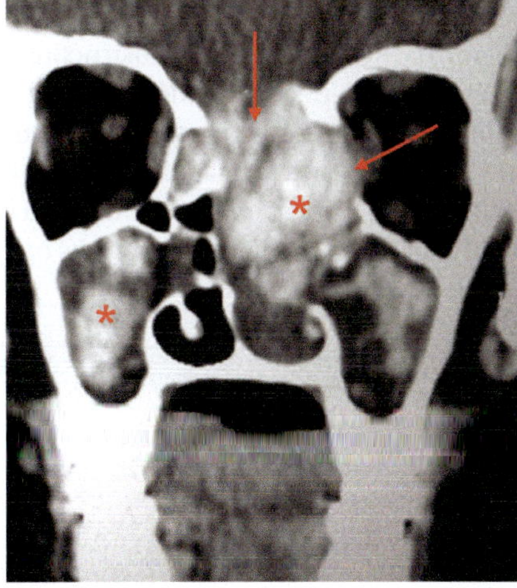

Fig. 10.3: Coronal CT scan of allergic fungal sinusitis showing double density sign (*) and loss of bone over ethmoid roof and left medial (arrows) orbital wall

common pathogen, the dematiaceous species of fungi like *Bipolaris, Curvularia, Alternaria,* etc. are also responsible for this condition. Raised fungal specific IgE antibodies are often seen in these patients. The CT scan findings with the classical double density sign are characteristic and occur due to the allergic mucin and fungus. The expansile exudate in the sinuses occasionally causes thinning and pressure necrosis of the bone over the skull base and medial orbital wall leading to exposure of the dura and the orbital periosteum (Fig. 10.3). The disease however almost always remains extradural and extra periosteal. Smear of the nasal secretions when examined under the microscope shows allergic mucin and fungal hyphae with Eosinophils and Charcot Leyden crystals. The disease is almost always extra mucosal without any tissue invasion. Treatment comprises of medical management in the form systemic steroids and topical steroid nasal sprays followed by surgical removal of all polyps, allergic mucin and fungus.

"Samter's triad" which comprises of nasal polyps, asthma and aspirin hypersensitivity is a condition where nasal polyps are extensive and recurrences common. This condition is accompanied by eosinophils in the bronchial and nasal secretions as well as in the peripheral blood. The patients may need continuous intranasal steroid therapy and very often require surgery. The asthma can be severe, chronic and persistent warranting long-term inhalation steroids and there can be associated hypersensitivity to other nonsteroidal anti-inflammatory drugs (NSAIDs) acting as cyclo-oxygenase inhibitors.[7] It is therefore mandatory to obtain a detailed history of asthma and drug hypersensitivity in patients with nasal polyposis and NSAIDs have to be avoided in such cases.

"Kartagener's syndrome" or more appropriately primary ciliary dyskinesia syndrome is an autosomal recessive disease comprising of male infertility, dextrocardia, situs inversus, obstructive airway disease and nasal polyposis. Although first described in the sperm, the ciliary abnormalities also affect mucus clearance from the bronchial tree, trachea, middle ear and nose. The electron microscopy shows lack of dynein arm on the cilia.[8] More recently reported ultrastructural abnormalities have included defective radial spokes, ectopic position of microtubules 3'7 with abnormal numbers of microtubules and transposition of outer microtubules to the central area.

"Young's syndrome" or the sinusitis-infertility syndrome is a triad of bronchiectasis, chronic rhinosinusitis and infertility. There is a vas deferens obstruction leading to obstructive azoospermia. Cystic fibrosis (CF) and primary ciliary dyskinesia as a differential diagnosis have to be excluded.[9] In this condition, sperms are produced but do not mix with the rest of the ejaculatory fluid due to a physical obstruction, resulting in non-existent levels of sperm in semen. In the nose and the paranasal sinuses, the basic problem lies in the sol-gel constitution of the mucus impeding its transport. The defective mucus clearance then leads to stagnation, infection and subsequent rhinosinusitis and polyp formation.

"Cystic fibrosis" (also known as CF or mucoviscidosis) is an autosomal recessive genetic disorder affecting most critically the lungs, the pancreas, liver, and intestine. It is characterized by abnormal transport of chloride and sodium across an epithelium, leading to thick, viscous secretions.[10] Mucus in the paranasal sinuses is equally thick and may also cause blockage of the sinus passages, leading to infection. Individuals with CF may develop overgrowth of the nasal tissue leading to nasal polyp formation due to inflammation from chronic sinus infections.[11] Recurrent sinonasal polyps can occur in as many as 10–25% of CF patients. These polyps can block the nasal passages and lead to increased breathing difficulties.[12]

SYMPTOMS

Nasal polyps cause symptoms which often impair quality of life (Table 10.2). "Nasal discharge" is a common complaint in most patients. The discharge may be initially thin or mucoid and may later turn purulent due to secondary bacterial infection. It is almost always bilateral. "Nasal obstruction" is an associated symptom and may get aggravated when the patient lies down due to obstruction of the choanae. "Itching" of the nose and eyes and "sneezing" may occur in patients with associated allergy. Other symptoms may include "headache" in the frontal and/or maxillary regions, "fullness in the ears" due to blockage of the eustachian tubes and "postnasal drip" with catarrh-induced irritation in the throat. Since polyps originate in the upper part of the nasal cavity and protrude from the middle or superior meatus, they block the airflow to the olfactory region and frequently lead to "anosmia or hyposmia." Occasional "epistaxis" may result in case of secondary infection. With extensive polyposis, "snoring" and obstructive sleep apnea may occur. If the polyps occur in early childhood before fusion of bones, there

may be expansion of the nasal bridge, "hypertelorism" or altered craniofacial structure. In case of spread to orbits, there may be "proptosis, diplopia" or sometimes even "reduced vision". Very rarely will there be a spread to the intracranial cavity giving rise to symptoms of raised intracranial tension.

SIGNS

Extensive polyps are easily visible on anterior rhinoscopy and appear as whitish, translucent structures. Very early polyps may be detected only following a diagnostic nasal endoscopy where their extent can be ascertained and the disease can be staged. The 3-tier staging system devised by Lund and Mackay is as follows:[13]

- 0, no polyps
- 1, confined to middle meatus
- 2, beyond middle meatus (Fig. 10.4).

Lildholdt and colleagues used a slightly varied system to assess the effect of multiple treatment methods. The 4-point system developed used the upper and lower edges of the inferior turbinate as a landmark to describe polyp extension. The highest score available extended to the inferior edge of the inferior turbinate, essentially contacting the floor and filling the nasal cavity.[14] The staging systems aid in determining effectiveness of conservative treatment and need for subsequent surgical intervention. A diagnostic nasal endoscopy is of special significance in case of complaints of nasal obstruction when anterior rhinoscopy appears apparently normal wherein polyps obstructing the choana can be detected. It also enables in determining the origin of a single unilateral polyp. A polyp in the middle meatus would in all probability be an "antrochoanal polyp" having its origin in the maxillary sinus while a polyp encountered between the septum and the middle turbinate will have its origin from the sphenoid sinus in most of the cases.

TABLE 10.2: Symptoms of nasal polyps
• Nasal discharge
• Nasal obstruction
• Itching
• Headache, facial pain
• Fullness in the ears
• Postnasal drip
• Anosmia or hyposmia
• Epistaxis
• Snoring
• Hypertelorism or altered craniofacial structure
Rarely:
• Proptosis, diplopia
• Reduced vision
• Symptoms of raised intracranial tension

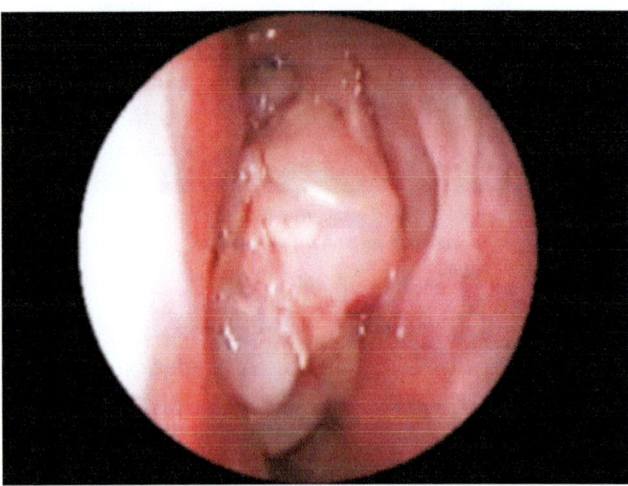

Fig. 10.4: Nasal polyps beyond middle meatus

On palpation nasal polyps appear soft, boggy and a probe can be passed around them which differentiates them from a tumor of the nasal cavity. It is important to determine whether one is dealing with a single or multiple polypi and whether the disease is unilateral or bilateral. The site of origin determines the therapeutic modality to be instituted. Ethmoidal polyps are primarily treated medically followed by surgical intervention in refractory cases whereas antrochoanal or sphenoidal polyps require surgical intervention.

DIFFERENTIAL DIAGNOSIS

Differential diagnoses exist and these need to be borne in mind especially in case of a unilateral nasal polyp. An "antrochoanal polyp" is the most common unilateral nasal polyp. It arises from the maxillary antrum enlarges in size, prolapses through either the natural or the accessory ostium of the maxillary sinus into the nasal cavity and then into the choana to achieve a trifoliate appearance (Figs 10.5 and 10.6). Polyps which bleed on touch need to be differentiated from hemangiomas (Fig. 10.7) and rhinosporidiosis. While an hemangioma commonly arises from the nasal septum, rhinosporidiosis is easily differentiated by its typically "strawberry" appearance. "Sphenoidal polyps" need differentiation from pituitary tumors, chordomas and craniopharyngiomas. An inverted papilloma may occasionally mimic an antrochoanal polyp and the diagnosis may be evident only on histopathology. Benign nasal tumors like angiofibroma, chondroma, and osteoma, malignant tumors like chondrosarcoma, osteosarcoma, esthesioneuroblastoma and adeno or squamous carcinomas form an important differential diagnosis of a unilateral nasal mass. While tumors are firm on palpation and may bleed on touch, occasionally polyps and tumors can coexist. In these cases, a polyp may occur as a result of a blocked sinus ostium due to an underlying tumor. Hence it is important to send all the material obtained at surgery for histopathology.

A rare differential diagnosis of a single unilateral nasal polyp is a "meningoencephalocele". It is therefore important to study the CT scan in detail in case surgical intervention is considered.

INVESTIGATIONS

Nasal polyposis is a clinical diagnosis and investigations are required when a differential diagnosis is suspected or if surgery is planned.

In allergic fungal sinusitis, fungal specific IgE antibodies may be elevated in the blood. Microscopic examination of the smear of nasal secretions can reveal presence of allergic mucin and fungal hyphae with eosinophils and Charcot-Leyden crystals.

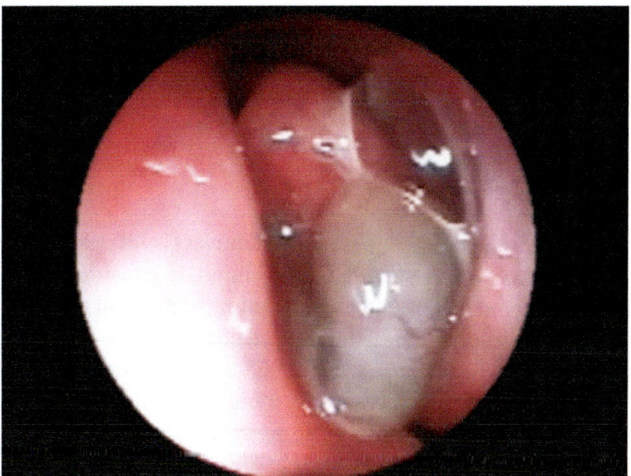

Fig. 10.5: Antrochoanal polyp in the left middle meatus

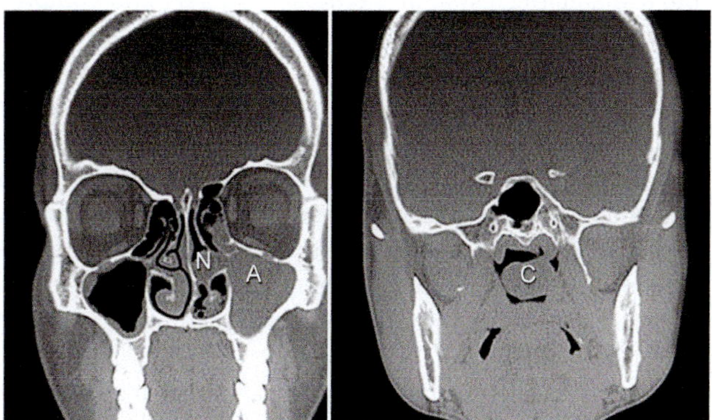

Fig. 10.6: Coronal CT scan showing the nasal (N), antral (A) and choanal (C) parts of the antrochoanal polyp

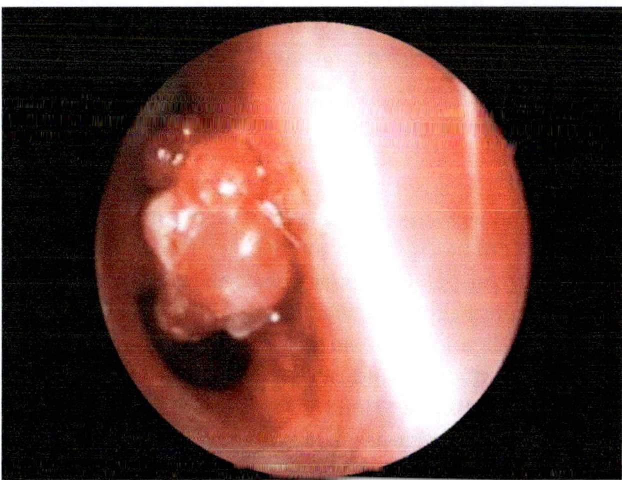

Fig. 10.7: Nasal septal hemangioma

In case of a Samter's triad when there is associated asthma a pulmonary function test may be warranted.

In suspected cystic fibrosis, sweat chloride levels may be evaluated.

Radiological Investigations

The CT scan of the paranasal sinuses is of paramount importance when surgical intervention is considered. The scans have to be done following optimum medical treatment when the exact extent of the disease not amenable to medical treatment will become evident. CT imaging remains in its ability an excellent diagnostic modality to provide a road map for surgical planning. The bony windows have to be in all three planes, i.e. axial, sagittal and coronal so that three-dimensional (3D) anatomy of the sinuses can be better understood. This is of particular significance in key areas like the frontal recess where understanding the anatomy of the frontal air cell system is crucial to surgery and complete disease removal is important. Soft tissue windows may be obtained in the coronal plane. A plain CT scan of the paranasal sinuses suffices to give all the relevant information in case of nasal polyposis. In case of suspected tumors one may need a scan with contrast. Nasal polyps appear as partial or complete opacification of the involved paranasal sinuses with infundibulum widening.[15] Expansion of the ethmoidal air cells may be evident and there may be thinning of the bony septae and margins in long standing disease (Figs 10.8 to 10.10).

An MRI is done in case of suspected orbital or intracranial extension of disease. MRI gives better soft tissue delineation and aids in differentiating between polyps, retro-obstructive sinusitis and tumors.

▍MEDICAL MANAGEMENT

Nasal polyps are considered as a local manifestation of a systemic problem. Appropriate and early treatment can bring notable benefits to patients and medical management forms the mainstay in the treatment of this condition.

Corticosteroids either oral or in the form of intranasal sprays are now the universally accepted drugs of choice and remain the mainstay of therapy for nasal polyposis. The mechanism of action involves the downregulation of inflammatory protein encoding genes by the activation of intracellular glucocorticoid receptors.[16,17]

Oral steroids are indicated in case of extensive disease, when hyposmia or anosmia are the main complaints or when surgical intervention is planned. They are very effective in reducing polyp size and improving symptoms and their use remains near universal in the treatment of nasal polyposis

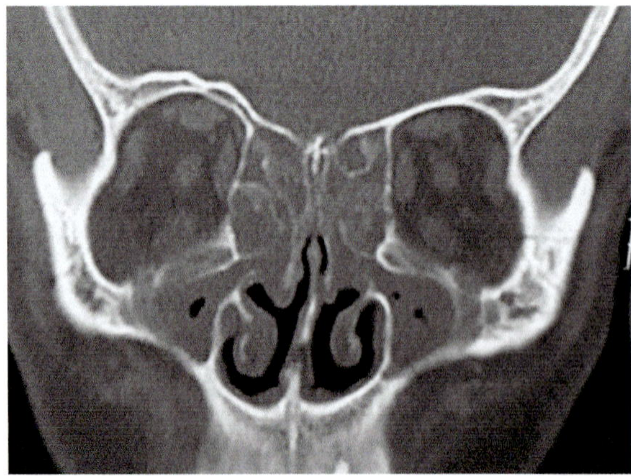

Fig. 10.8: Coronal CT scan bony windows showing opacification and expansion of ethmoid air cells by nasal polyps with widening of the infundibulum

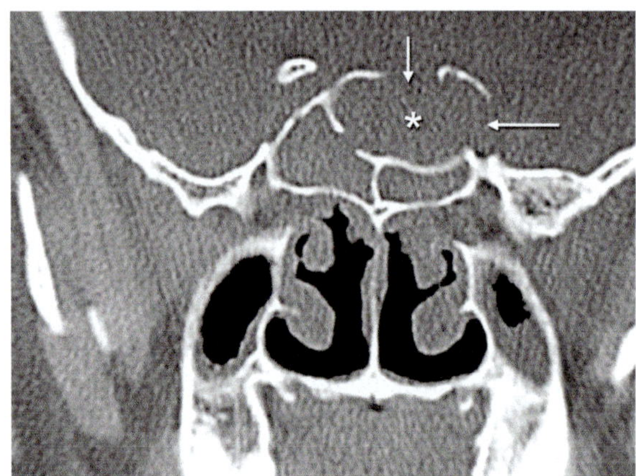

Fig. 10.9: Coronal CT scan bony windows showing expansion and opacification of an Onodi cell (*) with nasal polyps along with thinning out of its roof and (arrows) lateral wall

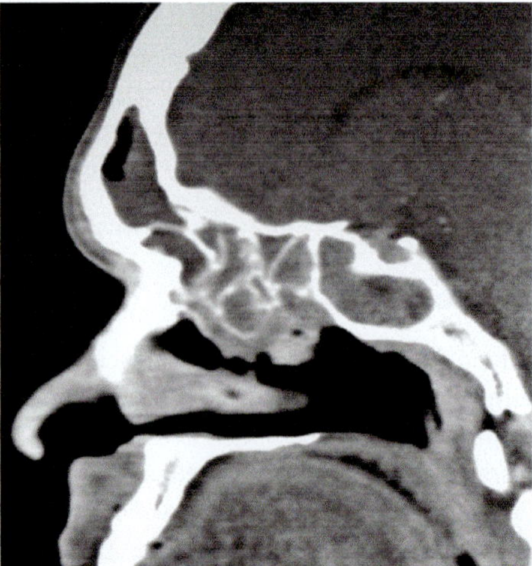

Fig. 10.10: Sagittal CT scan delineating anatomy of the frontal recess area

despite their well-documented side effects (Figs 10.11 and 10.12).

When surgery is planned, oral steroids have to be started 10–12 days prior. They cause reduction in the disease which in turn makes understanding of the anatomical landmarks better. There is reduced bleeding contributing significantly to easier surgery.

Dosage

Oral Prednisolone is administered in a dose of 1 mg/kg/day and is tapered over 10–12 days. Newer oral steroids such as methyl prednisolone have a greater anti-inflammatory

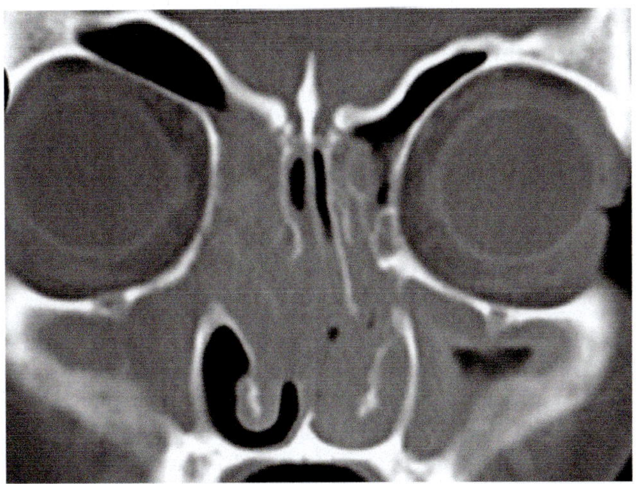

Fig. 10.11: Coronal CT scan with recurrent polyps in bilateral maxillary sinuses and operated ethmoid cavities

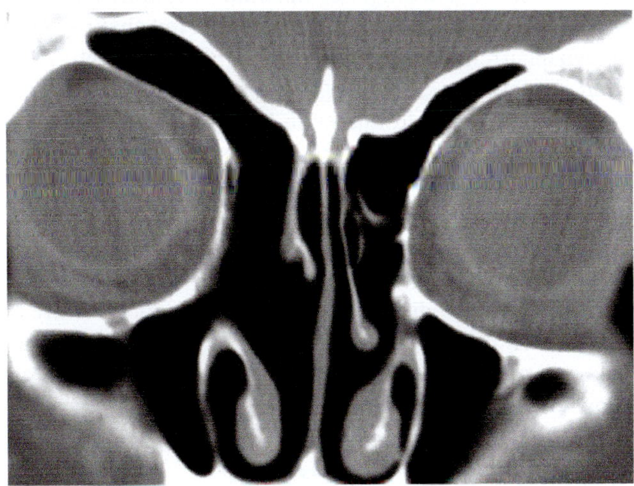

Fig. 10.12: Coronal CT scan of same patient after a course of oral steroids showing clear ethmoid and maxillary sinuses (medical polypectomy)

potency and a lesser tendency to induce sodium and water retention. Deflazacort has a lesser tendency towards induction of weight gain as well as lesser diabetes and osteoporosis inducing potential. The blood sugar needs to be monitored closely and calcium supplementation has to be given during the course of oral steroids.

Intranasal topical steroids sprays have made a tremendous impact on the treatment of nasal polyposis. They act locally by inhibiting the inflammatory cascade. Nasal topical steroids have been shown to decrease polyp size as well as improve nasal symptoms.[16] The use of these steroids postoperatively has also proved to reduce recurrence and the need for systemic therapy.[18] A wide range of steroid nasal sprays are now available, the most common being budesonide, momotasone and fluticasone.

Local decongestants like oxymetazoline or xylometazoline are prescribed when nasal blockage is the predominant symptom. Antibiotics may be needed in case of superadded bacterial infection when the nasal discharge is purulent and is accompanied by headache and facial pain.

Newer Drugs

Cysteinyl leukotriene receptor (LTR) antagonists, such as montelukast, function by blocking LTR sites. Multiple studies have shown clinical improvement in patients with chronic rhinosinusitis with nasal polyps wherein there is reduction in polyps, decreased steroid use and improvement in overall symptoms. These can therefore be used as an add-on therapy.[19-21]

Immunomodulators

Immunomodulators are being used with success in patients with eosinophilic asthma, otherwise known as patients with unified airway disease. In these patients, treatment with anti–IL-5 results in improved serum eosinophil levels, asthma control, and FEV1 levels.[22] Omalizumab is a humanized antibody which reduces serum levels of free IgE. Mepolizumab and Reslizumab are humanized monoclonal antibody against IL-5 which eliminate eosinophils from blood. Although the cost of immunomodulators limits their overall use, they can still be regarded as a crucial step in the individualized treatment of nasal polyposis.

Surgical Treatment

Endoscopic sinus surgery is the surgery of choice for nasal polyposis which is planned following optimal medical treatment. Surgery aims at decreasing the amount of inflammatory load making medical treatment more effective. It improves symptoms of nasal blockage, re-establishes ventilation and drainage of the sinuses and contributes considerably to an overall improvement in the quality of life. The patients however need to be counseled preoperatively as regards the recurrent nature of the disease.

Several hurdles like distortion of anatomy, loss of landmarks and bleeding may be encountered while operating on a patient with extensive nasal polyps.

Newer equipment like the microdebrider therefore has become indispensable in surgery for nasal polyposis. Continuous suction and irrigation keeps the field free of blood and improves visualization. Cutting blades having various angulations make it possible to reach different areas in the nose and allows disease to be removed therein. There is less tissue trauma which results in better postoperative healing.

Following adequate decongestion of the nose, the polyps in the nasal cavity are first removed or debrided so as to establish the constant landmarks. The standard steps of surgery for endoscopic sinus surgery are then followed. The uncinate process is removed along its entire vertical and horizontal extent. The maxillary sinus ostium is then identified and widened. Polyps within the maxillary sinus are removed. Angled instruments, curved debrider blades and angled scopes may be needed to access the lumen of the maxillary sinus in order to remove the disease lying therein. The frontal recess area is then tackled and the frontal sinus ostium is visualized. Following this, the anterior ethmoid sinuses are cleared. The ground lamella is identified and the posterior ethmoid sinuses are then cleared. After identifying the last posterior ethmoidal air cell, dissection is continued in the inferomedial direction to open the sphenoid sinus. In case there is difficulty in identifying the anterior wall of the sphenoid sinus due to presence of polyps, the sphenoid sinus can be accessed medially by passing the endoscope between the middle turbinate and the septum. The natural ostium of the sinus lies approximately 1.5 cm above the upper border of the choana. Utmost care has to be exercised while removing polyps from within the sphenoid sinus especially from its lateral wall since the carotid artery and the optic nerve are closely related to it. Complete disease removal is of utmost importance and goes a long way in preventing recurrences. Landmarks of the lamina papyracea laterally, orbital apex posterolaterally, skull base superiorly and the middle and superior turbinates medially have to be kept in mind and not violated. Close attention must be paid to mucosa preservation since it contributes towards better postoperative healing. Success in outcomes of ESS in patients with chronic rhinosinusitis with polyposis is heavily dependant on reducing postoperative scarring, edema, and crusting that can inhibit natural ciliary function and sinus drainage. Occasionally there may be difficulty in identifying the ostia of the maxillary or the sphenoid sinus due to extensive polyps blocking them. These can then be identified by visualizing air bubbles egressing from them which then guide the surgeon towards the ostia. Polyps near the skull base or lamina papyracea should never be pulled. The use of blunt curettes facilitates safe disease removal in these areas. Close attention has to be paid to preserve the integrity of the middle turbinate.

In the postoperative period, antibiotics and decongestants may be continued for a week to ten days. Regular nasal douching with saline is advised. Topical steroid nasal sprays may be started after a week.

Meticulous care of the operated nasal cavity in the immediate postoperative period has to be exercised. The patients may require two to three visits scheduled a week apart for cleaning the nose. During these visits crusts, fibrinous material and discharge are removed. Adhesions between the middle turbinate and lateral nasal wall if any need to be broken so as to keep the operated cavity open and well aerated. This prevents the development of dense synechiae postoperatively. Some amount of postoperative polypoidal changes in the mucosa are to be expected. This cobblestone appearance must not to be confused with recurrence of polyps and has to be left well alone wherein it settles down in due course of time.

RECURRENCE

Despite the best possible medical and surgical treatment, recurrence seems to be a common phenomenon associated with nasal polyps. Several studies have been conducted world over to determine factors leading to recurrence (Table 10.3). The most common factor identified is incomplete surgery with incomplete polyp removal. It is important to clear all the sinuses and remove all the polyps. The first surgery is usually the best time to do so. Formation of adhesions and scar tissue makes subsequent surgeries difficult. In a study conducted by Bassiouni and Wormald it was observed that persistent polyp recurrence occurred in 19.8% of patients after 6 months and increased to 22.7% after 12 months. Polyps first recurred in the area of the frontal sinus/ostium (55%) followed by the ethmoids (38%). Asthma and aspirin sensitivity were the most important variables affecting recurrence.[23] The other factor affecting recurrence is postulated to be mucosal eosinophilia. These patients had higher recurrence rate than those without.[24] Initial disease severity was also found to be another predictor of recurrence. The more severe the disease on preoperative CT scan, greater were the chances of recurrence.[25] Subjective olfactory change was also considered as an early marker of recurrent disease.[26]

Management of Recurrences

All patients with nasal polyps need a close follow-up to detect recurrences. Topical steroid nasal sprays are used to

TABLE 10.3: Factors contributing to recurrence

- Incomplete disease removal at first surgery
- Samter's disease
- Mucosal eosinophilia
- Evidence of extensive disease on preoperative CT scan
- Hyposmia/anosmia as presenting complaints

combat early and mild form of recurrences. Many clinicians utilize short-term oral steroids as rescue courses in more aggressive forms of recurrences in order to improve nasal patency. Recent studies have described the use of absorbable steroid-impregnated nasal dressings for the treatment of early recurrences. These are thought to deliver an effective concentration of corticosteroids in direct contact with polypoidal mucosa, while at the same time limiting systemic effects associated with steroids. The studies have concluded that targeted topical therapy offers an attractive alternative to short-course oral steroids by primarily avoiding their potential systemic side effects. Drug eluting stents impregnated with steroids which are placed in the middle meatus have also been recently described. One such study used Mometasone Furoate (MF) as the steroid. These stents are believed to be effective in improving wound healing, preserving sinus patency, reducing inflammation and minimizing adhesions via controlled local steroid delivery.[27]

SUMMARY

Nasal polyps occur as a result of a self-perpetuating inflammatory process. The origin is from the mucosa around the ostiomeatal complex. Differential diagnosis of other conditions associated with nasal polyps need to be borne in mind. This is more so in case of a unilateral polyp. The treatment is primarily medical and corticosteroids given either topically or systemically form the mainstay in the management of this condition. Surgery is reserved for extensive cases. Recurrence is a troublesome feature of this disease. Further research and guidelines are needed to specify optimum medical and surgical management.

REFERENCES

1. Vancil ME. A historical survey of treatment for nasal polyposis. Laryngoscope. 1969;79:435-45.
2. Settipane GA. Nasal polyps: pathology, immunology and treatment. American Journal of Rhinology. 1987;1:119-26.
3. Allan Knight. Rhinitis and polyps, general practice: Canadian Medical Association Journal. 1968;99:116-8.
4. European Academy of Allergology and Clinical Immunology. European position paper on Rhinosinusitis and Nasal polyps. EAACI Task force, Rhinology Supplement. 2005:18:1-87.
5. Hollender AR. Eye Ear Nose Throat Monthly. 1962;41:922.
6. Grove RC. Allergic rhinitis: relation to sinusitis and polyps. In: Samter M, Alexander HL (Eds). Immunological Diseases. Boston: Little, Brown & co. Inc; 1965. p. 573.
7. Niels M, Lund VJ. Nasal Polyposis in Scott Brown's Otolaryngology and Head and Neck Surgery, Vol. 2, 7th edition, pp. 1549-59.
8. Afzelius BA, Eliasson R, Johnsen O, et al. Lack of dynein arms in immotile human spermatozoa. J Cell Biol. 1975;66:225-329.
9. Goeminne PC, Dupont LJ. The sinusitis-infertility syndrome: Young's saint, old devil, Eur Respi Journal. 2010;35(3):698.
10. Yankaskas JR, Marshall BC, Sufian B, et al. Cystic fibrosis adult care consensus conference report. Chest. 2004;125(90010):1-39. DOI:10.1378/chest.125.1_suppl.1S. PMID 14734689.
11. Franco LP, Camargos PA, Becker HM, et al. Nasal endoscopic evaluation of children and adolescents with cystic fibrosis. Braz J Otorhinolaryngol. 2009; 75(6):806-13.
12. Ramsey B, Richardson MA. Impact of sinusitis in cystic fibrosis. J Allergy Clin Immunol. 1992;90:547-52.
13. Lund VJ, Mackay IS. Staging in rhinosinusitis. Rhinology. 1993;31:183
14. Lildholdt T, Rundcrantz H, Bende M, et al. Glucocorticoid treatment for nasal polyps: the use of topical budesonide powder, intramuscular betamethasone, and surgical treatment. Arch Otolaryngol Head Neck Surg. 1997;123(6):595-600.
15. Drutman J, Harnsberger HR, Babbel RW, et al. Sinonasal polyposis: Investigation by direct coronal CT. Neuroradiology. 1994;36(6):469-72.
16. Mullol J, Obando A, Pujols L, et al. Corticosteroid treatment in chronic rhinosinusitis: the possibilities and the limits. Immunol Allergy Clin North Am. 2009;29(4):657-68.
17. Pujols L, Mullol J, Torrego A, et al. Glucocorticoid receptors in human airways. Allergy. 2004;59(10):1042-52.
18. Rowe-Jones JM, Medcalf M, Durham SR, et al. Functional endoscopic sinus surgery: 5 year follow up and results of a prospective, randomised, stratified, double-blind, placebo controlled study of postoperative fluticasone propionate aqueous nasal spray. Rhinology. 2005;43(1):2-10.
19. Parnes SM. The role of leukotriene inhibitors in patients with paranasal sinus disease. Curr Opin Otolaryngol Head Neck Surg. 2003;11:184-91.
20. Ragab S, Parikh A, Darby YC, et al. An open audit of montelukast, a leukotriene receptor antagonist, in nasal polyposis associated with asthma. Clin Exp Allergy. 2001;31(9):1385-91.
21. Ulualp SO, Sterman BM, Toohill RJ. Antileukotriene therapy for the relief of sinus symptoms in aspirin triad disease. Ear Nose Throat J. 1999;78(8):604-6.
22. Parameswaran N, Pizzichini M, Kjarsgaard M, et al. Mepolizumab for prednisone-dependent asthma with sputum eosinophilia. N Engl J Med. 2009;360(10):985-93.
23. Bassiouni A, Wormald PJ. Role of frontal sinus surgery in nasal polyp recurrence. Laryngoscope. 2013;123(1):36-41.
24. Nakayama T, Yoshikawa M, Asaka D, et al. Mucosal eosinophilia and recurrence of nasal polyps: new classification of chronic rhinosinusitis. Rhinology. 2011;49(4):392-6.
25. Watelet JB, Annicq B, van Cauwenberge P, et al. Objective outcome after functional endoscopic sinus surgery: prediction factors. Laryngoscope. 2004;114:1092-7.
26. Senior BA, Kennedy DW, Tanabodee J, et al. Long-term results of functional endoscopic sinus surgery. Laryngoscope. 1998;108:151-7.
27. Murr AH, Smith TL, Hwang PH, et al. Safety and efficacy of a novel bioabsorbable, steroid-eluting sinus stent. Int Forum Allergy Rhinol. 2011;1:23-32.

CHAPTER 11

Rhinosinusitis

Arpit Sharma, Shraddha Deshmukh, JP Dabholkar

Rhinitis and sinusitis usually coexist and are concurrent in most individuals; thus, the correct terminology is now rhinosinusitis.

DEFINITION

The recent European Position Paper on Rhinosinusitis 2012[1], defines rhinosinusitis as:

Inflammation of the nose and the paranasal sinuses characterized by two or more symptoms, one of which should be either nasal blockage/obstruction/congestion or nasal discharge: ± facial pain/pressure, ± reduction or loss of smell and either:

- Endoscopic signs of:
  - Nasal polyps
  - Mucopurulent discharge primarily from middle meatus
  - Edema/mucosal obstruction primarily in middle meatus, or
- Computed tomography (CT) evidence of mucosal changes within ostiomeatal complex and/or sinuses.

DURATION OF THE DISEASE IN ADULTS

Acute: Less than 12 weeks.
Complete resolution of symptoms.

Chronic: More than or equal to 12 weeks' symptoms.
Without complete resolution of symptoms.
Chronic rhinosinusitis may also be subject to exacerbations.

ACUTE RHINOSINUSITIS

Definition

- Acute rhinosinusitis (ARS) in adults is defined as sudden onset of two or more symptoms, one of which should be either nasal blockage/obstruction/congestion or nasal discharge (anterior/posterior nasal drip):
  - ± facial pain/pressure
  - ± reduction or loss of smell
  - For less than 12 weeks
- Common cold/acute viral rhinosinusitis is defined as duration of symptoms for less than 10 days
- Acute postviral rhinosinusitis is defined as increase of symptoms after 5 days or persistent symptoms after 10 days with less than 12 weeks' duration.
- Acute bacterial rhinosinusitis (ABRS) is suggested by the presence of at least three symptoms/signs from the following:
  - Discolored discharge (with unilateral predominance) and purulent secretion in cavum nasi
  - Severe local pain (with unilateral predominance)

- Fever (> 38°C)
- Elevated erythrocyte sedimentation rate (ESR)/ C-reactive protein (CRP)
- Double sickening (i.e. a deterioration after an initial milder phase of illness).

Classification of Acute Rhinosinusitis

Acute rhinosinusitis can be divided into viral rhinosinusitis (common cold) and postviral rhinosinusitis. A small subgroup of the postviral rhinosinusitis is caused by bacteria (ABRS). Figure 11.1 shows the classification of ARS.

Predisposing Factors: Rhinosinusitis

Table 11.1 shows the predisposing factors for rhinosinusitis.

TABLE 11.1: Predisposing factors for rhinosinusitis

Environmental factors	Infection (bacteria, viruses, fungi)
	Allergy/asthma
	Air pollution/Smoking
Anatomic factors	Septal deviation
	Concha bullosa
	Mucociliary impairment
Systemic factors	Immunodeficiency state
	Pregnancy and endocrine states
	Laryngopharyngeal reflux
	Vasculitis
	Granulomatous diseases
	Aspirin sensitivity
Genetic factors	Ciliary motility disorders
Iatrogenic factors	Surgery, medications, nasal packing, nasogastric tube placement

Pathophysiology of Acute Rhinosinusitis

Acute bacterial rhinosinusitis begins with a viral upper respiratory tract infection in predisposed individuals. Viruses implicated are rhinovirus, coronavirus, influenza, parainfluenza, respiratory syncytial, adenovirus and enterovirus. Viral infection induces inflammatory response which in turn causes changes in nasal-sinus environment such as mucosal edema with obstruction of sinus ostia, impaired mucociliary transport, transudation of fluid into sinuses, changes in mucus which becomes more viscus. This leads to mucostasis and bacterial superinfection. Figure 11.2 displays the incidence of bacterial pathogens in acute maxillary sinusitis in an adult population.[2]

Diagnosis and Management of Acute Rhinosinusitis

Acute rhinosinusitis is very common and is usually self-limiting. Diagnosis is mainly on clinical grounds. It is characterized by acute onset of typical symptoms that include nasal blockage, discharge, facial pain or pressure and reduction in smell.

Viral rhinosinusitis is self-limiting, with symptoms peaking at day 2–3 and then waning with resolution of symptoms between 10 and 14 days after onset. If symptoms initially improve and then worsen, or if symptoms persist beyond 10 days, the probability of bacterial infection is increased and the diagnosis of ABRS can be made.[2-4]

Anterior rhinoscopy reveals hyperemia, purulence, pain on palpation of sinuses, pharyngeal irritation or postnasal discharge.

Sinonasal endoscopy is not considered necessary for an accurate diagnosis, although it should be utilized if available

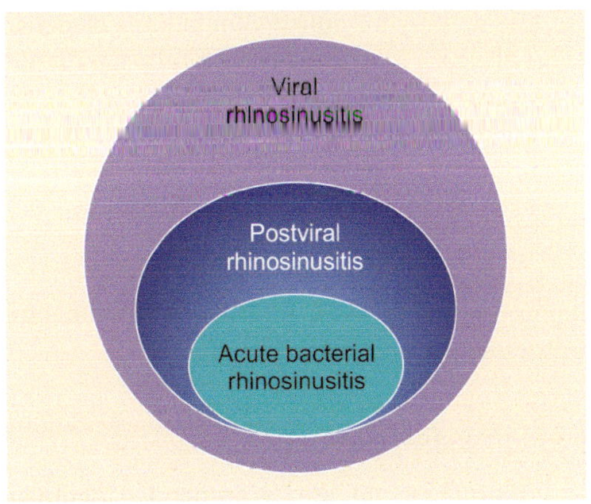

Fig. 11.1: Classification of acute rhinosinusitis

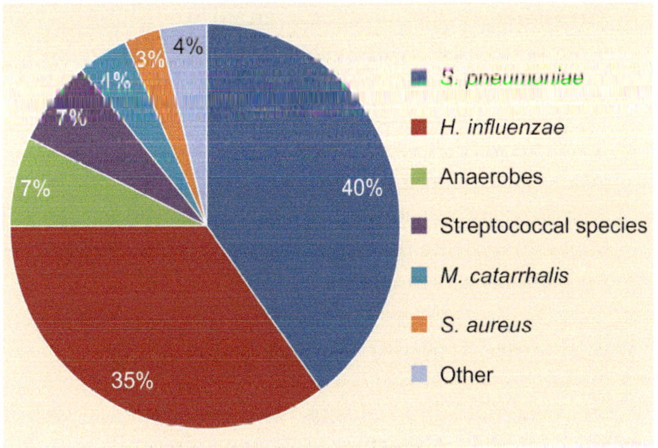

Fig. 11.2: The microbiology in ABRS in adults
[ABRS-Acute bacterial rhinosinusitis]

TABLE 11.2: Warning symptoms of complications in acute rhinosinusitis requiring immediate referral

- Periorbital edema
- Protrusion of eyeball
- Decreased vision
- Ophthalmoplegia, diplopia
- Altered consciousness
- Severe frontal headache
- Frontal swelling
- Signs of meningitis
- Neurological signs

TABLE 11.3: Treatment summary

- *Mild (viral, common cold):* Start with symptomatic relief (analgesics, saline irrigation, decongestants)
- *Moderate (postviral):* Additional topical steroids
- *Severe (including bacterial):* Additional topical steroids (consider IV antibiotics and surgery, if no improvement after 2–3 days)
- *Complicated sinusitis:* Hospitalization with IV antibiotics and/or surgery

as this enables to culture any purulence that is visualized. CT scans are not routinely recommended in ABRS and the role of CT scan is mostly for evaluation of suspected or impending complications such as orbital or intracranial involvement.

In patients with recurrent ARS, anatomical variations including Haller cells and septal deviation, nasal polyps, and choanal obstruction by benign adenoid tissue or odontogenic sources of infections should be considered.

Table 11.2 depicts the warning symptoms of complicated ABRS requiring urgent referral.

Other investigations:

- *Bacteriology:* Microbiological investigations are not routinely required, although they may be required in research settings and in more severe, recurrent or complicated presentations. In this case maxillary sinus tap culture remains gold standard though now endoscopic-directed sinonasal cultures can be taken to identify specific organisms for research. Middle meatal cultures can also be taken.
- *C-reactive protein:* CRP is a hematological biomarker and is raised in bacterial infection. Its use has been advocated in respiratory tract infection as an aid to targeting bacterial infection and so in limiting unnecessary antibiotic use.

    This is preliminary observation, and more research is needed before this test can be recommended as routine.
- *Erythrocyte sedimentation rate and plasma viscosity:* Markers of inflammation such as ESR and plasma viscosity are raised in ARS, may reflect disease severity and can indicate the need for more aggressive treatment in a similar way to CRP.

Treatment Strategy

Acute bacterial rhinosinusitis has microbial as well as inflammatory components. Treatment aims at controlling both. Table 11.3 shows the treatment summary.

Antimicrobial Therapy

Whether to start antibiotics? ARS resolves without antibiotic treatment in most cases. Symptomatic treatment and reassurance is the preferred initial management strategy for patients with mild symptoms.

It is clear, however, that antibiotics play an important role in reducing symptoms and speeding the time of recovery.

Today over prescription of antibiotics has resulted in emergence of resistance and hence warrants a judicious use of antibiotics.

Antibiotics may be withheld in patients with mild symptoms or in cases where bacterial etiology remains questionable and in cases where there are no comorbidities such as immunocompromise that makes an untreated ABRS intolerable.[5] On the other hand, antimicrobial agents should be started when symptoms are moderate to severe or comorbidities require quick resolution and clinical suspicion of bacterial etiology is high. According to recent EPOS (European position paper on rhinosinusitis and nasal polyps) guidelines, *antibiotic therapy should be reserved for patients with severe ARS, especially with the presence of high fever or severe (unilateral) facial pain.*[1]

What antibiotic to be prescribed? Most guidelines recommend high-dose amoxicillin, up to 4,000 mg/day for adults. In case of resistance, amoxicillin-clavulanate is a good alternative. Second-line therapy for amoxicillin failures or patients with penicillin allergies may include respiratory quinolones and ketolides. Cephalosporins are another alternative. Macrolide antibiotics (erythromycin, clarithromycin, azithromycin) have antimicrobial properties plus they also have anti-inflammatory effect which augments their clinical efficacy.

Length of therapy? Most ABRS antibiotic regimens aim for maintaining serum or tissue levels above minimal inhibitory concentrations for 7–10 days.

Role of Intranasal Steroids

Intranasal corticosteroids are recommended for the treatment of ARS, both in moderate (monotherapy) and severe (with oral antibiotics) disease.[1] Steroid nasal sprays when given with oral antibiotic in ABRS result in greater reduction of total symptoms.[6] The rationale for intranasal corticosteroid administration in ARS is based on the alleviation of inflammation and edema of the nasal mucosa, nasal turbinates, and sinus ostia. In patients with recurring ARS, steroid nasal sprays have been especially shown to improve obstruction related symptoms like headache, congestion and facial pain.[7]

Decongestant Therapy

These alpha adrenergic agents act on smooth muscle in mucosal vasculature, decreasing blood flow and thereby reducing mucosal edema. Topical decongestants may be helpful in relieving acute symptoms but must not be used for more than 3–5 days as they cause rhinitis medicamentosa. Prolonged topical use can cause atrophic rhinitis.

Antihistaminics

There is no indication for the use of antihistamines (both intranasal and oral) in the treatment of postviral ARS, except in coexisting allergic rhinitis.

Saline Administration

Saline administration via spray, aerosol, or irrigation is a simple and inexpensive means of softening viscous secretions and providing some relief from congestion.

CHRONIC RHINOSINUSITIS

Definition

Chronic rhinosinusitis (CRS), with or without nasal polyps in adults is defined as:[1]
- Inflammation of the nose and the paranasal sinuses characterized by two or more symptoms, one of which should be either nasal blockage/obstruction/congestion or nasal discharge (anterior/posterior nasal drip): ± facial pain/pressure, ± reduction or loss of smell.
For more than or equal to 12 weeks and either endoscopic signs of:
  - Nasal polyps, and/or
  - Mucopurulent discharge primarily from middle meatus and/or
  - Edema/mucosal obstruction primarily in middle meatus and/or
    o CT changes:
      - Mucosal changes within the ostiomeatal complex and/or sinuses

Chronic rhinosinusitis with nasal polyps (CRSwNP): CRS as defined above and endoscopically visualized polyps in middle meatus.

Chronic rhinosinusitis without nasal polyps (CRSsNP): CRS as defined above and no visible polyps in middle meatus, if necessary following decongestant.

Pathophysiology: CRS is an inflammatory disease and may or may not involve pathogenic organisms. It is characterized by mucosal inflammation of nose and paranasal sinuses of at least 12 consecutive weeks duration.

What mediates this prolonged inflammatory response? There are several, potentially coexisting, pathological factors implicated in the same which include ciliary dysfunction, immune deficiency, ostial obstruction, bacteria, fungi, superantigens, leukotriene abnormalities, biofilms,[8] osteitis and environmental factors.[1,9] In those patients with CRS who do have potential pathogenic bacteria, the most common organisms are *Staphylococcus aureus*, coagulase negative *Staphylococcus*, anerobic, Gram-negative bacteria and fungi.

Diagnosis

The symptoms of chronic rhinosinusitis can vary from local, regional or sytemic and are enumerated in Table 11.4.

Investigations

Primary Investigations

Nasal endoscopy and CT scan of paranasal sinuses form the foundation of CRS investigations.

Endoscopy: Mucosal edema, discharge, polyps and crusting form the cardinal endoscopic features of CRS. Endoscopy is useful to assess anatomy, to evaluate treatment response and if purulence is present a culture can be taken.

TABLE 11.4: Symptomatology of chronic rhinosinusitis		
Local	Regional	Systemic
Nasal obstruction and congestion	Sore throat	Malaise
Nasal discharge: anterior or posterior	Dysphonia	Fever
Facial pain	Cough	Anorexia
Facial fullness	Halitosis	Fatigue
Headache	Bronchospasm	
Smell dysfunction	Ear fullness or pain	
Anosmia	Eustachian tube dysfunction	
	Dental pain	

Computed tomography scan: It is the preferred radiologic test. It correlates fairly well with the extent of disease although it cannot distinguish between infection and inflammation. They have been useful in assessing severity of disease or response to treatment in CRS. A range of staging systems based on CT scanning have been described but the most commonly used is the Lund-Mackay system. CT is generally reserved for patients who have failed appropriate medical therapy and are being considered for surgery in uncomplicated rhinosinusitis.

Secondary investigations are not much relevant to general clinical practice and are more important for research purposes. These include various tests for olfaction, nasal airway assessment, ciliary dysfunction and certain blood tests.

Medical Management of Chronic Rhinosinusitis

Maximal medical therapy is the standard of care for CRS. Surgery is indicated in patients of CRS who have failed to respond to maximal medical therapy.

Aim of Treatment

The aim of medical treatment is to reduce mucosal inflammation and swelling, control infection, and restore aeration of the nasal and sinus mucosa thereby reducing signs and symptoms, improving patient's quality of life and preventing disease progression and/or recurrence.

Intranasal corticosteroids: CRS is best considered an inflammatory disease and intranasal corticosteroids are considered the mainstay and the first line of treatment in CRS patients. They reduce mucosal edema and inflammation.

Intranasal steroids causes reduction of obstructive symptoms, decrease in size of polyps and prevent postoperative polyp recurrence. When combined with antibiotic use, efficacy in symptom reduction was also found during acute exacerbations.[10] However, the benefit for nonpolypoid CRS has been harder to demonstrate.[11]

Various techniques of administration have been described in literature.[12] In the "cross-handed" technique patients are instructed to spray the right nostril with left hand and left nostril by right hand, this maximizes delivery to the inferior turbinate, a key structure in development of congestive symptoms and also increases the chance of medication reaching the middle meatus. Another technique is steroid instillation with vertex in dependent position, such as "Mecca position" and "Mygind position". Other methods of topical steroid application are nasal irrigation with steroid containing solution, nebulized steroids.

Systemic effects of topical steroids are negligible, local side effects include epistaxis, nasal dryness, crusting, pharyngitis and cough.

Systemic steroids: Systemic steroids are typically administered: (1) as part of a regimen of maximal medical therapy before considering a patient a candidate for surgery, (2) for use in perioperative period to reduce inflammation and to augment optimal healing postoperatively, (3) during exacerbation of CRS, (4) in management of comorbidities such as asthma or other allergic/inflammatory conditions.

Lennard and colleagues demonstrated the effects of steroids in inflammatory cytokines for patients with CRS by nasal biopsy before and after treatment. The authors found significant decreases in interleukin 6 (IL-6) levels after treatment, with tumor necrosis factor-α trending toward significance.[13]

Steroid treatment may also avert the need of surgery in some patients. Patients who fail maximal medical therapy, and those with diffuse sinonasal polyposis or AFS are candidates for surgery. Short courses of oral steroids are used in the treatment of CRS with nasal polyps but may also be used in cases of severe CRS when rapid symptomatic improvement is needed (Table 11.5).

Systemic steroids must be used with caution in patients with gastrointestinal ulcers, diabetes, cataract, glaucoma and osteoporosis.

Antibiotics: As seen previously chronic rhinosinusitis is more of an inflammatory disease rather than infective. The role of bacteria in pathogenesis is debatable nevertheless the commonly isolated bacteria are *Staphylococcus aureus*, coagulase negative *Staphylococcus*, anaerobic and Gram-negative bacteria. They should be advocated when

TABLE 11.5: Steroid regimens

	CRS without nasal polyposis	*CRS with nasal polyposis*
Treatment trial (as part of maximal medical therapy)	0.5 mg/ kg body weight tapered over 2 weeks	0.5 mg/ kg body weight tapered over 2 weeks
Before surgery	Not routinely required	0.5 mg/kg body weight over a week in tapering doses
Immediately after surgery	Not routinely required	0.5 mg/ kg body weight daily till resolution of disease on endoscopic examination, then tapered over 1–2 weeks
Acute exacerbation	0.5 mg/ kg body weight tapered over 2 weeks	0.5 mg/kg body weight tapered over 2 weeks

purulence is identified. Thus patients should be treated with at least 3 weeks of a culture-directed or broad spectrum oral antibiotics before considering surgery. Short-term treatment can be given in CRSsNP during exacerbations when the culture is positive.[1] Ideally a culture-directed antibiotic should be started. Antibiotics that can be selected include amoxicillin/clavulanate, quinolones, or combination therapy like clindamycin plus trimethoprim/sulfamethoxazole. A systemic course of at least 3 weeks is recommended although there is no general consensus regarding the duration of treatment.[14] Intravenous antibiotics may have a role in selected cases, such as in patients with orbital or intracranial complications (or pending complications), as well as those who manifest organisms resistant to oral antibiotics.

Topical antibiotics: Recent trends have explored the use of topical antibiotic delivery methods like nebulization and irrigation. The goal of topical antibiotic therapy is to deliver high concentrations of antibiotics directly to the site of infection with low systemic absorption and side effects. Most of the studies have utilized this modality in patients who have undergone prior functional endoscopy sinus surgery (FESS), as penetration of topical medications is minimal into sinuses that have not been surgically opened.[15] There is a paucity of controlled studies demonstrating the efficacy of these delivery methods. Some of the antibiotic solutions described are Tobramycin, which is utilized at a concentration of 80 mg/liter of normal saline, and patient is instructed to irrigate each nostril with 50 mL twice daily. Other antibiotics used are gentamycin, ceftazidime. Methicillin-resistant *Staphylococcus aureus* (MRSA) can be controlled by mupirocin irrigation. In a study, patients with surgically recalcitrant CRS who had positive nasendoscopically-guided cultures for *Staphylococcus aureus* were treated with twice-a-day nasal irrigation with 0.05% mupirocin in Ringer solution. 93% of patients had improved endoscopic findings, whereas 75% had symptom improvement.[16]

Duration of treatment with broad spectrum antibiotic is usually 3–4 weeks that may be extended up to 8–10 weeks.

Macrolide therapy: The use of long-term macrolide therapy originated in Japan, where it reduced the mortality rate of diffuse panbronchiolitis and concomitantly improved sinus symptoms.[17] Recent investigations have suggested that macrolides exhibit anti-inflammatory effects in addition to their antimicrobial properties. This modality decreases nasal obstruction, postnasal drip, reduces quantity and viscosity of nasal secretions[18] and also decreases size of polyps.[19] In

CRSsNP there is some evidence to use long-term, low-dose macrolide antibiotics for 12 weeks.[1] Selecting patients with normal serum IgE could improve response rate.[1] For now, long-term antibiotic treatment should be reserved for patients where nasal corticosteroids and saline irrigation has failed to reduce symptoms to an acceptable level. Data suggests that the populations with high serum IgE are less likely to respond to macrolide treatment and the ones with normal IgE more likely to do so.[20] At least 4 weeks of therapy is needed before symptomatic improvement is realized. Available evidence suggests that low-dose, long-duration macrolide therapy (erythromycin, clarithromycin and roxithromycin) is safe and can result in improvements in both subjective and objective measures of CRS in select patients.

Allergy management: Environmental control is important part of the management in those patients for whom allergy, pollution or mold exposures appear to be significant predisposing factors. Patients of CRS who exhibit features of allergic rhinitis are considered for allergy management which is shown to have a significant impact on patients' symptoms and outcomes. Treatment includes avoidance of allergen exposure, medical management and immunotherapy. Antihistaminics are very effective to control symptoms of nasal pruritus and rhinorrhea whereas congestive and obstructive symptoms are responsive to intranasal steroids. Mucolytics and oral decongestants are beneficial for acute exacerbation and topical decongestants should be used judiciously. Immunotherapy should be a strong consideration in CRS patients, who exhibit significant allergies.

Antifungals in CRS: The use of antifungals in CRS is debatable. There is no confirmed benefit of topical antifungal over saline irrigation[21,22] Oral antifungals have been proposed as a treatment option for select patients with allergic fungal sinusitis[23-25] and nonallergic eosinophilic fungal sinusitis,[24] diseases considered to be similar to allergic bronchopulmonary aspergillosis (ABPA).

Nasal Saline Irrigation and Saline Nasal Spray

Intranasal saline is a safe and effective treatment modality, often used along with intranasal corticosteroid in the management of CRS. Improvements in quality of life, reduction in postnasal drip, and mediators within nasal secretions have been observed. It promotes mucociliary clearance by flushing out mucus, crusts and irritants. Saline sprays are also effective in the same. Benefits of nasal saline irrigation include enhanced ciliary beat activity, removal of antigen, biofilm or inflammatory mediators, and a protective role on sinonasal mucosa.[26] It also allows local steroid spray to act better. It is also useful after endoscopic sinus surgery to clear crusts and thick mucus that are common postoperatively.[12] Nasal lavage can be done using nasal lavage pot, syringe, bulb.

Decongestants, mucolytics and antihistaminics: Decongestants are α-adrenergic agonists that induce the release of norepinephrine from sympathetic nerves leading to vasoconstriction of the nasal vasculature. Topical decongestants will usually reduce symptoms and speed recovery in patients with rhinosinusitis. However, topical decongestants should not be used for longer than 3 days to avoid rebound nasal congestion and rhinitis medicamentosa.

Mucolytics: Mechanical drainage can also be improved with a mucolytic. Guaifenesin is the most commonly used medication to thin mucus secretions.[27] Antihistaminic therapy should be considered in patients with CRS with allergic component.

Leukotriene inhibitors: Leukotriene inhibitors like montelukast cause significant reduction in absolute eosinophil count in patients with allergic rhinitis and asthma. The observation that leukotriene levels are increased in the nasal secretions of people with asthma with aspirin sensitivity and nasal polyposis raised the possibility that antileukotriene therapy could benefit patients with CRS with nasal polyps.[28] At this time, more research is required to determine which subset of patients with CRS will benefit most from leukotriene inhibitors.

Aspirin desensitization: Aspirin sensitivity is usually associated with nasal polyposis and asthma (Samter's triad). These patients have intense inflammatory disease with poor response to surgery and have frequent relapse. Aspirin sensitive patients should be considered for aspirin desensitization. Patients are treated with increasing doses of Aspirin followed by daily maintenance therapy. This has been shown to improve nasal and chest symptoms and reduces acute exacerbations.

Maximal medical therapy should be given for a period of 4–6 weeks. It comprises of oral steroid in tapering doses, intranasal steroids, oral antibiotics at least for 3 weeks and saline irrigation. Endoscopic sinus surgery is indicated in patients of CRS who have failed to respond to maximal medical therapy.

SUMMARY

- Rhinosinusitis is a group of disorders characterized by inflammation of mucosa of nose and paranasal sinuses
- Diagnosis of ARS is best made on clinical grounds with little role of imaging
- Acute rhinosinusitis is mainly viral in origin and tends to be self-limiting. Antibiotic therapy is usually not needed until 7–10 days after the onset of symptoms in an upper respiratory tract infection
- Resistance is developing amongst pathogenic bacteria in part due to overprescription and injudicious use of antibiotics.
- It is now clear that CRS is a heterogeneous group of disorders characterized by inflammation rather than infection
- Medical treatment of CRS is intended to reduce signs and symptoms, improve quality of life and prevent disease progression and/or recurrence
- Maximal medical therapy should be given in all patients of CRS for at least 4–6 weeks, surgery is indicated in those patients who fail to respond to maximal medical therapy.
- The goal of preoperative preparation for surgery is to reduce the inflammation and to optimize the nasal mucosa
- A significant postoperative care is required to achieve the goals of surgery and to ensure long-term results and to prevent recurrences.

REFERENCES

1. Fokkens WJ, Lund VJ, Mullol J, et al. European position paper on rhinosinusitis and nasal polyps. Rhinology. 2012;50(Suppl 23):1-305.
2. Gwaltney JM, Scheld WM, Sande MA, et al. The microbial etiology and antimicrobial therapy of adults with acute community-acquired sinusitis: a fifteen year experience at the University of Virginia and review of other selected studies. J Allergy Clin Immunol. 1992;90:457-62.
3. Rosenfeld RM. Clinical practice guideline on adult sinusitis. Otolaryngol Head Neck Surg. 2007;137:365-77.
4. Gwaltney JM, Hendley JO, Simon G, et al. Rhinovirus infections in an industrial population. Characteristics of illness and antibody response. JAMA. 1967;202:494-500.
5. Acute Rhinosinusitis in adults. 2005 (cited 2007). [online] Available from: http://cme.med.umich.edu/pdf/guideline/rhino05.pdf. [Accessed August 2013].
6. Nayak AS, Settipane GA, Pedinoff A, et al. Effective dose range of mometasone furoate nasal spray in the treatment of acute rhinosinusitis. Ann Allergy Asthma Immunol. 2002;89(3):271-8.
7. Meltzer EO, Charous BL, Busse WW, et al. Added relief in the treatment of acute recurrent sinusitis with adjunctive mometasone furoate nasal spray. The Nasonex Sinusitis Group. J Allergy Clin Immunol. 2000;106(4):630-7.
8. Harvey RJ, Lund VJ. Biofilms and chronic rhinosinusitis: systematic review of evidence, current concepts and directions for research. Rhinology. 2007;45(1):3-13.
9. Benninger MS, Ferguson BJ, Hadley JA, et al. Adult chronic rhinosinusitis: definitions, diagnosis, epidemiology, and pathophysiology. Otolaryngol Head Neck Surg. 2003;129 (Suppl 3):S1-S32.
10. Statham MM, Seiden A. Potential new avenues of treatment for chronic rhinosinusitis: an anti-inflammatory approach. Otolaryngol Clin North Am. 2005;38:1351-65.

11. Kalish LH, Arendts G, Sacks R, et al. Topical steroids in chronic rhinosinusitis without polyps: a systemic review and meta-analysis. Otolaryngol Head Neck Surg. 2009;141:674-83.

12. Benninger MS, Hadley JA, Osguthorpe JD, et al. Techniques of intranasal steroid use. Otolaryngol Head Neck Surg. 2004;130: 5-24.

13. Lennard CM, Mann EA, Sun LL, et al. Interleukin-1 beta, interleukin-5, interleukin-6, interleukin-8, and tumor necrosis factor-alpha in chronic sinusitis: response to systemic corticosteroids. Am J Rhinol. 2000;14:367-73.

14. Dubin MG, Kuhn FA, Melroy CT. Radiographic resolution of chronic rhinosinusitis without polyposis after 6 weeks vs. 3 weeks of oral antibiotics. Ann Allergy Asthma Immunol. 2007;98:32-5.

15. Hwang PH, Woo RJ, Fong KJ. Intranasal deposition of nebulized saline: a radionuclide distribution study. Am J Rhinol. 2006; 20:255-61.

16. Uren B, Psaltis A, Wormald PJ. Nasal lavage with mupirocin for the treatment of surgically recalcitrant chronic rhinosinusitis. Laryngoscope. 2008;118:1677-80.

17. Amsden GW. Anti-inflammatory effects of macrolides—an underappreciated benefit in the treatment of community-acquired respiratory tract infections and chronic inflammatory pulmonary conditions? J Antimicrob Chemother. 2005;55: 10-21.

18. Majima Y. Clinical implications of the immunomodulatory effects of macrolides on sinusitis. Am J Med. 2004;117(Suppl 9A):20-5.

19. Gotfried MH. Macrolides for the treatment of chronic sinusitis, asthma, and COPD. Chest. 2004;125(Suppl 2):52-61.

20. Haruna S, Shimada C, Ozawa M, et al. A study of poor responders for long-term, low-dose macrolide administration for chronic sinusitis. Rhinology. 2009;47(1):66-71.

21. Ponikau JU, Sherris DA, Weaver A, et al. Treatment of chronic rhinosinusitis with intranasal amphotericin B: a randomized, placebo controlled double-blind pilot trial. J Allergy Clin Immunol. 2005;115:125-31.

22. Ebbens FA, Scadding GK, Badia L. Amphotericin B nasal lavages: not a solution for patients with chronic rhinosinusitis. J Allergy Clin Immunol. 2006;188:1149-56.

23. Chan KO, Genoway KA, Javer AR. Effectiveness of itraconazole in the management of refractory allergic fungal rhinosinusitis. J Otolaryngol Head Neck Surg. 2008;37:870-4.

24. Seiberling K, Wormald PJ. The role of itraconazole in recalcitrant fungal sinusitis. Am J Rhinol Allergy. 2009;23:303-6.

25. Rains BM, Mineck CW. Treatment of allergic fungal sinusitis with high-dose itraconazole. Am J Rhinol. 2003;17:1-8.

26. Harvey RJ, Schlosser RJ. Local drug delivery. Otolaryngol Clin North Am. 2009;42:829-45.

27. Suh JD, Kennedy DW. Treatment options for chronic rhinosinusitis. Proc Am Thorac Soc. 2011;8:132-40.

28. Gillespie MB, Osguthorpe JD. Pharmacologic management of chronic rhinosinusitis, alone or with nasal polyposis. Curr Allergy Asthma Rep. 2004;4:478-85.

CHAPTER 12

Invasive Fungal Sinusitis

Kashmira Chavan, Gauri Mankekar, Bachi Hathiram, Milind V Kirtane

INTRODUCTION

Fungal sinusitis was a rare entity and rarely encountered. In recent years, however, the incidence of fungal sinusitis has been on the rise. Fungal infection of the maxillary sinus was first reported in 1791 by Plaignaud.[1] Schubert, in 1885, gave a description of sinus aspergillosis.[2] Later, in 1897, Oppe reported a case of invasive aspergillosis of the sphenoid sinus with cerebral extension.[3] Hora in 1965, classified fungal sinusitis as invasive and noninvasive varieties.[4]

Based on histopathological examination, fungal sinusitis can be broadly classified into invasive and noninvasive types. Fungal sinusitis is labeled as invasive when fungal invasion of the sinus mucosa, submucosa, blood vessels, bone, etc. is seen on histopathology.[5]

The invasive form of fungal sinusitis is usually seen in immunocompromised individuals. Factors predisposing to the development of invasive fungal sinusitis include:[5-9]

- Systemic disorders
  - Diabetes mellitus
  - Hematological disorders, e.g. leukemias, lymphomas, aplastic anemia
  - Iron overload
  - Acquired immunodeficiency syndrome (AIDS)
- Iatrogenic immunosuppression
  - Systemic steroid therapy
  - Chemotherapy
- Post organ transplantation.

Rarely, invasive disease may be seen in immunocompetent individuals too.[5,9,10] Noninvasive fungal disease may progress to invasive disease if the immunological status of a patient changes.

CLASSIFICATION

The disease is defined as acute when the duration is less than 4 weeks, while disease of more than 4 weeks duration is said to be chronic.[8] Depending on the course and duration of the disease, invasive fungal sinusitis has been further subclassified as:[5]

- Acute fulminant invasive fungal sinusitis
- Chronic invasive fungal sinusitis
- Granulomatous invasive fungal sinusitis.

Acute Fulminant Invasive Fungal Sinusitis

Acute fulminant invasive fungal sinusitis is a rapidly progressing invasive disease usually seen in immunocompromised patients.[5] The disease can have a rapid downhill course over a few days to weeks. Rapid spread of the infection occurs as a result of vascular invasion by the fungus, leading to vascular thrombosis and tissue infarction.

Chronic Invasive Fungal Sinusitis

Chronic invasive fungal sinusitis is a relatively rare type of invasive fungal sinusitis seen usually in diabetic patients, with disease progression occurring over weeks to a few months.[5,11]

Granulomatous Invasive Fungal Sinusitis

Granulomatous invasive fungal sinusitis also has an indolent course and is usually seen in immunocompetent individuals, with patients usually presenting with proptosis. This type of fungal sinusitis has been reported from Sudan, India, Pakistan.[5,11] Histopathology in this condition is characterized by a granulomatous inflammation.[5]

MICROBIOLOGY[5,6,8,11,12]

A variety of fungi can lead to acute fulminant invasive fungal sinusitis; however, members of the class *Zygomycetes (Mucor, Rhizopus)* and *Aspergillus* are the most common causative organisms. Other fungi that can cause invasive fungal sinusitis include *Rhizomucor, Absidia, Cunninghamella, Pseudallescheria boydii*, etc. Chronic invasive fungal sinusitis is usually caused by *Aspergillus fumigatus* while *Aspergillus flavus* has been identified as the organism causing granulomatous fungal sinusitis. *Aspergillus fumigatus*,[13] *Rhizopus*,[14] *Schizophyllum commune*,[15] *Scytalidium dimidiatum*,[16] *Paecilomyces lilacinus*[17] have been reported to cause invasive fungal sinusitis in immunocompetent individuals.

PATHOGENESIS

The progression and spread of fungal disease depends upon immune status of the host and local tissue conditions. Invasive fungal sinusitis is usually seen in immunocompromised individuals, although the chronic and granulomatous forms of the disease usually affect immunocompetent hosts. Fulminant disease has also been rarely reported in apparently immunocompetent individuals.[5,9,10] Mucormycosis commonly affects patients with diabetes mellitus. Hyperglycemia and acidosis provide ideal conditions for fungal growth and tissue invasion. Also, ketoacidosis has been shown to adversely affect phagocytic activity.[18] Once the organism invades the sinuses, disease progression may occur, with arterial invasion followed by venous and lymphatic invasion. Vasculitis and thrombosis occurs leading to tissue ischemia, infarction and necrosis. Vascular invasion results in a fulminant course with direct spread to adjacent structures such as the orbit, palate and oral cavity. Involvement of the orbit may lead to third, fourth and sixth cranial nerve palsies. Fifth and seventh cranial nerves may be involved in advanced disease. Intracranial spread may occur either through the cribriform plate, via the orbital apex or, via septic emboli. Once the ophthalmic and other orbital arteries are involved, infection can further reach the cavernous sinus and carotid artery. Acute subdural hematoma, cavernous sinus thrombosis and internal carotid artery thrombosis may occur in rhinocerebral mucormycosis. Invasion of the carotid arteries can rapidly lead to cerebral ischemia and death.[6,19]

CLINICAL FEATURES

Diagnosis of invasive fungal sinusitis needs a high degree of clinical suspicion, along with microbiological and histopathological evidence for further definitive management.

Symptoms

The following symptoms, especially in an immunocompromised patient should arouse the suspicion of fungal disease:
- Fever with spikes, not responding to antibiotics, may be the initial presentation
- Nasal blockage with mucopurulent or blood-stained serosanguineous nasal discharge
- Facial or periorbital swelling, facial pain, numbness, headache may be seen as disease progression occurs
- *Orbital symptoms:* Proptosis, ptosis, visual abnormalities
- Cranial nerve palsies especially second, third, fourth, fifth, sixth and seventh nerve
- Central nervous system (CNS) symptoms such as altered conscious, delirium, convulsions, hemiparesis, hemiplegia or coma may be seen in patients with intracranial involvement.

Examination

- *Diagnostic nasal endoscopy:* Although the physical examination in cases of invasive fungal sinusitis may occasionally not be very obvious, a change in the appearance of the nasal mucosa should always be looked for. Crusting, whitish discoloration (due to tissue ischemia) or black discoloration with eschar formation (due to tissue necrosis) may be visualized.[20] Granulation or ulceration of the nasal mucosa may also be present. These changes have been most commonly found to occur on the middle turbinate, followed by the septum, palate and inferior turbinate.[9] Decreased nasal mucosal bleeding on account of tissue ischemia or infarction may be noticed. Swabs and biopsy can be taken from suspected areas of the middle and inferior turbinate during a diagnostic nasal endoscopy and the tissue sent for microbiological and histopathological examination.
- Decreased facial or nasal mucosal sensations may be present even in early stages of the disease before development of other signs and symptoms.
- Facial and/or periorbital edema and erythema may be present
- Gingival or palatal eschars or ulceration may be found.

- Spread of disease to the orbit may lead to chemosis, proptosis, ptosis, decreases vision and ophthalmoplegia.
- Fifth and seventh cranial nerve involvement may occur with spread of infection.

Persistence of fever of unknown origin for more than 48 hours inspite of appropriate antibiotic therapy, in the presence of localized sinonasal symptoms in an immunocompromised patient, warrants nasal endoscopy and imaging studies.[8,9,21]

INVESTIGATIONS

Rapid confirmation of a diagnosis of acute fulminant invasive fungal sinusitis is necessary so that immediate treatment can be initiated.

Microbiology

Fungal Stains and Microscopy[22]

A nasal swab or tissue from the suspected region should be sent for an urgent microbiological examination. Potassium hydroxide (KOH)—calcoflour white method is a highly sensitive method to detect fungal hyphae. It gives results within a few hours and thus an early diagnosis. KOH dissolves human tissue while calcoflour white, an optic brightener, binds to the cell wall of the fungal hyphae and helps in their identification. Fungal cell walls and hyphae can be identified on fluorescence microscopy.

Fungal Cultures

Fungal cultures may take days to weeks to yield positive results, but may be required in unresponsive cases where antifungal sensitivity testing is needed.[6,22]

Histopathology

Histopathologic examination of tissue using hematoxylin-eosin staining and special stains such as periodic-acid Schiff (PAS) and Gomori—methenamine silver staining can be used to differentiate between species.[5,6,22] Gomori methenamine has been described to be the most sensitive of the commonly used stains and it has been recommended that a negative diagnosis should not be given unless a silver stain has been performed.[22] A frozen section should be performed at the time of initial biopsy so that immediate treatment can be initiated.[23] On histopathology, Mucor hyphae are large (6–50 m), irregular, nonseptate with branching at right angles, and show obliterative vascular invasion. Aspergillus hyphae on the other hand, are narrower (2.5–5 m), septate with branching at 45°. They may demonstrate vascular invasion which is nonobliterative in nature.[8,9] A histiocytic or giant cell reaction to fungal hyphae is the chief histologic feature seen in rhinocerebral aspergillosis.[24] However both frozen section and special stains may be at times unable to provide a definite differentiation between fungal species.[6,12] A classification system for invasive fungal sinusitis based histopathology has been proposed by deShazo et al.[5] (Table 12.1).

Imaging

Imaging studies provide information about the extent of disease and guide the surgeon in deciding the extent of surgical debridement (Figs 12.1 to 12.4).

Computed Tomography

A computed tomography (CT) scan of the paranasal sinuses with thin slices in the axial and coronal planes should be

TABLE 12.1: Classification of invasive fungal sinusitis (deShazo et al.)[5]

Syndrome	Previous name(s)	Histopathological features	Immunocompetence
Granulomatous invasive fungal sinusitis	Chronic invasive, indolent, primary paranasal *Aspergillus* granuloma in Sudan	Granuloma composed of multinucleated giant cells, variable numbers of lymphocytes, and plasma cell; center of granuloma may be composed of eosinophilic material surrounded by fungus, giant cells, and pallisading nuclei	Apparently immunocompetent
Chronic invasive fungal sinusitis	Invasive, fulminant invasive	Tissue necrosis with little inflammatory infiltrate, dense hyphal accumulation resembling mycetoma may be present; fungi breach the mucosal barriers to invade blood vessels and cause tissue necrosis	Diabetes mellitus
Acute fulminant invasive fungal sinusitis	Acute fulminant, rhinocerebral mucormycosis, invasive *Aspergillus* sinusitis	Fungal vascular invasion with vascular thrombosis and tissue infarction; centrifugally spreading necrotizing reaction with minimal cellular infiltrate; often have necrotic nasal ulcer (eschar)	Usually immunocompromised because of cancer, therapeutic immunosuppression, poorly controlled diabetes mellitus, protein calorie malnutrition, or iron overload; case reports in immunocompetent patients

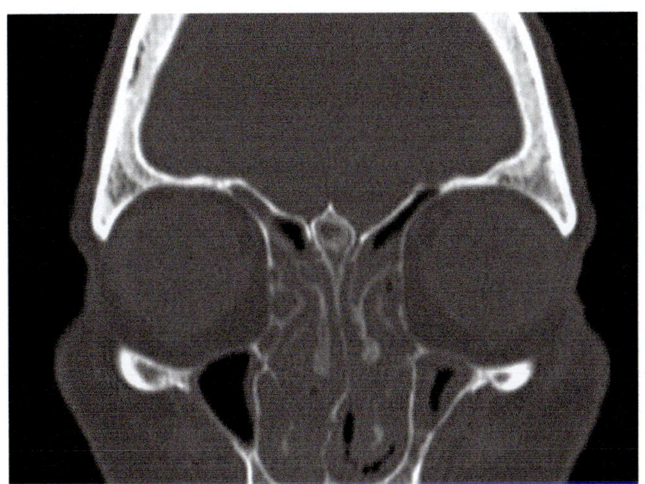

Fig. 12.1: Coronal computed tomography scan of the paranasal sinuses in a 55-year-old leukemia patient with mucormycosis

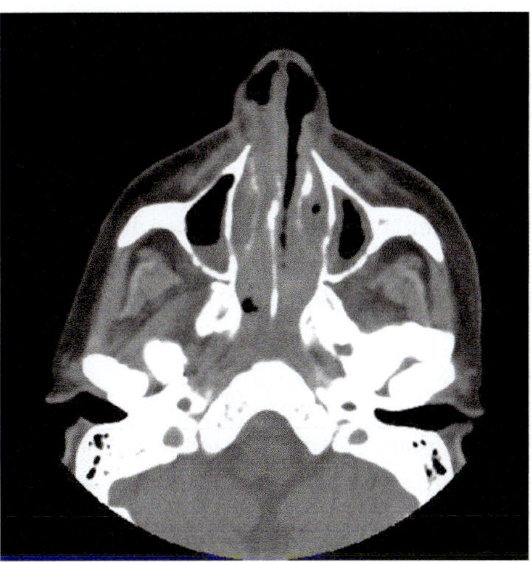

Fig. 12.2: Axial computed tomography scan of the paranasal sinuses showing fat stranding in the infratemporal fossa in a 55-year-old leukemia patient with mucormycosis

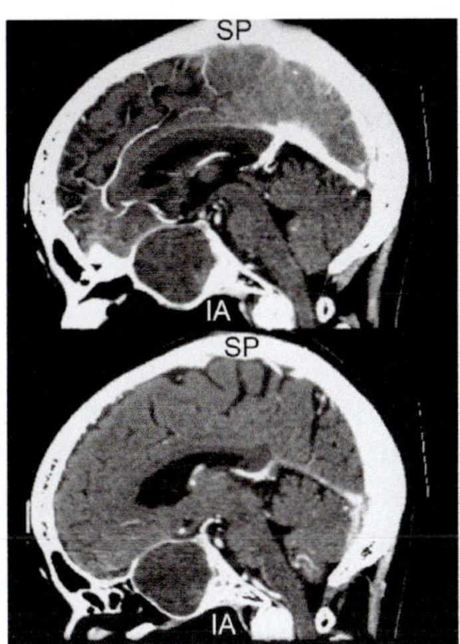

Fig. 12.3: Magnetic resonance imaging showing isolated sphenoid *Pseudoallescheria boydii*

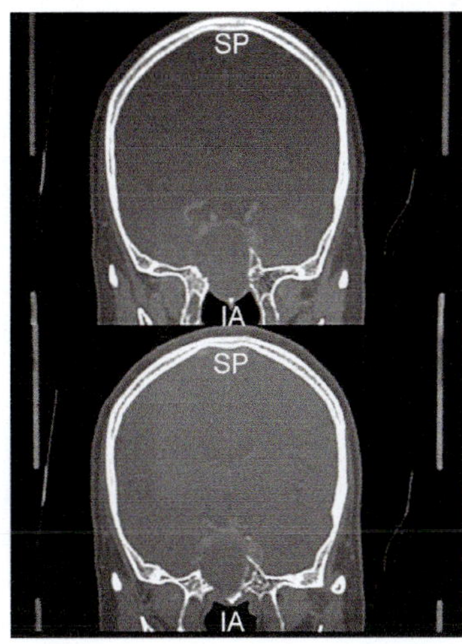

Fig. 12.4: Coronal computed tomography scan of the paranasal sinuses showing isolated sphenoid *Pseudoallescheria boydii*

obtained in suspected cases of invasive fungal sinusitis. Additional orbital and intracranial cuts should also be obtained to look for any spread of disease. Intravenous contrast is required if intracranial or intraorbital spread is suspected on the initial evaluation. Cases with early disease may only reveal thickening of the nasal mucosa or with or without periantral fat plain involvement.[25] Mucosal thickening, air fluid levels within the sinuses, bony erosion and soft tissue infiltration may be seen on CT scan. Erosion of the lamina papyracea may be seen when the disease involves the orbit. Involvement of the superior ophthalmic vein and ophthalmic artery have been described as specific radiologic signs to diagnose orbital apex syndrome secondary to mucormycosis.[26] Although CT scans provide useful details about the bony anatomy and act as a guide for surgical planning, magnetic resonance imaging (MRI) is a more superior study to determine soft tissue involvement and intracranial extension.[6]

Magnetic Resonance Imaging

Magnetic resonance imaging is a useful modality to evaluate soft tissue involvement, intraorbital, intracranial spread and vascular invasion such as involvement of the cavernous sinus. Intravenous contrast administration may be required if involvement of the orbital apex or intracranial extension is suspected. Enhancement of the involved soft tissue (such as superior ophthalmic vein and ophthalmic artery in orbital apex involvement) is seen. However in acute cases with orbital apex involvement the superior ophthalmic vein and ophthalmic artery may not reveal any enhancement.[27]

Magnetic Resonance Angiography

Magnetic resonance angiography may be occasionally required in cases with vascular involvement or pseudo-aneurysm formation.[27]

Diagnostic criteria for invasive fungal sinusitis based on histopathology and imaging has been proposed by deShazo et al:[5]

- Mucosal thickening or air fluid levels compatible with sinusitis on imaging.
- Histopathological evidence of hyphal forms within the sinus mucosa, submucosa, blood vessel or bone. Concomitant stains for mycobacteria should be negative, and fungal elements within tissue, provoking a granulomatous response with giant cells must be present, to diagnose granulomatous invasive fungal sinusitis.

The character of the cellular infiltrate is otherwise not considered as a component of deShazo et al's. proposed criteria. Necrosis of bone has also not been included in this criteria, as necrosis could occur either as a result of the pressure effects of polypoidal tissue or due to bony expansion (as seen in allergic fungal sinusitis) or due to infarction (as seen in invasive fungal sinusitis). Hence necrosis of bone cannot be relied upon to diagnose invasive fungal sinusitis.[5] Immune status has also not been included, as invasive fungal sinusitis can rarely occur in immunocompetent individuals.

Cerebrospinal Fluid Examination

Examination of cerebrospinal fluid (CSF) may be performed in rhinocerebral fungal sinusitis. The findings are however usually nonspecific. CSF pressure may be elevated slightly, with mild increase in protein levels. Cellular examination may show some amount of pleocytosis with about 50% polymorphonuclear cells.[27,28]

Nonculture-based Tests

1. Galactomannan enzyme-linked immunoassay is a surrogate marker for diagnosis of invasive aspergillosis.[29-37] Serial assessment of galactomannan antigenemia may facilitate therapeutic monitoring.[38,39] However, duration of therapy should be determined not solely by normalization of antigenemia, but also by resolution of clinical and radiological findings.
2. Beta-D-glucans detection by Tachypleus or Limulus assay or Fungitell assay. The presence of beta-D-glucan in serum signifies the presence of fungal invasion but is not specific for *Aspergillus* species.[40]
3. Polymerase chain reaction (PCR) based diagnosis which amplifies *Aspergillus* specific fungal genes has also shown promise for invasive aspergillosis.[41,42]

TREATMENT

Invasive fungal sinusitis requires a rapid initiation of different modalities of therapy. The principles of management of invasive fungal sinusitis are:

- Control/correction of any underlying predisposing condition (e.g. diabetes mellitus, neutropenia, iron overload, etc.)
- Wide surgical debridement of the involved tissues and ensuring adequate sinus drainage
- Intravenous antifungal therapy
- Continuous monitoring to look for residual/recurrent disease.

Medical Management

Antifungal Therapy

Systemic amphotericin B is the drug of choice in treatment of most cases of invasive fungal sinusitis. Intravenous amphotericin B in a dose of 0.25–1.0 mg/kg/day up to a total dose of 2–4 grams over 6–8 weeks can be administered.[6] Continuous monitoring of the patient is required as amphotericin B administration is known to be associated with side effects such as chills, fever, headache, nausea, vomiting and thrombophlebitis. Other long-term adverse effects include hypokalemia, bone marrow suppression, and ototoxicity. Monitoring the patient's renal function is also necessary as the drug is nephrotoxic and can lead to renal tubular acidosis.[6,43,44] In patients developing renal toxicity or other severe side effects, amphotericin B may have to be withheld or substituted with liposomal amphotericin B (*Dose:* 3–5 mg/kg/day), which has lower systemic side-effects.[45] However, this drug is expensive and hence should only be reserved for clinically proven invasive fungal sinusitis patients in whom amphotericin B cannot be given or in those whom disease progression occurs inspite of amphotericin B therapy.[6]

Another antifungal agent, voriconazole has been shown to have better results and improved survival rate as compared to amphotericin B in cases of invasive aspergillosis.[46]

A loading dose of 6 mg/kg intravenous (IV) every 12 hours for two doses is recommended for intravenous voriconazole, followed by a maintenance dose of 4 mg/kg every 12 hours. Oral voriconazole has good bioavailability and can be given in a dose of 200 mg every 12 hours. The optimum duration of therapy however, has not been defined. As voriconazole has a more rapid clearance in children, higher doses may be required. The recommended maintenance dose in children is 7 mg/kg twice daily. However no standard recommendations for loading doses in children are available due to lack of sufficient studies. Adverse effects noted with voriconazole include visual disturbances (photopsia), hepatotoxicity, which may be dose-limiting (elevated serum bilirubin, alkaline phosphatase, and hepatic aminotransferase enzyme levels may be present), skin rashes and visual hallucinations. Intravenous voriconazole needs to be administered with care in patients with altered renal function.[47]

Posaconazole in a dose of 200 mg thrice a day orally is used for salvage treatment,[48] especially in patients with renal insufficiency or refractory invasive fungal infections.[49] The Food and Drug Administration (FDA), USA has approved prophylactic posaconazole use in prevention of invasive aspergillosis in neutropenic patients receiving remission induction chemotherapy for acute myelogenous leukemia or myelodysplastic syndrome and for hematopoietic stem cell transplant recipients with graft versus host disease.[47] Itraconazole 400 mg/day is recommended for indolent nonmeningeal aspergillosis.[50] But amphotericin B is preferred if the infection involves bone and is more extensive. Caspofungin may be administered to patients with proven or probable invasive aspergillosis who are refractory to or cannot tolerate other therapies.[47] The recommended dose is a single 70 mg loading dose on day 1, followed by 50 mg/day thereafter administered by slow IV infusion over 1 hour. In adults with compromised liver function, a dose of 35 mg should be given. The pediatric dose of caspofungin is 50 mg/m^2/day.[47]

Surgical Management

Aggressive surgical debridement is required in cases of invasive fungal sinusitis especially in those with fulminant disease. Debridement helps in slowing disease progression and in decreasing the fungal load so as to improve the effectiveness of antifungal therapy.[6,9,27] Surgery alone may suffice in some cases of granulomatous invasive fungal sinusitis without the need for antifungal therapy.[5] The extent of surgical debridement depends on the extent of the disease. Debridement of the tissues is performed until disease-free mucosa with bleeding edges is identified, and may be performed either endoscopically, via an external approach or a combined approach, depending on the disease extent and the surgeon's experience. Frozen section may be of assistance during debridement to differentiate between diseased and nondiseased tissues. Orbital exenteration may have to be carried out in the presence of ophthalmoplegia or orbital apex involvement or to prevent intracranial spread. An attempt may be made to preserve the orbit if the vision is unaffected in the presence of minimal orbital invasion, by performing conservative orbital debridement along with local amphotericin B irrigations.[51] Adequate data about the same is however unavailable. Radical resections such as a radical maxillectomy or craniofacial resection may have to be performed if the disease spreads beyond the sinonasal cavity.[9,52] Repeated debridements and a repeat biopsy may be required if persistent disease is suspected.

Repeated follow-up nasal endoscopies along with repeated swabs, biopsy and imaging studies are required to identify residual or recurrent disease till the patient is disease free and till cell counts are normal in patients with neutropenia. Thereafter a follow-up of once a month for atleast 6 months is recommended.[9]

Adjunctive Treatment

Desferroxamine

Host iron availability is fundamental to the pathogenesis of mucormycosis. There are reports[53,54] of desferroxamine being used as adjunctive therapy in invasive mucormycosis in the dose of 5–20 mg/kg body weight/day for 14–21 days for iron chelation.

Hyperbaric Oxygen

Hyperbaric oxygen therapy has been tried as adjunctive treatment in patients with invasive fungal sinusitis, especially mucormycosis. There are few reports of it being used in invasive aspergillosis. Oxygen in sufficient concentrations is fungicidal and decreases acidosis, which leads to improved phagocytosis by the leukocytes and macrophages, thus increasing tissue survival.[55,55a] There is no clinical data to suggest appropriate pressures and duration of therapy. It is usually started during the acute phase of the illness and not as salvage therapy, at 2.4–3.0 ATA range of pressures twice daily depending on the patient's general condition and ability to tolerate the pressures. In some successful cases, up to 30 treatments have been reported.[56]

Other Adjunctive Therapies

Granulocyte transfusions[57] and granulocyte colony-stimulating factors (G-CSF)[58] have been used as adjunctive therapy in patients with neutropenia.

PROGNOSIS

Older studies had reported high mortality rates for cases of acute fulminant invasive fungal sinusitis (50–80%). Recent studies however place the rates at about 20%.[6,8] However in cases with symptomatic intracranial involvement, mortality may reach 100%.[52,59,60] Also, mortality is higher in patients with invasive mucormycosis than in those with invasive aspergillosis.[60] Higher mortality is seen in diabetic patients with invasive fungal sinusitis due to *Mucor* being the causative organism more commonly than *Aspergillus* in these patients.[61] Patients with extensive disease such as those with orbital apex involvement and intracranial extension are less likely to respond to extensive surgical debridement and thus have a poorer prognosis.

Fungal sinusitis is more common than what was previously thought. Diagnosing invasive fungal disease requires a high index of clinical suspicion. Early diagnosis and treatment along with regular follow-up is the key to effective management of invasive fungal sinusitis.

REFERENCES

1. Plaignaud M. Observation sur un fungus du sinus maxillare. J Chir (Paris).1791;1:111-6.
2. Schubert P. Zur Casuistik der Aspergillusmykosen. Dtsch Arch Klin Med. 1885;36:162-79.
3. Oppe W. Zurr Kentnis der schimmelmykosen bei den Menschen. Zbl Allg Path. 1897;8:301-6.
4. Hora JS. Primary aspergillosis of the paranasal sinuses and other areas. Laryngoscope. 1965;75:768-73.
5. deShazo RD, O'Brien M, Chapin K, et al. A new classification and diagnostic criteria for invasive fungal sinusitis. Arch Otolaryngol Head Neck Surg. 1997;123(11):1181-8.
6. Epstein VA, Kern RC. Invasive fungal sinusitis and complications of rhinosinusitis. Otolaryngol Clin N Am. 2008;41:497-524.
7. Stringer SP, Ryan MW. Chronic invasive fungal rhinosinusitis. Otolaryngol Clin North Am. 2000;33(2):375-87.
8. Ferguson BJ. Definitions of fungal rhinosinusitis. Otolaryngol Clin North Am. 2000;33(2):227-35.
9. Gillespie MB, O'Malley BW. An algorithmic approach to the diagnosis and management of invasive fungal rhinosinusitis in the immunocompromised patient. Otolaryngol Clin North Am. 2000;33(2):323-34.
10. Sridhara SR, Paragache G, Panda NK, et al. Mucormycosis in immunocompetent individuals: an increasing trend. J Otolaryngol. 2005;34(6):402-6.
11. Sant K. Invasive Fungal Sinusitis: An Overview. Otolaryngol Clin. 2009;1(1):45-7.
12. deShazo RD. Fungal sinusitis. Am J Med Sci. 1998;316(1):39-45.
13. Mylona S, Tzavara V, Ntai S, et al. Chronic invasive sinus aspergillosis in an immunocompetent patient: a case report. Dentomaxillofac Radiol. 2007;36:102-04.
14. Scharf JL, Soliman AM. Chronic rhizopus invasive fungal rhinosinusitis in an immunocompetent host. Laryngoscope. 2004;114(9):1533-5.
15. Premamalini T, Ambujavalli BT, Anitha S, et al. "Schizophyllum commune a causative agent of fungal sinusitis: a case report," Case Reports in Infectious Diseases. 2011;2011:4. Article ID 821259, doi:10.1155/2011/821259
16. Ikram A, Hussain W, Satti ML, et al. Invasive infection in a young immunocompetent soldier caused by Scytalidium dimidiatum. J Coll Physicians Surg Pak. 2009;19(1):64-6.
17. Wong G, Nash R, Barai K, et al. Paecilomyces lilacinus causing debilitating sinusitis in an immunocompetent patient: a case report. J Med Case Rep. 2012;6:86
18. Abramson E, Wilson D, Arky RA. Rhinocerebral phycomycosis in association with diabetic ketoacidosis. Ann Int Med. 1967;66:735-42.
19. Lehrer RI, Howard DH, Sypherd PS, et al. Mucormycosis. Ann Intern Med 1980;93:93-108.
20. Idris N, Lim LH. Nasal eschar: a warning sign of potentially fatal invasive fungal sinusitis in immunocompromised children. J Pediatr Hematol Oncol. 2012;34(4):e134-6.
21. Park AH, Muntz HR, Smith ME, et al. Pediatric invasive fungal rhinosinusitis in immunocompromised children with cancer. Otolaryngol Head Neck Surg 2005;133(3):411-6.
22. Schell WA. Histopathology of fungal rhinosinusitis. Otolaryngol Clin North Am. 2000;33(2):251-76.
23. Kohn R, Helper R. Management of limited rhino-orbital mucormycosis without exenteration. Ophthalmology. 1985;92: 1440-4.
24. Lowe J, Bradley J. Cerebral and orbit *Aspergillus* infection due to invasive aspergillosis of the ethmoid sinus. J Clin Pathol.1986;39:774-8.
25. DelGaudio JM, Swain RE, Kingdom TT, et al. Computed tomographic findings in patients with invasive fungal sinusitis. Arch Otolaryngol Head Neck Surg 2003;129(2):236-40.
26. Gamba JL, Woodruff WW, Djang WT, et al. Craniofacial mucormycosis: assessment with CT. Radiology. 1986;160:207-12.
27. Dhong HJ, Lanza DC. Fungal Rhinosinusitis. In: Kennedy DW, Bolger WE, Zinreich JS, (Eds). Diseases of the Sinuses: Diagnosis and Management, Part 611. 1st edition. Canada: BC Decker; 2001. pp. 179-96.
28. Lehrer RI, Howard DH, Sypherd PS, et al. Mucormycosis. Ann Intern Med. 1980;93:93-108.
29. Francis P, Lee JW, Hoffman A, et al. Efficacy of unilamellar liposomal amphotericin B in treatment of pulmonary aspergillosis in persistently granulocytopenic rabbits: the potential role of bronchoalveolar lavage D-mannitol and galactomannan as markers of infection. J Infect Dis. 1994;169: 356-68.
30. Herbrecht R, Letscher-Bru V, Oprea C, et al. *Aspergillus galactomannan* detection in the diagnosis of invasive aspergillosis in cancer patients. J Clin Oncol. 2002;20:1898-906.
31. Maertens J, Verhaegen J, Lagrou K, et al. Screening for circulating galactomannan as a noninvasive diagnostic tool for invasive aspergillosis in prolonged neutropenic patients and stem cell transplantation recipients: a prospective validation. Blood. 2001;97:1604-10.
32. Marr KA, Balajee SA, McLaughlin L, et al. Detection of galactomannan antigenemia by enzyme immunoassay for the diagnosis of invasive aspergillosis: variables that affect performance. J Infect Dis. 2004;190:641-9.

33. Mennink-Kersten MA, Donnelly JP, Verweij PE. Detection of circulating galactomannan for the diagnosis and management of invasive aspergillosis. Lancet Infect Dis. 2004;4:349-57.

34. Mennink-Kersten MA, Verweij PE. Non-culture-based diagnostics for opportunistic fungi. Infect Dis Clin North Am. 2006;20:711-27.

35. Patterson T, Miniter P, Ryan J, et al. Effect of immunosuppression and amphotericin B on aspergillus antigenemia in an experimental model. J Infect Dis. 1988;158:415-22.

36. Stynen D, Goris A, Sarfati J, et al. A new sensitive sandwich enzyme-linked immunosorbent assay to detect galactofuran in patients with invasive aspergillosis. J Clin Microbiol. 1995;33:497-500.

37. Sulahian A, Tabouret M, Ribaud P, et al. Comparison of an enzyme immunoassay and latex agglutination test for detection of galactomannan in the diagnosis of aspergillosis. Eur J Clin Microbiol Infect Dis. 1996;15:139-45.

38. Boutboul F, Alberti C, Leblanc T, et al. Invasive aspergillosis in allogeneic stem cell transplant recipients: Increasing antigenemia is associated with progressive disease. Clin Infect Dis. 2002;34:939-43.

39. Anaissie EJ. Trial design for mold-active agents: time to break the mold—aspergillosis in neutropenic adults. Clin Infect Dis. 2007;44:1298-306.

40. Pickering JW, Sant HW, Bowles CA, et al. Evaluation of a (1->13)-beta-D-glucan assay for diagnosis of invasive fungal infections. J Clin Microbiol. 2005;43:5957-62.

41. White PL, Linton CJ, Perry MD, et al. The evolution and evaluation of a whole blood polymerase chain reaction assay for the detection of invasive aspergillosis in hematology patients in a routine clinical setting. Clin Infect Dis. 2006;42:479-86.

42. Lass-Florl C, Gunsilius E, Gastl G, et al. Clinical evaluation of *Aspergillus*-PCR for detection of invasive aspergillosis in immunosuppressed patients. Mycoses. 2005;48(Suppl 1):12-7.

43. Jones E, Goldman M. Lipid formulations of amphotericin B. Cleve Clin J Med. 1998;65(8):423-7.

44. Walsh TJ, Whitcomb P, Piscitelli S, et al. Safety, tolerance, and pharmacokinetics of amphotericin B lipid complex in children with hepatosplenic candidiasis. Antimicrob Agents Chemother. 1997;41(9):1944-8.

45. Walsh TJ, Goodman JL, Pappas P, et al. Safety, Tolerance, and Pharmacokinetics of High-Dose Liposomal Amphotericin B (AmBisome) in Patients Infected with *Aspergillus* Species and Other Filamentous Fungi: Maximum Tolerated Dose Study. Antimicrob Agents Chemother. 2001;45(12):3487-96.

46. Herbrecht R, Denning DW, Patterson TF, et al. Voriconazole versus amphotericin B for primary therapy of invasive aspergillosis. N Engl J Med. 2002;347(6):408-15.

47. Walsh TJ, Anaissie EJ, Denning DW, et al. Treatment of aspergillosis: clinical practice guidelines of the Infectious Diseases Society of America. Clin Infect Dis. 2008;46:327-60.

48. Alexander BD, Perfect JR, Daly JS, et al. Posaconazole as salvage therapy in patients with invasive fungal infections after solid organ transplant. Transplantation: 2008;86(6):791-6.

49. Mullane K, Toor AA, Kalnicky C, et al. Posaconazole salvage therapy allows successful allogeneic hematopoietic stem cell transplantation in patients with refractory invasive mold infections. Transpl Infect Dis. 2007;9(2):89-96.

50. Luna B, Drew RH, Perfect JR. Agents for treatment of invasive fungal infections. Otorhinolaryngol Clin of North Am. 2000;33:2:277-99.

51. Seiff SR, Choo PH, Carter SR. Role of local amphotericin B therapy for sino-orbital fungal infections. Ophthal Plast Reconstr Surg. 1999;15(1):28-31.

52. Kennedy CA, Adams GL, Neglia JP, et al. Impact of surgical treatment on paranasal fungal infections in bone marrow transplant patients. Otolaryngol Head Neck Surg. 1997;116(6 Pt 1):610-6.

53. Spellberg B, Ibrahim AS, Chin-Hong PV, et al. The Deferasirox-AmBisome Therapy for Mucormycosis (DEFEAT Mucor) study: a randomized, double-blinded, placebo-controlled trial. J Antimicrob Chemother. 2012;67(3):715-22.

54. Spellberg B, Andes D, Perez M, et al. Safety and outcomes of open-label deferasirox iron chelation therapy for mucormycosis. Antimicrob Agents Chemother. 2009;53(7):3122-5.

55. Kajs-Wyllie M. Hyperbaric oxygen therapy for rhinocerebral fungal infection. J Neurosci Nurs. 1995;27(3):174-81.

55a. Segal E, Menhusen MJ, Shawn S. Hyperbaric oxygen in the treatment of invasive fungal infections: a single-center experience. IMAJ. 2007;9:355-7.

56. Neuman TS, Thom SR (Eds). Physiology and rationale of hyperbaric oxygen therapy. Saunders Elsevier. 2008.

57. Carter KB, Loehrl TA, Poetker DM. Granulocyte transfusions in fulminant invasive fungal sinusitis. Am J Otolaryngol. 2012;33(6):663-6.

58. Sahin B, Paydaş S, Coşar E, et al. Role of granulocyte colony-stimulating factor in the treatment of mucormycosis. Eur J Clin Microbiol Infect Dis. 1996;15(11):866-9.

59. Gillespie MB, O'Malley BW, Francis HW. An approach to fulminant invasive fungal rhinosinusitis in the immuno-compromised host. Arch Otolaryngol Head Neck Surg. 1998;124(5):520-6.

60. Denning DW. Therapeutic outcome in invasive aspergillosis. Clin Infect Dis. 1996;23(3):608-15.

61. Parikh SL, Venkatraman G, DelGaudio JM. Invasive fungal sinusitis: a 15-year review from a single institution. Am J Rhinol. 2004;18(2):75-81.

CHAPTER 13

Instrumentation in Functional Endoscopy Sinus Surgery

Samir Bhargava

INTRODUCTION

The dramatic changes in treatment of sinusitis and nasal problems have been due to the tremendous leap in instrumentation. The single greatest advance in rhinology till date is probably the introduction of the rigid endoscope. The ability to access the nooks and corners of the ethmoidal labyrinth has been thanks to the sophisticated technology of endoscopes. Conventional instruments were grabbing and pulling instruments and resulted in denuding mucosa and subsequent scarring in the healing process. The need for precision surgery to not only tackle the problem, but also to deliver superior results led to development of instrumentation which enabled one to get there. As the endoscopist gained proficiency in dealing with sinonasal pathology, he embarked on accessing adjacent intracranial cavity and orbit pathology which necessitated the development of tools that ensured safe removal of significant amount of bone in a faster and controlled fashion. Quite often, technology drives new technique. The microdebrider was the first introduction of a powered sinus instrument. Several other powered tools like the endoscopic drill, coblator and ultrasonic aspirator have also been used in special circumstances, though like the microdebrider these may also one day become mainstay of the surgical arsenal.

OPERATION THEATER LAYOUT

The surgeon is seated or standing on the right side of the patient. The anesthesiologist is at the foot-end of the patient. The assistant and the scrub nurse stands on the left side of the patient along with the instrument trolley. An instrument trolley carrying the endoscopes and antifogging solution is positioned at the head end of the patient.

The video stack housing the monitor, the camera system, recording system and the xenon light source is stationed opposite the surgeon (Fig. 13.1). The height of the monitor should be just above the eye level of the surgeon. A second monitor is desirable for the assistant and scrub nurse.

A computerized tomography (CT) scan viewing screen must be present in the operating room so that the surgeon can inspect the CT scan before and during the procedure.

ENDOSCOPES

Harold Hopkins in the early 1950s developed the rod optic endoscope. 0° 4-mm endoscopes were the first to be manufactured. They enabled the endoscopist to do majority of work, but the nooks and corners of the maxillary sinus, the frontal recess or the lateral recess of the sphenoid needed a more angled telescope. Further development led to introduction of endoscopes with angled views ranging from 30°, 70°, 90° and 120°. A 30° telescope gives a wider view and is an excellent diagnostic tool permitting us to see a little more than the 0°. 45° or 70° is required when one wishes to operate inside the maxillary sinus or frontal recess with increased visibility (Figs 13.2A and B). Pediatric scopes of 2.7 mm may be required in very small children.

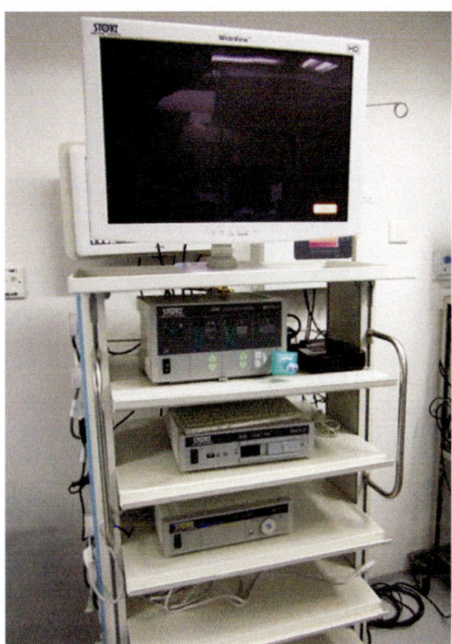

Fig. 13.1: Video stack with monitor, camera and recording system

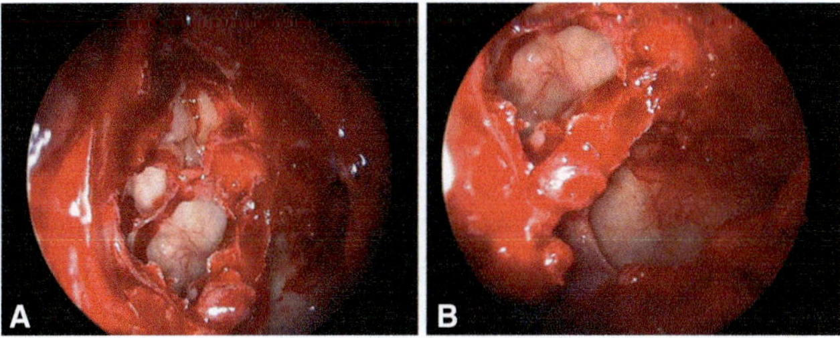

Figs 13.2A and B: Same view using 0° and 45° telescope showing increased visibility of maxillary sinus

Cyclops

This endoscope has been developed to avoid the need to repeatedly remove one endoscope and replace it with another to view certain specific areas with one endoscope. One can view from 10° to 90° without the need to withdraw the endoscope.

Traditionally the light cable attachment is 180° from the direction of the lens angle. Newer endoscopes have repositioned this attachment to 0° or 90° from the angle of view thereby enabling the surgeon more freedom in surgical field during introduction of instruments.

Some systems come with lens cleaning sheaths that help to provide the clearest view possible during surgery. The software automatically adjusts forward and reverse flows to clean the lens.

The scopes can be used with a handle holder which helps to stabilize the endoscope and provide better comfort while operating.

CAMERA

Most surgeons now operate viewing the monitor. Operating with the naked eye down the endoscope provides a good image but can result in the operator developing neck problems over a period of time. A beam splitter reduces the quality of the image. Hence, working off the monitor screen is recommended. The monitor should be positioned at a level just above the plane of the visual axis of the surgeon so that the surgeon can maintain a good posture and prevent long-term neck and back posture problems. A large-sized monitor with high resolution is preferred.

A good camera is now an essential part of the equipment. Single chip cameras were used for many years. But a three-chip camera provides a much better and more detailed image. Digital cameras have chips to process the color information. Single chip cameras process all color information together and hence they have limitation in contrast and balance. Three-chip cameras have chips to process each of the three primary colors, i.e. red, blue and green which enhances video quality. High definition camera improves the image quality and results in better attention to detail.

A halogen light source of at least 250 W is required. A xenon light source of 180 W or 300 W provides a better light particularly in the event of bleeding.

SUCTION TIPS

Straight-ended suction tip with fenestration and bent down the shaft are needed. Sizes needed are 2–4 mm. The suction can be used also to locate the sphenoid sinus adjacent to the septum and to make an opening into the ground lamella.

Curved olive-ended suction tips of different angles are needed (Figs 13.3A to C). The rounded ends can be used to probe the ostia or check if there is space behind partitions before these are removed. The curved right angle suction is used for the maxillary sinus. The obtuse suction, which is narrower, is used for the frontal recess. The curved suction allows suctioning of the contents inside the sinus. A malleable suction which can be bent can also be used to probe and suck the more lateral and deeper areas of the sinus.

SICKLE KNIFE

It is used to incise the uncinate process at its attachment to the frontal process of the maxilla (Figs 13.4A and B). One must ensure that there is sufficient space between the uncinate and the orbit before this incision is made. The movement of the knife is from above downward cutting through the two layers of mucosa anterior and posterior to the uncinate bone. The sickle knife can also be used to incise a concha bullosa as well as making an incision for the dacryocystorhinostomy (DCR) operation on the frontal process of maxilla.

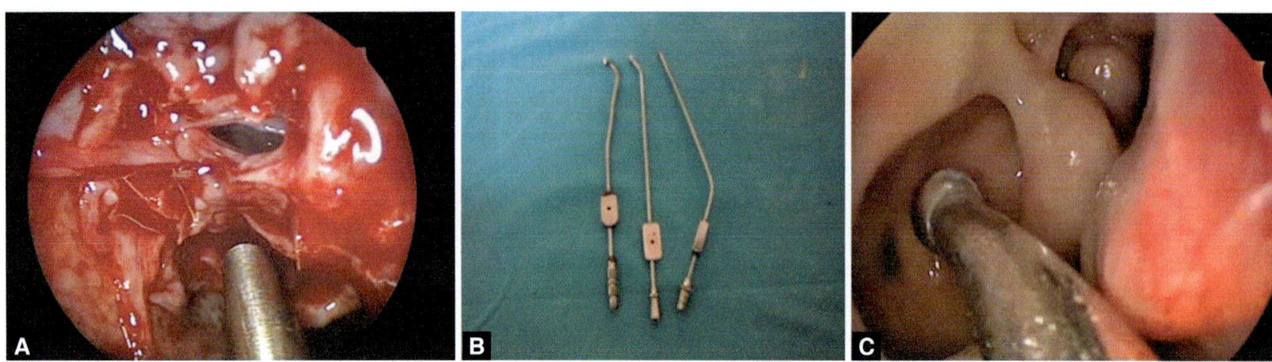

Figs 13.3A to C: Straight and curved olive tipped

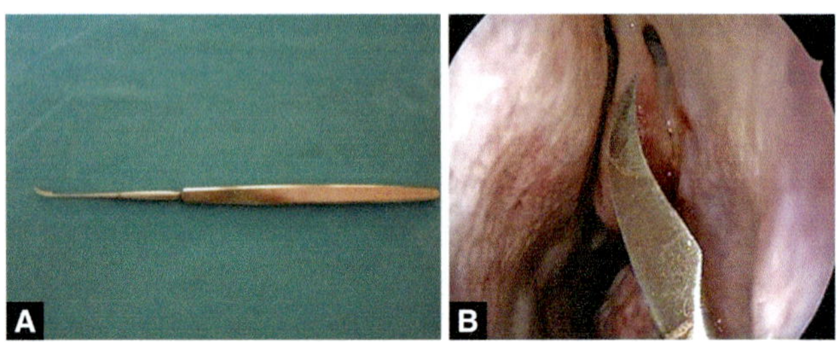

Figs 13.4A and B: Sickle knife

FREER ELEVATOR

This instrument is used for medializing or lateralizing the middle turbinate gently to visualize the structures beyond using the blunt midsection and not the end (Figs 13.5A to C). It is also used to elevate mucoperiosteum or mucoperichondrium while doing a septoplasty or DCR operation. The elevator can also be used to negotiate the sphenoid ostium by gently sliding it along the nasal septum. It can also be used to slide in the cotton patties to decongest the mucosa. Cottonoid strips or patties are made from soft roll cotton pads of size 3 × 1.5 cm with a black silk or white cotton thread about 12 inches long. These cottonoids are dipped in 4% xylocaine with adrenaline and are used for decongestion.

BALL PROBES

Ball probes can be used to probe the frontal recess (also called Kuhn probe) (Figs 13.6A and B). They can be used to dissect the mucosa off the uncinate process and off the agger nasi cell before the bone fragment is removed (submucosal dissection). They are also used to probe behind the septa to determine the level of the base skull before removing the ridges. Some ball probes have a reverse end which allows bony fragments to be retrieved that have been pushed inadvertently into the maxillary sinus or frontal recess.

CURETTES: STRAIGHT AND CURVED CURETTES

Curettes help in controlled removal of bone. Curettes are used to break partitions and separations in the frontal recess area and agger nasi cells (Figs 13.7A and B). The bulla ethmoidalis can also be curetted from behind forward so that its attachment to lamina papyracea is completely fractured and then can be removed with forceps. The straight curette can be used to open the ground lamella and to widen the opening before the curved curette is used to remove the cells upto the fovea ethmoidalis.

BLAKESLEY FORCEPS

It is used for removing polyps with bony septa, removing the uncinate process, making an opening on the bulla or ground lamella (Figs 13.8A to C). The forceps when removing polyps or mucosa do tend to tear resulting in exposure of bone and stripping of the mucosa. Hence its use should be combined with a microdebrider. The sharp tip of the forceps must be used carefully while close to the lamina papyracea or the skull base. While working close to the lamina, the side of the forceps must be used.

The upturned forceps can be used to judge the space behind the bony partitions near the skull base before removing the septa. The 90° forceps must be used carefully as the blade's end may not be completely in view while operating. But the forceps gives a tactile feedback which may be absent while using a microdebrider.

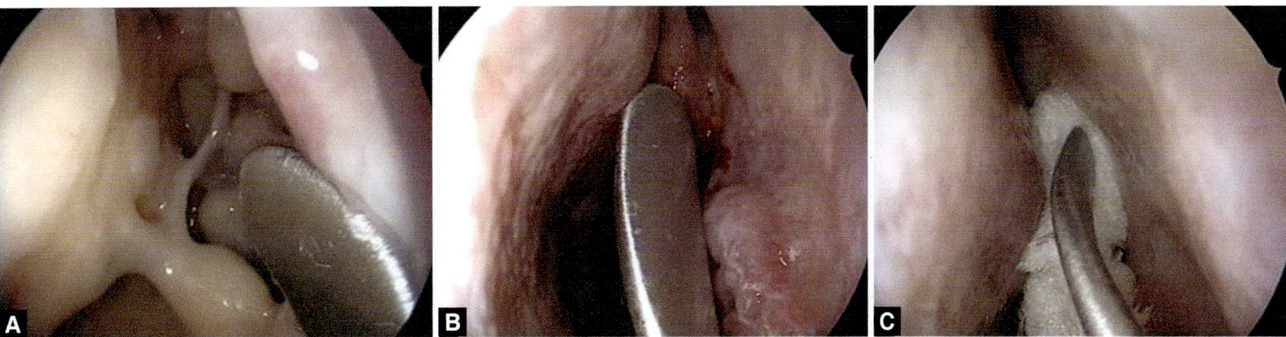

Figs 13.5A to C: Freer elevator

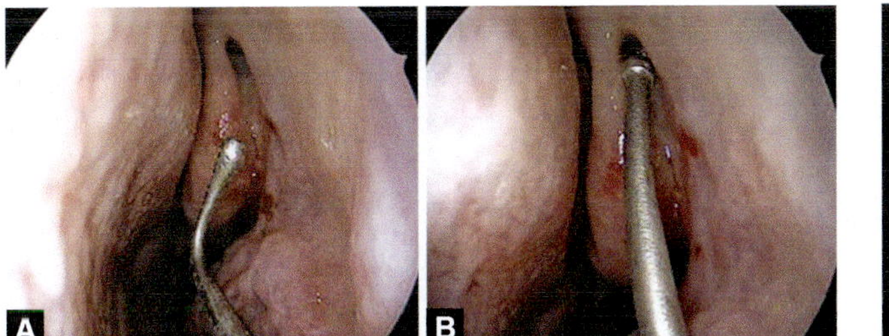

Figs 13.6A and B: Double-ended ball probe and curette

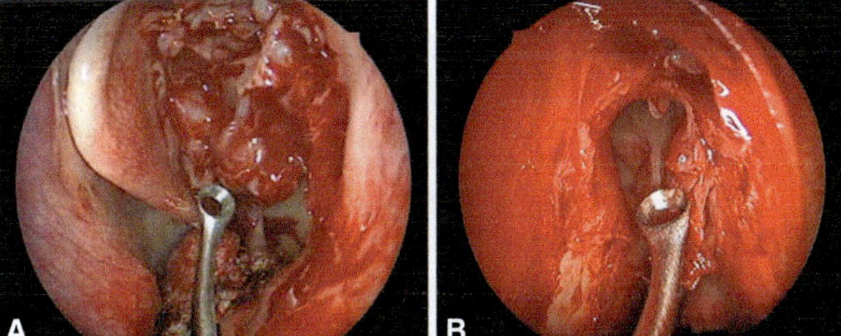

Figs 13.7A and B: Ring curette

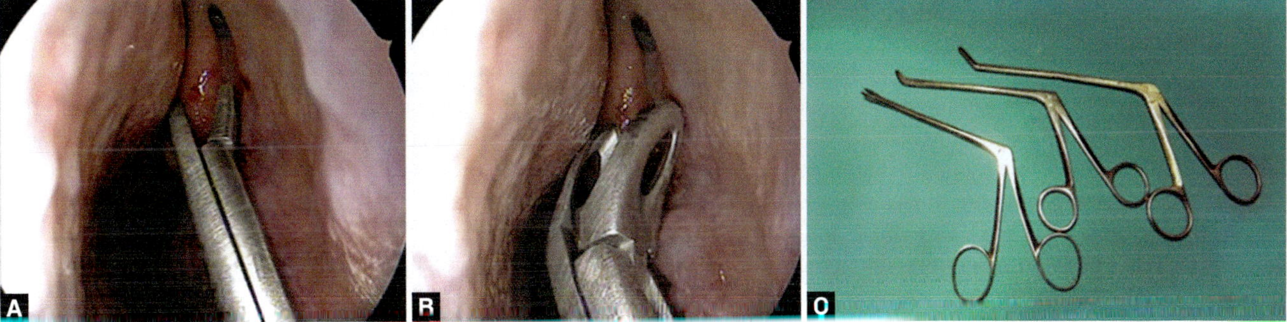

Figs 13.8A to C: Blakesley forceps straight and upturned

THROUGH-CUTTING INSTRUMENTS: RHINOFORCE BLAKESLEY

These are used for making precise cuts and removal of bony fragments and mucosa precisely (Figs 13.9A and B). They prevent tearing of mucosa unlike the traditional forceps avoiding unnecessary raw bone exposure. The removal of tissue is more controlled resulting in less trauma to mucosa and surrounding tissue with lesser bleeding and better healing. These forceps are also used by first gauging the space available behind the bony septa and then engaging the bone to make a precise cut. Through cutting instruments are available as straight and 45 upturned.

TOBEY REVERSE CUTTING FORCEPS AND STAMMBERGER ANTRUM PUNCH

Tobey forceps are used to make a small window into the intermediate part of the uncinate process before the uncinate

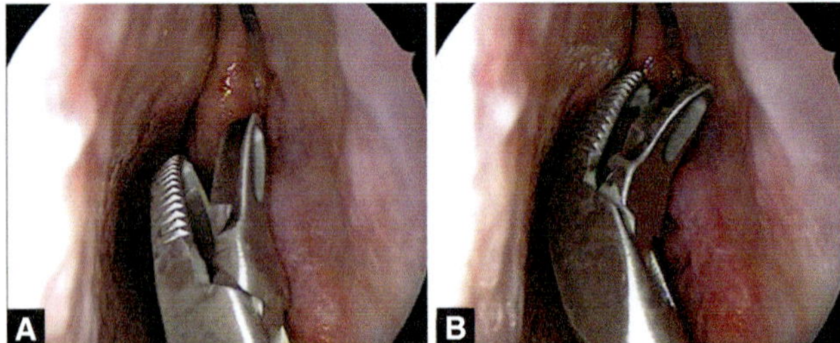

Figs 13.9A and B: Through cut forceps straight and upturned

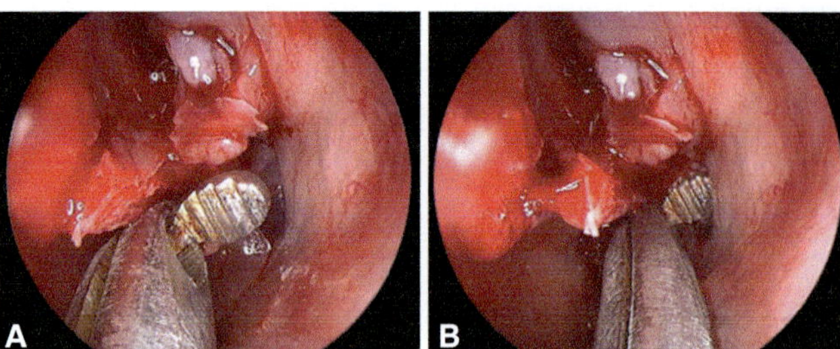

Figs 13.10A and B: Tobey reverse cutting forceps

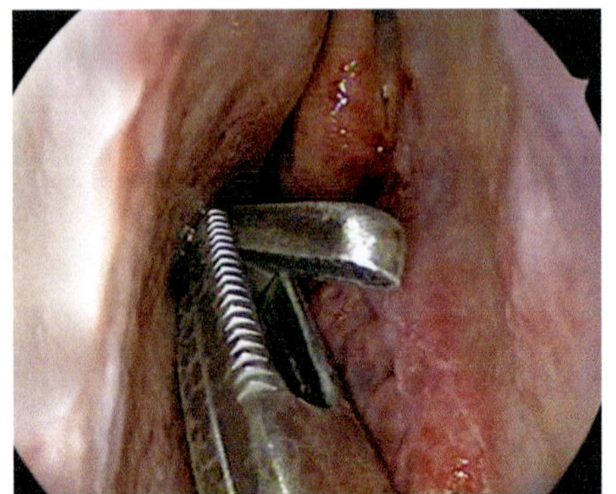

Fig. 13.11: Stammberger antrum punch

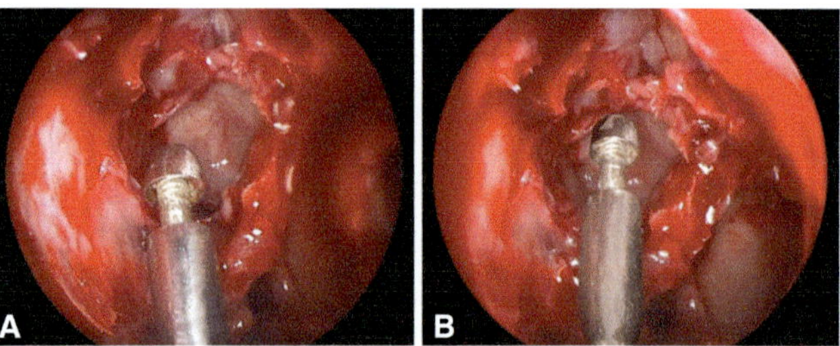

Figs 13.12A and B: Stammberger mushroom punch

process is removed using a punch or microdebrider (Figs 13.10A and B). The instrument is introduced in a closed position along the inferior turbinate and then opened to engage the junction of the vertical and horizontal portion of the uncinate process to back bite till one feels the attachment of the uncinate process. Separate "reverse cutting" punch is available for the left and right side.

The larger Stammberger antrum punch can also be used for the uncinectomy along with the widening of the maxillary ostium anteriorly (Fig. 13.11). One must stop short at tough bone so that the nasolacrimal duct is not at risk to be injured.

STAMMBERGER MUSHROOM PUNCH

It is used to safely widen the sphenoid ostium or frontal recess. The blunt top of the punch prevents any trauma to distal tissues. It can punch only small pieces as compared to the Hajek punch and hence several bites are required. The angled-mushroom punch is used for the frontal recess (Figs 13.12A and B).

KERRISON PUNCH

It is useful for removal of bone like in widening the sphenoid ostium or even removing the uncinate process, or agger nasi cells (Figs 13.13A and B). During an endonasal DCR frontal

process of maxilla or lacrimal crest can be removed using the punch. The punch can only remove bone that its leading beak can negotiate which makes it very safe.

BELLUCCI SCISSORS

These are used for cutting the tags of mucosa that are attached to uncinate process or concha so as to avoid tearing the mucosa. They are also used for widening the maxillary ostium posteriorly or making flaps in the lacrimal sac in a DCR (Figs 13.14A and B).

HEUWIESER ANTRUM GRASPING FORCEPS

These are used for grasping polyps or diseased mucosa from the floor of the maxillary sinus. The longer blade helps in reaching the depth of the floor and the sharp end prevents avulsion of polyps and exposing too much bone (Figs 13.15A and B).

GIRAFFE FORCEPS (KUHN)

These are angled forceps to remove small fragments of bone or polyps high up in the frontal recess. They are forward and

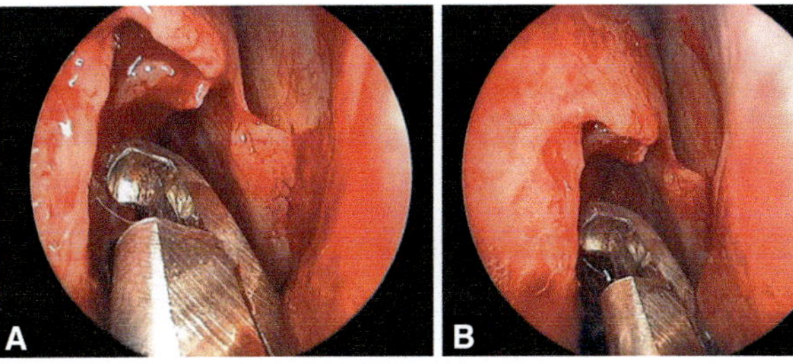

Figs 13.13A and B: Kerrison punch

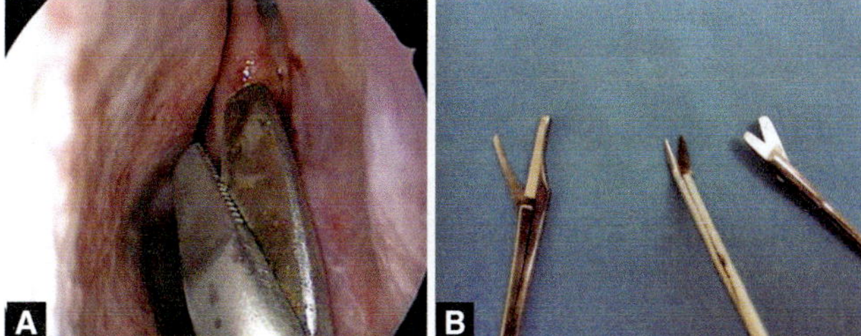

Figs 13.14A and B: Bellucci scissors

side grasping depending upon the positioning of the tissue that needs removal.

STAMMBERGER SIDE-BITING PUNCH FORCEPS

These are used to widen a middle meatal antrostomy inferiorly. Care must be taken not to bite through the base of the inferior turbinate which can sometimes result in bleeding from a branch of the sphenopalatine artery.

MICRODEBRIDER POWER SHAVERS

Setliff and Parsons in 1994 introduced the microdebrider in nasal surgery.

The microdebrider has been one of the premier innovations in instrumentation for endoscopic sinus surgery. The advantage of using the microdebrider includes improved precision, sparing adjacent mucosa and better visualization due to real time suction and quick tissue removal. This results in less bleeding, better tissue healing and less scarring and synechae (Figs 13.16A and B).

These are essentially two types:
1. Soft tissue shavers for removing polyps and redundant mucosa.
2. Bone cutting drills.

The microdebrider system consists of a cylinder with electrically powered shaver with continuous suction. There is an outer fixed cannula with a port on the side of the tip with an inner rotating or oscillating inner cannula. Soft tissue is sucked into the port and the trapped tissue is sheared off between the outer and inner cannulas. A dedicated suction machine is required for the microdebrider.

Microdebrider blades are available with various angulations besides the straight blade so as to gain better access. Some microdebriders are designed in such a way that the blade can be rotated on their axis so that the port is oriented toward the tissue. Some microdebriders allow a 360 up rotation facilitated by a wheel on the handpiece. Besides

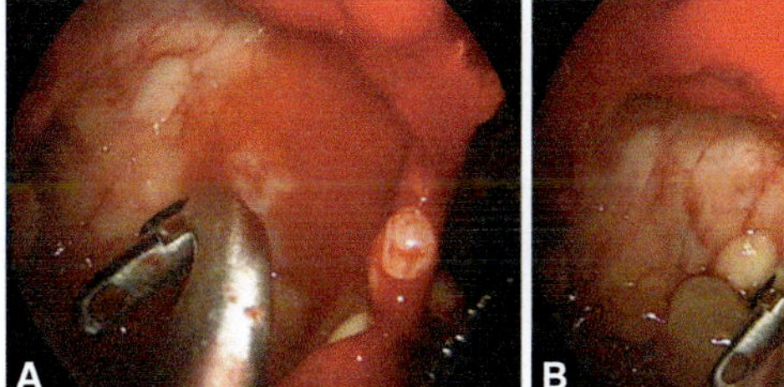

Figs 13.15A and B: Heuwieser antrum grasping forceps

the angulated blades, specialized blades for the submucous resection of the inferior turbinate and removal of adenoid tissue are also available. The microdebrider generally is able to remove the thin bony partitions but when the bone is tougher and thicker, drills enable the surgeon to do a more controlled and faster bone removal. The drill can be used for bone removal during DCR, drilling the maxillary crest, widening the sphenoidotomy laterally or resecting the floor of the frontal sinus and nasofrontal beak during modified Lothrop procedure. Endoscopic drills are slimmer than otologic drills and have a protective sheath with suction and irrigation function. The drills have a longer shank and long burrs which allow drilling without abrading the surrounding mucosa. The speed with which the drill takes down bone depends on the number of flutes on the burr. Lesser the flutes, faster is the bone removal. Diamond burrs are less aggressive than cutting burrs and are used to minimize risk of damage while close to delicate structures (Figs 13.17A to C).

The disadvantage of the microdebrider is that if a complication occurs it tends to progress faster because of the powered instrumentation and suction capability of the instrument. The other disadvantage is the recurring cost of the disposable blade besides the basic cost of the equipment.

NASAL PACKING

Removal nasal packing has been designed to tamponade mucosal bleeding, prevent lateralization of middle turbinate and prevent adhesion formation. Various packing materials

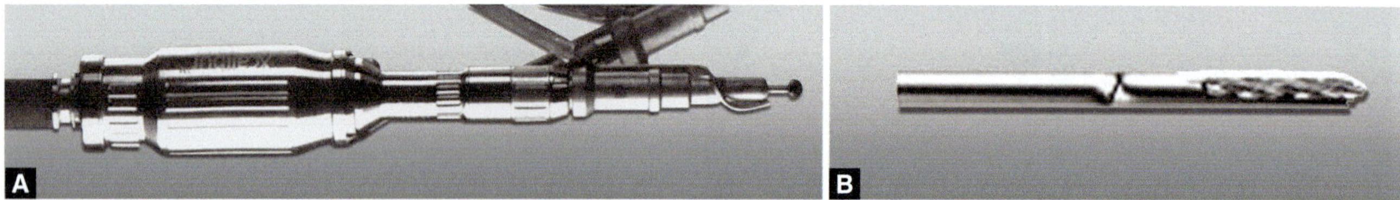

Figs 13.16A and B: (A) Microdebrider handpiece and (B) burr

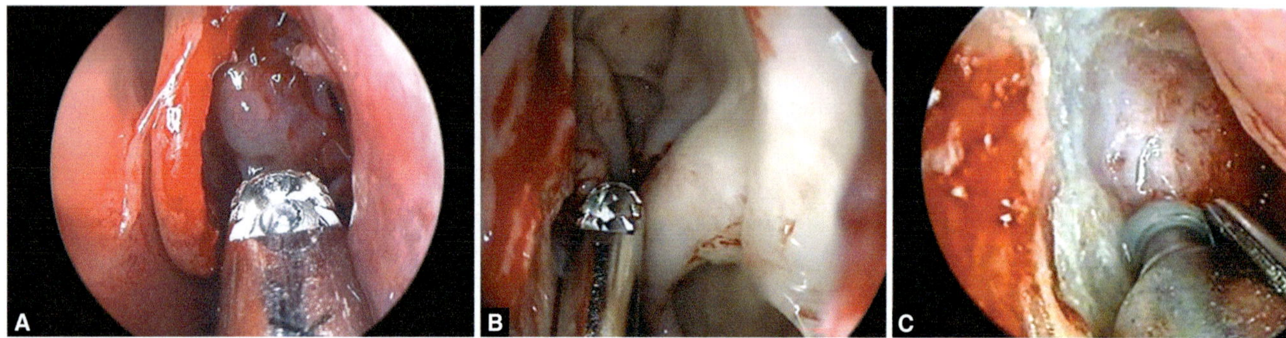

Figs 13.17A to C: Microdebrider blade and burr

like vaseline-soaked ribbon gauze, fingerstall packs, polyvinyl acetate sponge (Merocel) (Figs 13.18A and B) have been used.

Removal of the packs can be accompanied by significant pain and bleeding. Other complications include pack dislodgement, toxic shock syndrome and transient impairment of mucociliary clearance.

DISSOLVABLE NASAL PACKING

It can be used to absorb drainage, control minimal bleeding and prevent middle turbinate from lateralizing. They eliminate the need for packing removal, which can be quite painful. These contain hyaluronic acid to keep surgical site moist, reduce adhesions and decrease healing time after surgery.

SUCTION DIATHERMY

Unipolar Cautery

The insulated suction cautery helps in cauterization at the required site only. The suction channel helps in keeping the site free of blood and removal of smoke (Fig. 13.19A).

The unipolar suction is used for bleeding from the branches of the sphenopalatine artery. The unipolar cautery should not be used to coagulate the anterior ethmoidal artery for risk of tearing the dura and starting a cerebrospinal fluid (CSF) leak when the anterior ethmoidal artery exits the lateral lamella.

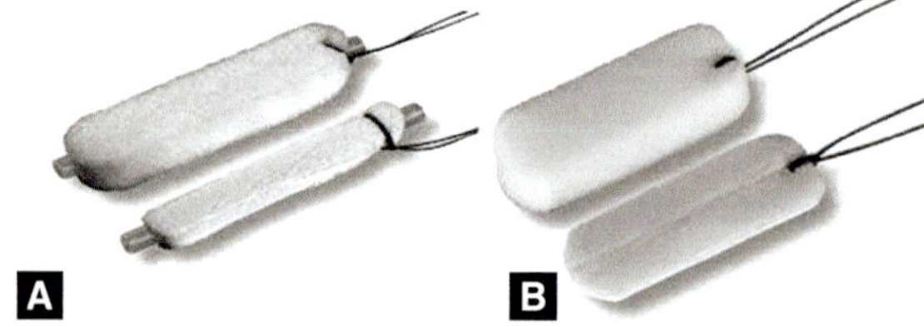

Figs 13.18A and B: Nasal packs with and without tubes

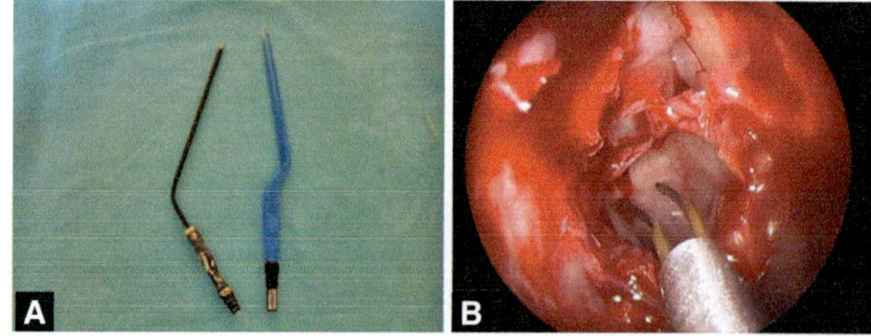

Figs 13.19A and B: Mono- and bipolar diathermy

Bipolar Suction Diathermy

It is used when cauterizing the anterior ethmoidal artery or in tumor surgery (Fig. 13.19B).

BALLOON CATHETER

Balloon catheter-based technology is a relatively new and novel tool to dilate sinus ostia in patients with chronic

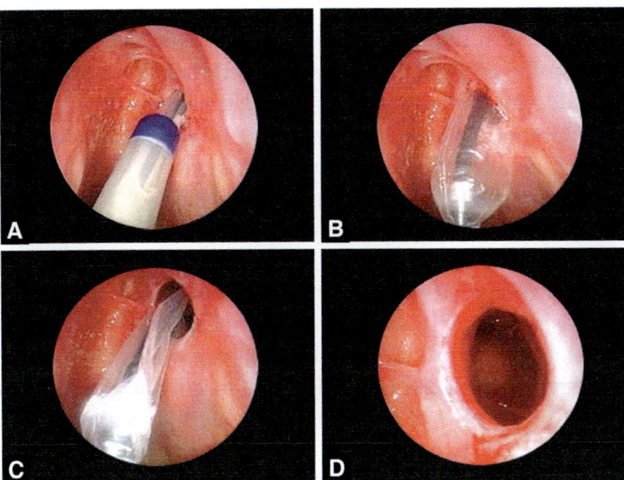

Figs 13.20A to D: Balloon dilatation—preoperative and postoperative

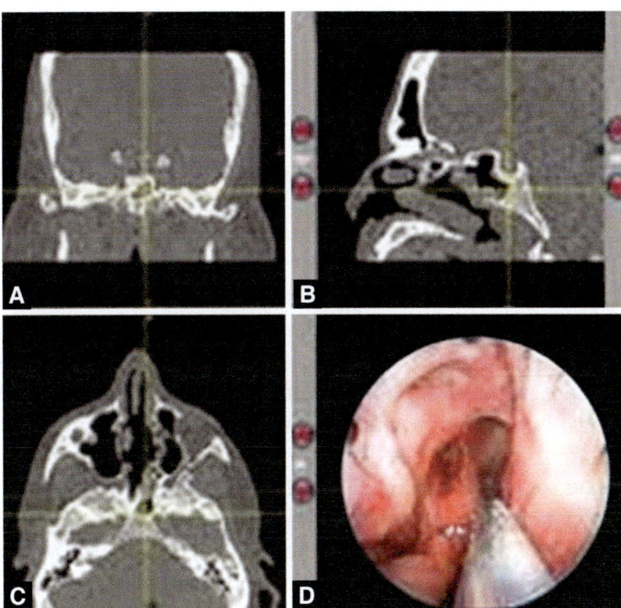

Figs 13.21A to D: Image-guided view on monitor

rhinosinusitis while preserving the mucosa and its surrounding structures (Figs 13.20A to D). The transnasal balloon catheter dilatation system that can be used during endoscopic sinus surgery for minimally invasive treatment of chronic sinus disease was introduced by Acclarent, Inc. in 2005.

The system has three components:

1. Guide catheter
2. Guidewire
3. Balloon catheter.

The sinus guide catheter which is either straight at the tip (for sphenoid sinus) or curved (for maxillary and frontal sinus) is a rigid translucent tube which is first introduced. Then a transillumination guidewire called Luma is threaded into the sinus. Previously, confirmation of entry into the sinus was performed by fluoroscopy. Though the radiation dose to patient and surgeon is extremely less during fluoroscopy use, transillumination completely avoids this risk.

Direct sinus illumination confirms the location of the guidewire.

A balloon catheter is then inserted over the guidewire into the sinus. The balloon is then inflated with air which results in fracture dilatation of the sinus ostia. Balloon catheters are designed for multiple sinus use in a single patient. The balloon dilatation can be performed on all sinuses viz. frontal, sphenoid and maxillary outflow tracts. The guidewire is then withdrawn. Irrigation catheter is then introduced and the sinuses are washed. The catheter guide is then withdrawn. In some patients, a hybrid procedure can be done which entails a traditional endoscopic ethmoidectomy in addition to balloon ostial dilatation.

Balloon dilatation has been shown to be a very safe procedure with negligible complication rate. In years to come, balloon dilatation may not replace conventional endoscopic sinus surgery in treatment of chronic sinusitis but will be a safe and effective tool in treating select patients. There are studies going on for use of temporary stents with drugs to be placed in the ethmoid sinus.

IMAGE-GUIDANCE SYSTEMS

Endoscopic surgery is mostly conducted viewing a two-dimensional magnified image. Whenever there is extensive disease, intraoperative bleeding or distorted anatomy, better visualization for safer surgery is desired. Surgical navigation technology is being used to determine the exact location of important and critical structures during an operation.

Navigation systems help to identify anatomical landmarks by tracking position of specialized instruments and projecting the instrument location onto patient specific CT (or MRI) image that has been acquired preoperatively and displaying that on the screen in all three anatomic planes (coronal, axial and sagittal planes) (Figs 13.21A to D). Image-guided sinus surgery helps to navigate each patient's unique anatomy to do safer surgery when operating near crucial structures like brain, orbit or carotid artery. Image-guidance systems are being used for revision surgery, for base skull and tumor surgeries, extensive polyposis or cases with distorted anatomy.

PROCEDURE

The CT (or MRI) scan is done preoperatively. The CT or MRI data is transferred to the computer in the operation room. Caliberation of the instruments is mandatory prior to the operation to verify the accuracy. The data from the preoperative axial CT scan is reformatted to reconstruct images in the coronal, sagittal and axial planes at the same time. The surgeon can view the CT projections and the endoscopic-navigated view simultaneously. The endoscopy picture can be viewed on a larger screen and the surgeon can refer to the CT projected view whenever required to confirm the position of the instrument.

Before starting the procedure, registration is performed. This process establishes the relationship between the previously obtained images and the system used to describe every point in the surgical field. Once this is done, the navigation system is ready for translating any point on the patient to the same point on the CT image. Three types of registrations are available: paired point, automatic and contour-based registration. Automatic registration requires a head set which has metal fiducials embedded to be worn by the patient at the time of the CT or MRI and during the surgery. In the paired point method the surgeon designates fiducial points on the patient and imaging data (generally 6–10).

Tracking the movement and location of the instrument in relation to the patient can be done by either of the two tracking systems, i.e. optical and electromagnetic-based systems.

The electromagnetic system utilizes a radiofrequency transmitter within the headset and a receiver which is positioned in the instruments. The headset has to be worn during the preoperative CT scan and during the operation. Metallic instruments within the field can distort or create interference. The optical system utilizes infrared light and a camera positioned above the patients head to track instruments. During the course of the surgery, the surgeon may need to confirm the accuracy of the image-guided system.

Image-guided surgery or surgical navigation can be of significant use in patients with advanced disease, distorted anatomy or unusual pathology. It can be considered in patients where the disease is close to critical structures as the orbit or base of the skull or in revision surgeries with significant disease. It is an excellent teaching tool for the trainee surgeon. Some systems allow customization for each surgeon including procedure-specific pathways for functional endoscopy sinus surgery and lateral or anterior skull base.

Use of surgical navigation technique increases the time duration of the surgery besides increasing the cost due to use of advanced instrumentation. Image-guided surgery though a useful tool in select cases is definitely not a substitute for thorough knowledge of anatomy, extensive surgical training and sound operative technique.

CHAPTER 14

Endoscopic Sinus Surgery in Orbital Lesions

Hetal Marfatia Patel

INTRODUCTION

The lesions of orbit were always dealt conventionally by team approach using the microscope. The ophthalmologists, otolaryngologists and neurosurgeons approached these lesions either by transconjunctival, transcranial, external ethmoidectomy or transantral approach.[1] With the advent of endoscopic sinus surgery and excellent illumination provided by it, the medial orbital lesions can be dealt endoscopically by experienced surgeon.

ENDOSCOPIC APPROACH

The endoscopic approach to the orbit may be attempted for resection or biopsy of the lesion. It gives excellent exposure to medial wall of the orbit, orbital apex and the optic canal.[1] While, the inferomedial wall of the orbit can be approached from the widened maxillary ostium. The procedure is done under general anesthesia. Adequate nasal decongestion is performed using patty soaked in 4% xylocaine adrenaline. Two percent lignocaine with adrenaline is infiltrated. Then uncinotomy is done, maxillary ostium is identified and widened. After that anterior and posterior ethmoid cells are cleared. Even sphenoid sinus is opened and widened. Thus complete sphenoethmoidectomy is performed. The medial wall of orbit, i.e. lamina papyracea is skeletonized. The orbit is deliberately entered with the help of a periosteum elevator (Fig. 14.1) The lamina papyracea should be entered below

the level of anterior ethmoidal artery.[2] If there is a need to go above that level then anterior ethmoidal artery must be cauterized with the bipolar cautery and cut to prevent retrobulbar hemorrhage and vision loss. Entire lamina papyracea is removed in the medial direction to prevent injury to the periorbita. The lesion in the medial extraconal region is exposed and dealt with.

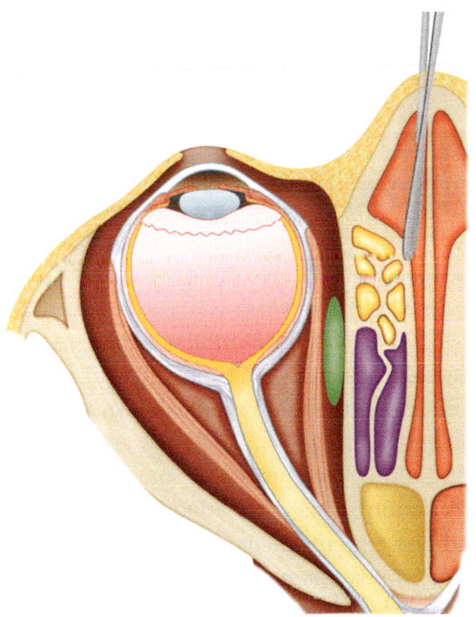

Fig. 14.1: Complete ethmoidectomy with deliberate opening of lamina papyracea

Use of endoscope for resection or biopsy of the lesions located on medial extraconal aspect of orbit and orbital apex is well accepted. However, resection of intraconal lesion is still limited by poor exposure, accessibility and instrumentation. Intraconal lesions of orbit are fairly uncommon and surgical treatment is challenging due to close proximity to intraocular muscles and optic nerve itself. Temporary medialization of the medial rectus muscle facilitates exposure to the orbital cone.[3] This is technically challenging and is done by applying transseptal sutures.[3] In case of intraconal lesions the dissection must be done between the muscles.[2] This technique can be done safely in selected cases only by the experienced hand.

Expanded endonasal four-handed approach may be done to address the lesion medial to optic nerve.

ORBITAL ABSCESS

Orbital complication of sinusitis results in orbital abscess. There is cellulitis and edema of the eye with proptosis. Nose is congested, inflamed and there is pus in the middle meatus. The orbital abscess is commonly secondary to ethmoidal sinusitis. The pus may enter the orbit through the congenital dehiscence in lamina papyracea or may go through the breach in lamina papyracea.[4,5] Figure 14.2 is showing diagrammatic representation of extraconal orbital abscess. Usually there is extraconal periorbital collection of pus which can be dealt endoscopically. Figure 14.3 is showing diagrammatic representation of orbital abscess being drained after the deliberate entry in the orbit following lamina papyracea removal.

The only challenge is bleeding due to acute inflammation, which demands surgical experience.

ORBITAL DECOMPRESSION OF GRAVES' ORBITOPATHY

The endoscopic orbital decompression was first described in 1990. It allows excellent visualization and decompression of medial wall of orbit up to orbital apex. It can be extended to inferomedial decompression too. Thyroid manifestations of Graves' disease are treated medically with steroids, low dose radiation and surgery.

During the procedure it is mandatory to widen the maxillary ostium. This gives adequate access to the floor of orbit and prevents maxillary sinus blockage from prolapsed orbital fat. Care is taken to prevent bone removal superiorly in the region of frontonasal recess. The periosteum may be incised using a sickle knife, or no. 11 blade or no. 12 blade. Care should be taken to prevent burying the tip of the knife

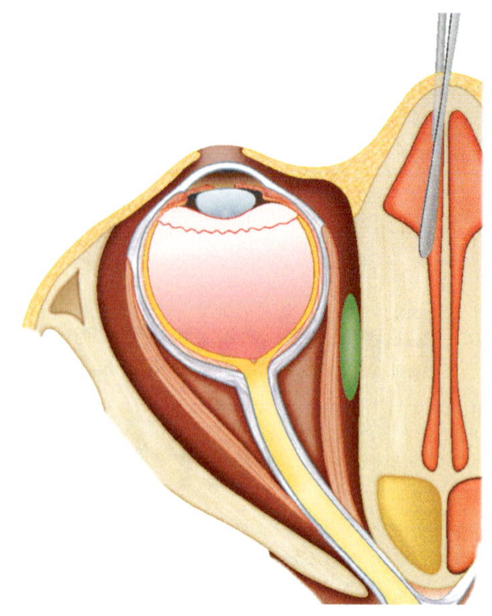

Fig. 14.2: Diagrammatic representation of extraconal orbital abscess

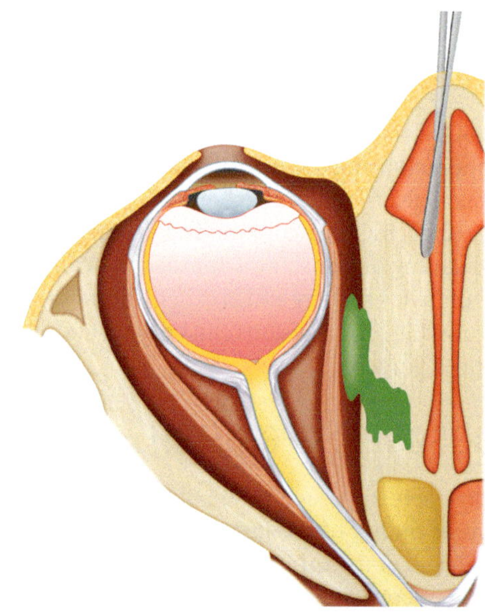

Fig. 14.3: Orbital abscess being drained after the deliberate entry in the orbit following removal of lamina papyracea

for which Steri-Strip may be used 2 mm proximal to the tip as a marker.[6] This prevents the injury to underlying structure especially the medial rectus muscle. Parallel incision is taken along the roof of ethmoid and floor of orbit in the postero-anterior direction so that the prolapsed fat does not obscure the vision. A sling of fascia overlying the medial rectus muscle is preserved to decrease the incidence of diplopia.[7]

As far as possible the medical line of treatment is preferred. The cases do not respond to long term steroid therapy and show vision deterioration, and those with exposure keratitis are the main indications. The orbital decompression may result in increase in lid retraction and exacerbates diplopia for which strabismus correcting surgery may be required.

ORBITAL HEMATOMA

It can occur following blunt trauma to the orbit. This may present as black eye with proptosis and painful ocular movement.

The connective tissue of peripheral nervous system may show fluid level in the orbit (Fig. 14.4).

If the hematoma is small, it may get absorbed. But if it is causing proptosis and visual disturbance then the orbit should be decompressed.

After complete sphenoethmoidectomy, lamina papyracea is entered and medial orbital wall is decompressed right up to the orbital apex and hematoma is drained. Figure 14.5 shows right eye proptosis in a child following a cricket ball injury and Figure 14.6 shows postoperative result.

Iatrogenic Orbital Hematoma

It may occur during endoscopic sinus surgery, by accidental breach of lamina papyracea or due to retraction of the anterior ethmoid artery. This retracted artery may bleed within the orbit causing periorbital, intraorbital or retrorbital hematoma.[8] The latter can cause optic nerve compression and vision loss. Within no time there is proptosis, black eye, conjunctival edema and restriction of eye ball movement. The most important is to assess the vision of the patient. If the vision is deteriorating immediate intervention in the form of lateral canthotomy should be done, the orbital septum should be detached to relieve the pressure on the optic nerve. This relieves pressure on the optic nerve and gives some time to arrange for the orbital decompression. Meanwhile, intranasal pack must be removed and gentle massage on the eyeball may be given to prevent the organization of the hematoma. This massage may allow the blood to come out of the orbit through breech in the lamina papyracea[8] (Fig. 14.7).

BLOW OUT FRACTURE OF THE ORBIT

It involves the inferior wall of the orbit and can result in entrapment of the inferior rectus muscle. This can cause restriction of the ocular movement and forced duction test may be positive. Patient may present with periorbital ecchymoses and subconjunctival hemorrhage. On CT scan

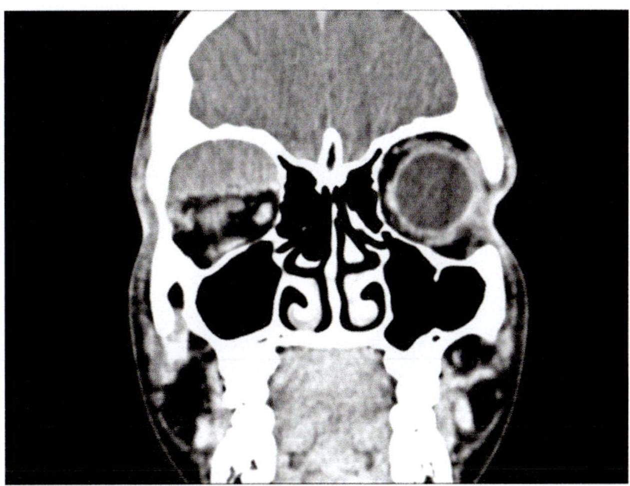

Fig. 14.4: Orbital hematoma—preoperative CT

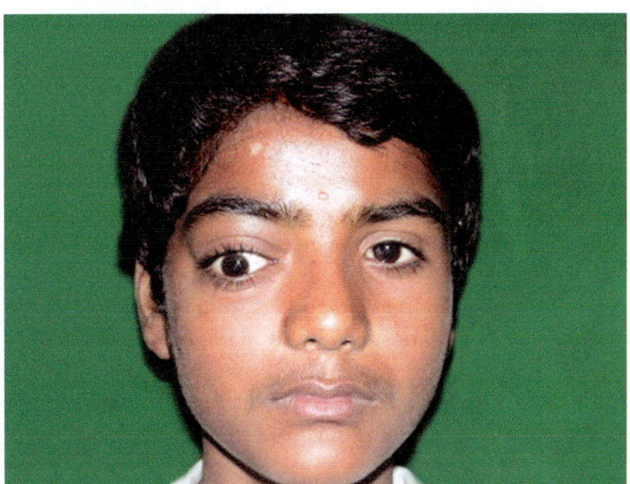

Fig. 14.5: Orbital hematoma

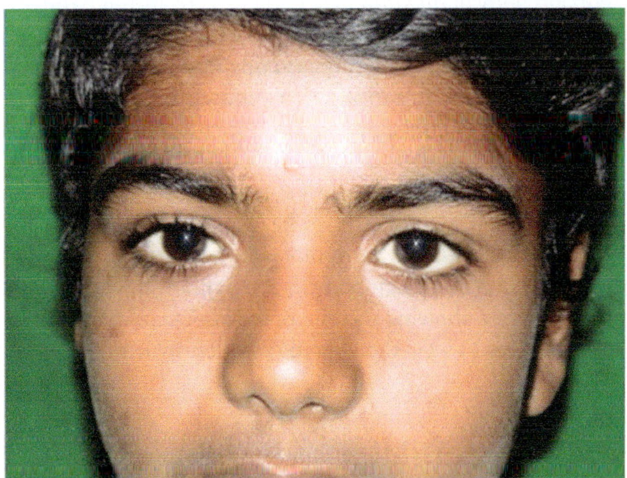

Fig. 14.6: Orbital hematoma—postoperative

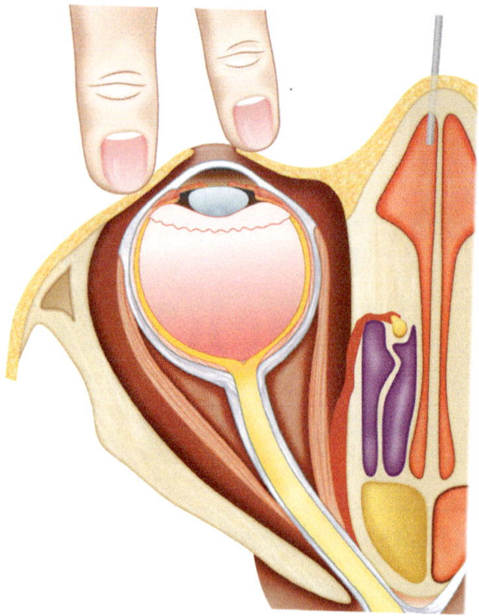

Fig. 14.7: Orbital massage

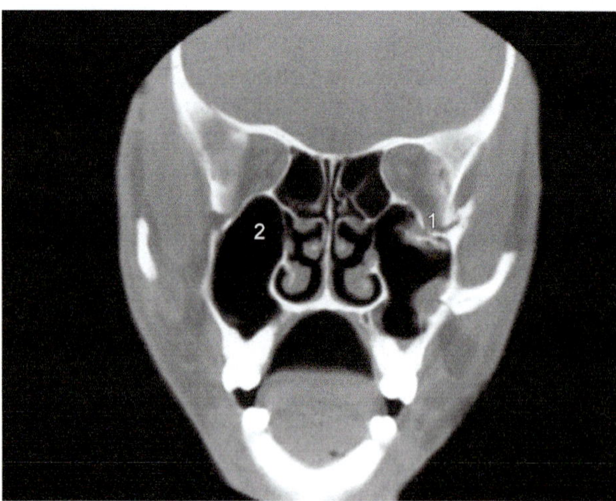

Fig. 14.8: Fracture of floor of left orbit. [1–Fracture of left infra-orbital wall with tear drop sign; 2–Normal right maxillary sinus for the comparison]

one can see fracture of the floor of orbit and there may be tear drop sign. Figure 14.8 is showing fracture of floor of the orbit. The infra orbital fracture can be approached through widened maxillary ostium. The fracture is reduced and entrapped muscle is released. Bony fragments from the fracture site are removed. Orbital floor may be supported by Foleys catheter inflated with air or water, which may be kept in place for 2 weeks. If there is a large segment then transconjunctival silastic sheet may be introduced to prevent exophthalmos.[9]

FOREIGN BODY OF THE ORBIT

Foreign body of the orbit may enter directly through the orbit or indirectly from the surrounding structures, e.g. skin or the paranasal sinuses if the foreign body is stipulated in medial part then it is feasible to access it endoscopically.

After adequate preparation, uncinectomy was done then anterior and posterior ethmoidal cells were cleared. Following complete sphenoethmoidectomy, foreign body was identified. Medial orbital wall was removed. Foreign body was removed gently. Figure 14.9 is showing congestion of the right eye due to foreign body in the right orbit, Figures 14.10 and 14.11 are showing CT scan of the foreign body of the right orbit. Figure 14.12 is showing the wooden stick removed from orbit.

ORBITAL TUMOR

Endoscopic approach to tumors of the orbit is used for tumor resection or biopsy; medially or inferomedially situated

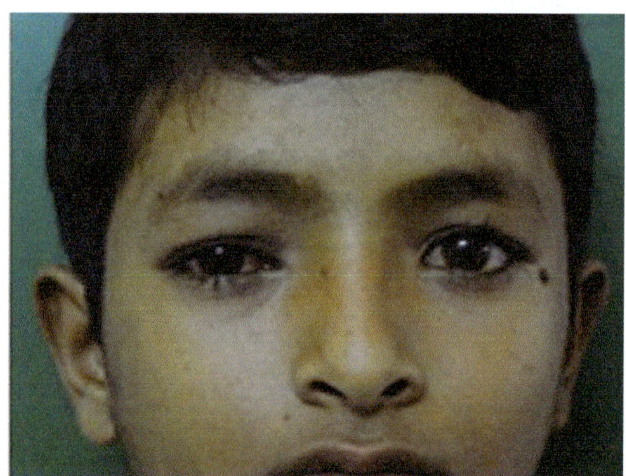

Fig. 14.9: Congestion of the right eye due to foreign body in the right orbit

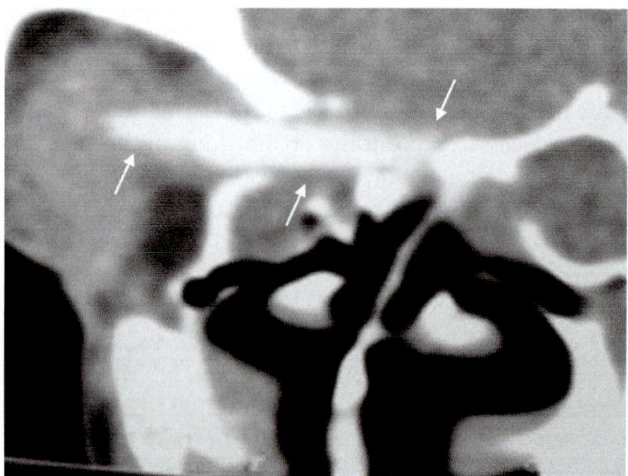

Fig. 14.10: Foreign body right orbit: wooden stick

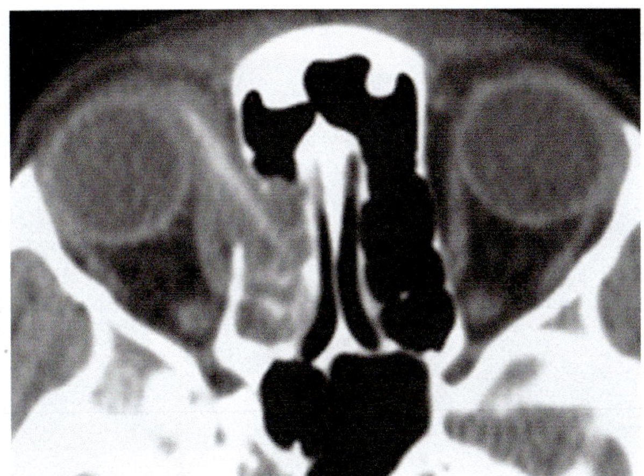

Fig. 14.11: Foreign body right orbit: wooden stick (axial cut)

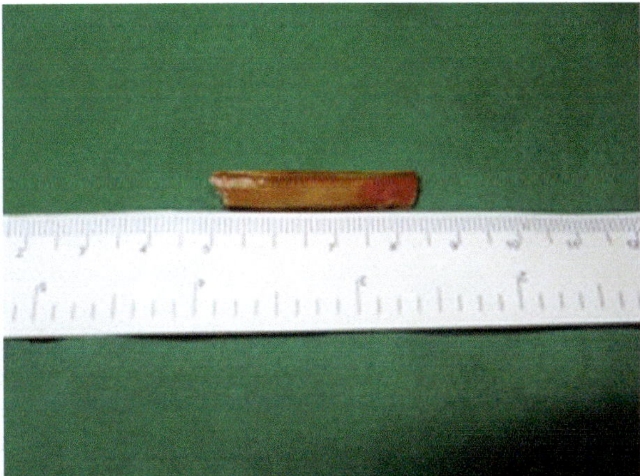

Fig. 14.12: Foreign body right orbit: wooden stick (coronal)

tumors are amenable to resection. Same principle is used to approach the tumor. After complete sphenoethmoidectomy, lamina papyracea is removed. Orbital periosteum is incised and blunt instrument, viz. ball point is used to dissect the tumor all around. External counter pressure is applied to the orbit to facilitate the dissection. If the need arises then extraocular muscles can be identified with the help of ophthalmologists by passing a sling through the muscle and giving a small pull.[2,9] Figures 14.13 and 14.14 (CT coronal and sagittal sections) are showing the orbital hemangioma.

ENDOSCOPIC ASSISTED ORBITAL LESION

Intraconal lesion can be dealt by combined approach, e.g. endoscopic assisted external ethmoidectomy approach. This can be done using a Lynch Howarth incision. The orbit is exposed and periorbita is incised to approach the intraconal pathology. Here, the endoscope allows excellent visualization within the orbit and avoids excessive manipulation and retraction there by preventing injury to muscles and optic nerve.

Figure 14.15 shows a 4-year-old child with air gun pellet in the left orbit. This was approached through Lynch Howarth's approach. Endoscope was used for excellent illumination and documentation and with the help of magnet we tried lifting the pellet however since it was not magnetic we had to use artery forceps to lift the pellet without much manipulation to prevent pressure on the optic nerve. The air gun pellet (Fig. 14.16) was removed successfully and the vision was preserved.

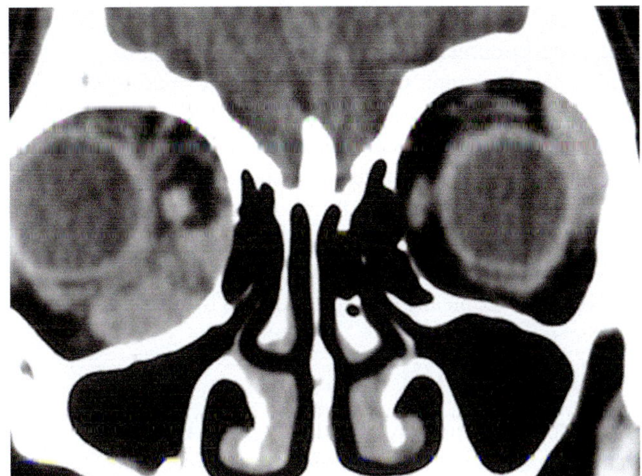

Fig. 14.13: CT coronal section showing the orbital hemangioma

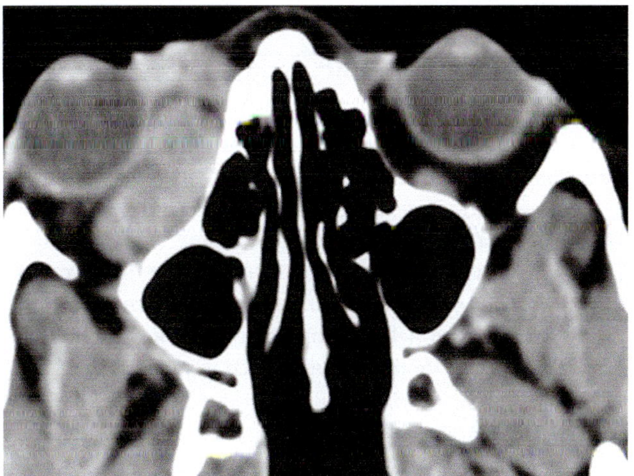

Fig. 14.14: Axial CT scan showing the orbital hemangioma

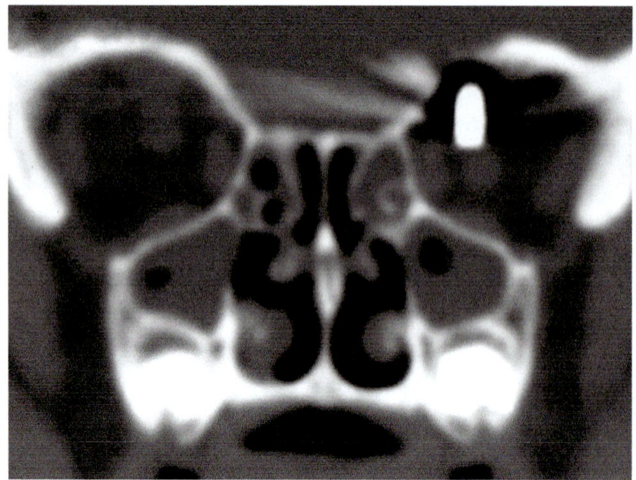

Fig. 14.15: Bullet in the left orbit

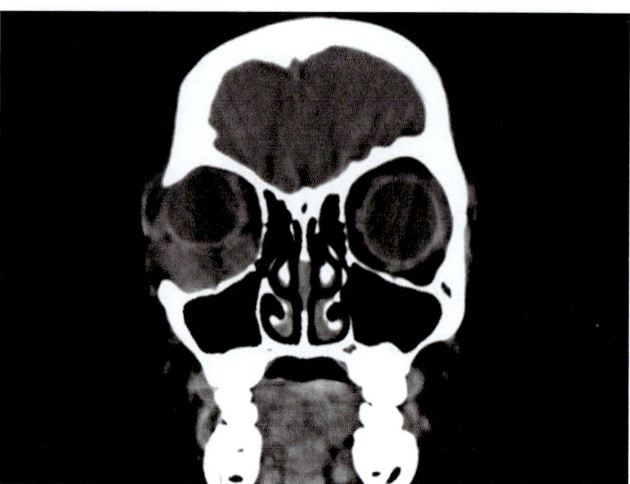

Fig. 14.17: Coronal CT of the right orbital mass occupying inferior half of the orbit

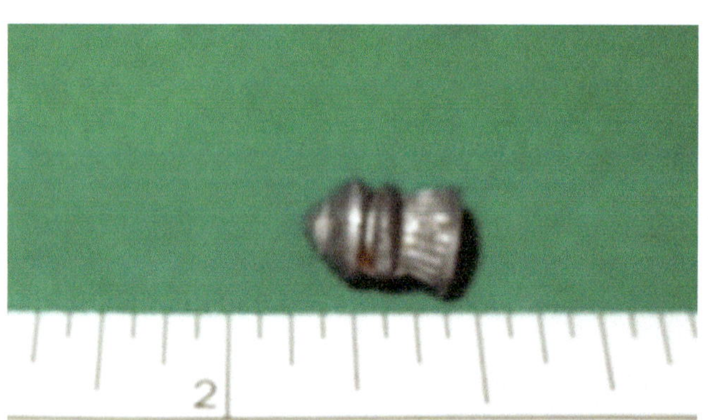

Fig. 14.16: Bullet from the left orbit

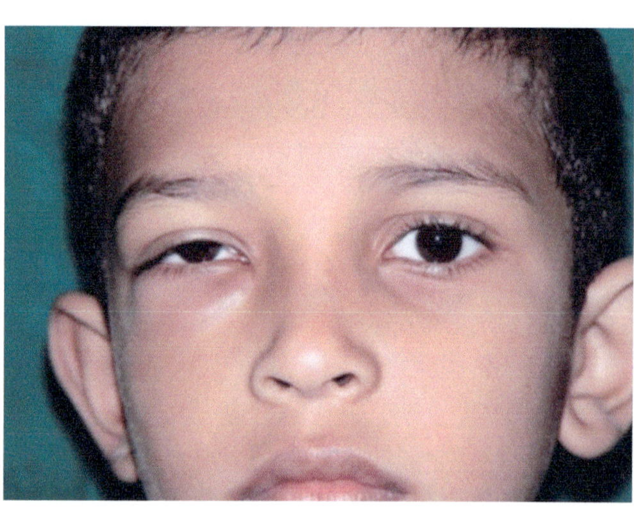

Fig. 14.18: Right orbital mass occupying inferior half of the orbit

TIPS AND PEARLS

- All patients must be thoroughly examined by ophthalmologists for the acuity of vision and field of vision.
- Computed tomography scan and MRI must be done to know exact size, shape extent and relation to the extra-ocular muscles and optic nerve.
- For all cases ophthalmologists should be involved as at times they can pass a stitch through the muscle and giving a gentle tag to help identify the muscle intra-operatively. It is also safe for medicolegal purpose.

LIMITATIONS

If one draws an imaginary line passing through the pupil then only those lesions lying medial to that line can be dealt endoscopically the most favorable being the lesions in inferomedial quadrant and others may require combined approach. At no point of time the optic nerve should be crossed and hence, suprolateral and infrolateral lesions cannot be addressed endoscopically.

Figures 14.17 and 14.18 have tumor extending lateral to imaginary line passing through pupil, shows limitation that was not amenable to resection and only biopsy, which was taken endoscopically through widened ostium.

CONCLUSION

Endoscopic approach to orbit is safe and effective. It is cosmetically superior as there is no scarring. It is very precise and being minimally invasive there is less morbidity. The excellent illumination and magnification obtained by the endoscope allows meticulous surgery within the narrow space of the orbit. The approach to intraconal orbital lesion is challenging but it is safe in appropriately selected cases by experienced surgeon.

REFERENCES

1. Cebula H, Lahlou A, De Battista JC. Endoscopic approaches to the orbit. Neurochirurgie. 2010;56(2-3):230-5.
2. McKinney KA, Snyderman CH, Carrau RL, et al. Seeing the light: Endoscopic endonasal intraconal orbital tumor surgery. Otolaryngol Head Neck Surg. 2010;143(5):699-701.
3. Tomazic PV, Stammberger H, Habermann W, et al. Intraoperative medialization of medial rectus muscle as a new endoscopic technique for approaching intraconal lesions. Am J Rhinol Allergy. 2011;25(5):363-7.
4. Page EL, Wiatrak BJ. Endoscopic versus external drainage of orbital subperiosteal abscess. Arch Otolaryngol Head Neck Surg. 1996;122(7):737-40.
5. Wormald PJ. Endoscopic orbital decompression for exopthalmos, acute orbital hemorrhage and orbital subperiosteal abscess. In: Wormald PJ (Ed.) Endoscopic sinus surgery: Anatomy, three-dimensional reconstruction and surgical technique. Stuttgart: Thieme Medical Publishes, Inc; 1996.pp.135-40.
6. Pletcher SD, Sindwani R, Metson R. Endoscopic Orbital and Optic Nerve Decompression. Otolaryngol Clin North Am. 2006; 39(5):943-58.
7. Metson R, Samaha M. Reduction of diplopia following endoscopic orbital decompression: the orbital sling technique. Laryngoscope. 2002;112:1753-7.
8. Sharma S, Wilcsek GA, Francis IC, et al. Management of acute surgical orbital haemorrhage: an otorhinolaryngological and ophthalmological perspective. J Laryngol Otol. 2000;114(8): 621-6.
9. Ikeda K, Suzuki H, Oshima T, et al. Endoscopic endonasal repair of orbital floor fracture. Arch Otolaryngology Head Neck Surg. 1999;125:59-63.

CHAPTER 15

Endoscopic Decompression for Post-traumatic Optic Neuropathy

Milind V Kirtane, Roshni Nambiar

INTRODUCTION

Historically, surgical decompression of the optic nerve has been one of the main treatments advocated for traumatic optic neuropathy.[1-3] In recent years, the definitive role of surgery in these patients has been questioned.[4,5] However, traumatic nerve injury still remains one of the most frequent indications for optic nerve decompression (OND).[1] Endonasal endoscopic decompression of the optic nerve offers many advantages including excellent visualization, preservation of olfaction, rapid recovery time, lack of external scars, and less operative stress in patients who may have multisystem trauma.[1,6-8]

HISTORICAL ASPECTS

Hippocrates noted the association of trauma just above the eyebrow with gradual vision loss. In 1879, Berlin described the first pathologic examination of the optic nerve after head trauma. In 1890, Battle first distinguished penetrating direct optic nerve injuries from nonpenetrating indirect injuries. The 20th century saw significant progress in defining the classification, pathophysiology, and management of traumatic optic nerve injuries.[9]

Traditional surgical approaches for OND include transorbital, extranasal transethmoidal, transantral, intranasal microscopic, and craniotomy approaches.[2]

In the early 1900s, transcranial unroofing of the optic canal was the surgical procedure of choice for traumatic optic neuropathy treatment. This procedure was used sparingly because of the inherent risks of intracranial surgery.[9]

In the 1920s, Sewell performed a transethmoidal optic canal decompression by removing the lamina papyracea and medial wall of the optic canal. This technique was refined by progressive advances in transnasal, transantral, transorbital, and external paranasal sinus surgery. However, the surgery was not performed routinely until the 1960s in Japan and the 1980s in the United States.[9]

With advances in technology and endoscopic surgery, surgical techniques for management of traumatic optic neuropathy have undergone a change over a period of time.

Currently, endonasal endoscopic OND via an intranasal and transethmoidal or transsphenoidal approach is the preferred surgical approach in traumatic optic neuropathy.[1,3,4,9]

SURGICAL ANATOMY

The course of the optic nerve may be divided into three segments:
1. Intraorbital
2. Intracanalicular
3. Intracranial

The orbital portion of the optic nerve is about 20–30 mm in length with a slightly sinuous course to allow for movements of the eyeball.[10] Several authors have divided this portion of the optic nerve into an intraocular segment measuring about 1 mm and an intraorbital segment separately.[11,12]

As the nerve enters the optic canal, its dural sheath becomes continuous with that lining the orbit and the optic foramen. In the optic foramen, the ophthalmic artery usually lies below and lateral to the nerve. This segment of the optic nerve measures about 10 mm in length. Traumatic optic neuropathy mainly involves this intracanalicular segment.[12]

The intracranial portion of the optic nerve is about 10–14 mm in length.[10]

The goal of OND is to relieve compressive forces within the intracanalicular portion of the optic nerve.[1]

PATHOPHYSIOLOGY

Traumatic optic neuropathy can be classified as direct or indirect, based on the type of nerve injury.

- Direct traumatic optic neuropathy refers to injuries where the optic nerve is crushed, impinged or transected. This is usually seen with extensive craniofacial trauma, associated with penetrating injuries, or extensive crush injuries with displaced cranio-orbital fractures.
- Indirect traumatic optic neuropathy occurs in the absence of direct nerve injury. It is believed that compression forces from the site of trauma are transferred via the orbital bones to the orbital apex and optic canal. Contusion of the intracanalicular optic nerve axons and pial microvasculature produces localized optic nerve ischemia and edema. The edematous ischemic axons result in further neural compression within the fixed-diameter bony optic canal, precipitate a positive feedback loop, and trigger the development of an intracanalicular compartment syndrome.[2,9]

Medical or surgical intervention or a combination of both may be indicated in the management of a patient with traumatic optic neuropathy. In the Cochrane database of systematic reviews, no randomized controlled trials were identified for either the use of corticosteroids or surgical treatment for traumatic optic neuropathy.[13,14] Currently, there is no absolute indication for surgical intervention, which has been validated by controlled outcome studies. Hence the decision to proceed with surgery or high-dose corticosteroids depends on the clinical judgment and surgical skills of the surgeon, as well as informed consent of the patient to appreciate the benefits and risks of both treatments.[13,14] Patients with traumatic optic neuropathy may also present with non-ocular comorbidities such as closed head injury or multi-organ trauma. The evaluation and treatment of traumatic optic neuropathy begins after all life-threatening injuries have been stabilized and basic lifesaving protocols have been fulfilled.[9]

PREOPERATIVE WORK-UP

The diagnosis of traumatic optic neuropathy is mainly clinical. Although most patients will present with obvious craniofacial or neurosurgical comorbidities, some may show minimal or no external sign of injury. The typical site of injury is the lateral frontotemporal region (Figs 15.1A and B).[15]

OPHTHALMIC EXAMINATION

A comprehensive ophthalmic examination is necessary in all patients in whom traumatic optic neuropathy is suspected and should include the following assessments:

- *Examination of the orbital adnexa:* To look for signs of orbital fractures, extraocular muscle dysfunction, orbital edema, enophthalmos, or proptosis.

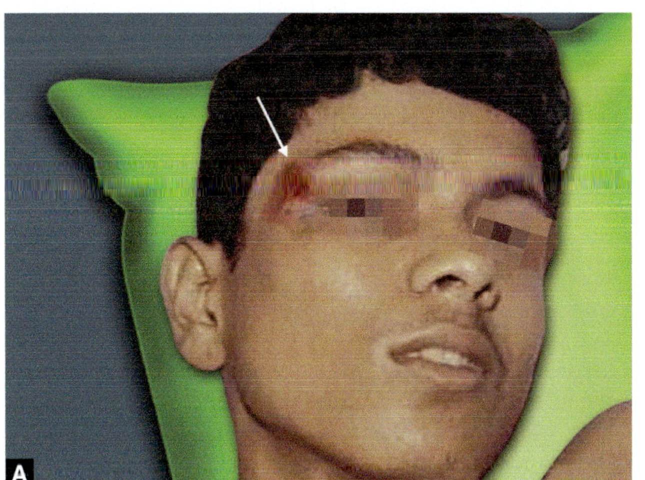
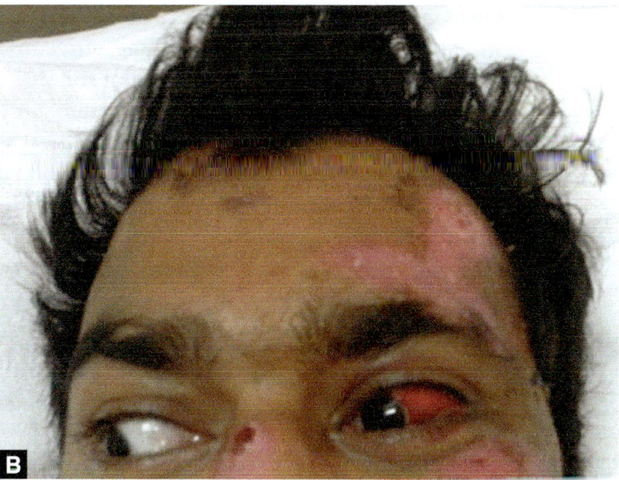

Figs 15.1A and B: (A) Minor injury to the outer part of the right brow (white arrow) in a case of traumatic optic neuropathy and (B) Post-traumatic optic neuropathy
Site of injury: Left zygoma and temporal region

- *Visual acuity:* Visual acuity should be tested immediately on presentation, and then repeated 24 hours later to check for cases of delayed optic neuropathy. Almost 50% of patients will present with a visual acuity of light perception only, or no light perception. However about 20% may have a visual acuity of 20/200 or better.
- *Pupillary reaction:* An afferent pupillary defect (APD) is a necessary condition for the diagnosis of traumatic optic neuropathy. Light in the affected eye causes only mild or no constriction of both pupils, whereas light in the unaffected eye causes normal constriction in both pupils. On alternating the light between each eye every 2–3 seconds, the pupil of the affected eye will dilate with direct light and constrict with light in the unaffected eye. This is also known as the Marcus Gunn pupil.[12,16]
- *Intraocular pressure:* Intraocular pressure may be raised when there is an associated orbital hematoma, diffuse orbital hemorrhage, orbital emphysema, or soft tissue edema.
- *Ophthalmoscopy:* Ophthalmoscopy is performed to evaluate the retinal and choroidal circulation, optic nerve head morphology, and the presence of hemorrhage near the optic nerve head.
- *Visual field perimetry:* Although visual field defects are not necessarily pathognomonic of traumatic optic neuropathy, quantification of visual field defects is useful to assess convalescent visual improvements.

IMAGING

Computed tomography (CT) scanning can provide adequate imaging of orbital soft tissue and is better than MRI at delineating bony defects. Fractures through the optic canal can be best depicted with high resolution CT scanning (1.5 mm cuts with 1 mm intervals). A thin-section CT scan also provides an intraoperative road map for the surgeon in patients undergoing surgical decompression (Fig. 15.2).[16]

The decision for surgical decompression should still be based primarily on the clinical examination findings and not the CT scan findings. Small-review series have also found that sometimes the extent of bony canal injury documented at surgery was underestimated by CT scan findings.[9]

MEDICAL THERAPY

Currently the most widely accepted management for traumatic optic neuropathy includes observation, steroids, and surgical decompression. There have been concerns about the use of corticosteroids in patients with acute brain trauma. The corticosteroid randomization after significant head injury (CRASH) trial in 2005 showed a significantly increased risk of mortality in patients that received mega dose

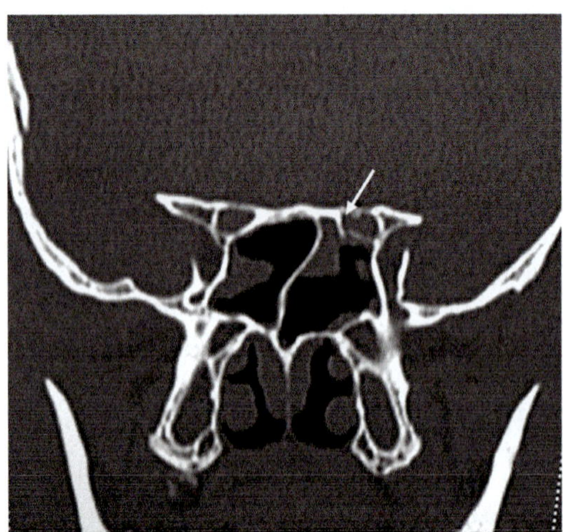

Fig. 15.2: Coronal CT scan showing fracture lines (white arrow) at the left optic canal

steroids at their 6-month follow-up when compared with the placebo group.[17] Lack of a prospective large-scale clinical trial perpetuates controversy as to the optimal treatment for traumatic optic neuropathy.[4] The timing and type of decompression procedure and selected use and optimal dosing of perioperative corticosteroids have also been widely reported, but have not been validated by controlled outcome trials.[18]

Based on the current evidence, a therapeutic role for corticosteroids in the management of traumatic optic neuropathy is unsubstantiated. If steroids are considered, they should not be used in cases with concomitant traumatic brain injury or in patients that present 8 hours or more after initial injury.[4,18]

SURGICAL MANAGEMENT

The rationale for surgical therapy in traumatic optic neuropathy is to decompress the optic nerve at the site of injury, which is often the intracanalicular segment. Surgical decompression is thought to help reduce optic nerve compression and subsequent vascular compromise that may occur as a result of the indirect injury. Additionally, surgery has been advocated to remove bone fragments that may be impinging on the optic nerve within the optic canal. Patients with no light perception on visual acuity testing, treated surgically within 7 days of injury had a better improvement degree than patients managed medically.[6-8]

An intranasal endoscopic approach is favored because of the proximity of the optic nerve to the sphenoid sinus and Onodi cell. Advantages of this approach include lack of external scars, preservation of olfaction, decreased morbidity, and faster recovery time.[6-8]

Preoperative Care

Imaging studies are obtained to delineate the exact anatomical relationship of the optic nerve and carotid artery to the posterior ethmoid cells and sphenoid sinus. If the patient has been receiving systemic corticosteroids, it may be continued at a tapered dosage. If the patient has completed a preoperative corticosteroid trial, a loading dose of dexamethasone 1.5 mg/kg (or equivalent) may be given a few hours preoperatively. The steroid's anti-inflammatory effect reduces the inflammation induced by surgery. Preoperative systemic antibiotics may be initiated once surgery is scheduled to suppress any pre-existing chronic rhinosinusitis.[9,16,19]

Procedure

The patient is placed in a supine position under general anesthesia. The area around the nose is prepared and draped as with standard endoscopic sinus procedures and the eyes are exposed in the surgical field. The nasal cavity is decongested adequately using pledgets soaked in saline with adrenaline. Normal saline with 1:1,00,000 adrenaline is used for local infiltration.

A complete sphenoethmoidectomy is performed. The anterior wall of the sphenoid sinus (or the sphenoid face) is opened wide. The bulge of the optic nerve is identified along the lateral wall of the sphenoid sinus, superior to the carotid artery. The lamina papyracea is then fractured approximately 1 cm anterior to the optic canal. Care is taken to avoid penetrating the periorbita, as herniation of periorbital fat will obscure the surgical field.[1] The bone is carefully removed in a posterior direction. As the optic canal is approached, the thin lamina bone is replaced by thick bone of the lesser wing of the sphenoid. It is often necessary to thin this bone with the help of a drill, before removal with a curette. Removal of bone

for a distance of 1 cm posterior to the face of the sphenoid is usually sufficient in most cases, and the bony opening is widened to expose at least a 120° circumference of the nerve (Figs 15.3A and B). Longitudinal opening of the annulus of Zinn and optic nerve sheath may be performed, although the indications for this still remain controversial.[16] Once the procedure is complete, intranasal packing is avoided to prevent compression of the exposed nerve.

Postoperative Care

The systemic steroid therapy started preoperatively is continued every 8 hours for 24 hours. This may be continued at a tapered dosage for 1–2 weeks.

Postoperative antibiotic therapy has no known role, except in patients with preoperative chronic rhinosinusitis.

The patient is asked to start saline nasal irrigations twice a day on discharge. These irrigations are continued for a few weeks, until normal mucociliary function resumes.[9]

Recovery of visual function is measured based on serial assessment of multiple visual function parameters (e.g. visual acuity, visual field).

A check CT scan is usually performed 3 months postoperatively.

▍ COMPLICATIONS

- Breach of periorbita during removal of the lamina papyracea can cause injury to the globe, extraocular muscles and the optic nerve.
- Injury to the anterior ethmoidal artery with its retraction into the orbit can produce an orbital hematoma and further aggravate compression of the optic nerve.
- There is an increased risk of CSF leaks and meningitis with OND surgery as compared to standard endoscopic sinus surgery.

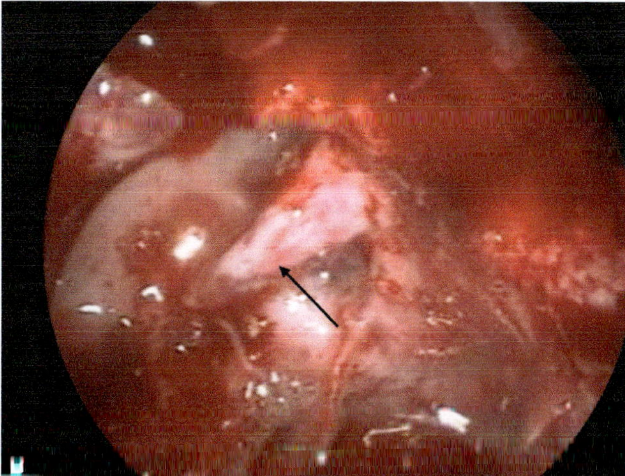

Figs 15.3A and B: *Intraoperative picture:* Left optic nerve decompression (OND). (A) Fracture fragment (white arrow) being removed. (B) Decompressed optic nerve (black arrow)

- Massive intracranial bleeding and stroke may follow injury to the intracranial internal carotid artery.
- Visual acuity may worsen in some cases after OND surgery.

To date, no standardized evidence exists to guide the management of traumatic optic neuropathy. A better delineation of surgical indications and the standardization of operative technique will better the outcome in these patients.[9] Till such a time, therapeutic decisions in traumatic optic neuropathy will have to be made on an individual patient basis.[4,8,16] The decision to proceed with surgery should depend on the clinical judgment and surgical skills of the surgeon as well as informed consent of the patient to appreciate the benefits and risks of the surgery.

▌REFERENCES

1. Metson R, Pletcher SD. Endoscopic orbital and optic nerve decompression. Otolaryngol Clin North Am. 2006;39(3):551-61.
2. Thaker A, Tandon DA, Mahapatra AK. Surgery for optic nerve injury: should nerve sheath incision supplement osseous decompression? Skull Base. 2009;19(4):263-71.
3. Cook MW, Levin LA, Joseph MP, et al. Traumatic optic neuropathy. A meta-analysis. Arch Otolaryngol Head Neck Surg. 1996;122(4):389-92.
4. Levin LA, Beck RW, Joseph MP, et al. The treatment of traumatic optic neuropathy: the International Optic Nerve Trauma Study. Ophthalmology. 1999;106(7):1268-77.
5. Levin LA, Baker RS. Management of traumatic optic neuropathy. J Neuroophthalmol. 2003;23(1):72-5.
6. Kong DS, Shin HJ, Kim HY, et al. Endoscopic optic canal decompression for compressive optic neuropathy. J Clin Neurosci. 2011;18(11):1541-5.
7. Peng A, Li Y, Hu P, et al. Endoscopic optic nerve decompression for traumatic optic neuropathy in children. Int J Pediatr Otorhinolaryngol. 2011;75(8):992-8.
8. Yang QT, Zhang GH, Liu X, et al. The therapeutic efficacy of endoscopic optic nerve decompression and its effects on the prognoses of 96 cases of traumatic optic neuropathy. J Trauma Acute Care Surg. 2012;72(5):1350-5.
9. O'Brien EK, Leopold D, Gigantelli JW, et al. (2003) Optic nerve decompression for traumatic optic neuropathy.[online] E medicine Journal. Available from http://emedicine.medscape.com/article/868252. [Accessed September 2013].
10. Gray H. Anatomy of the human body, 20th edition. Bartleby.com; 2000.pp.557-8.
11. Miller NR, Newman NJ, Biousse V. Walsh and Hoyt's Clinical Neuro-ophthalmology, 6th edition. Lippincott Williams & Wilkins; 2004.
12. Selhorst JB, Chen Y. The optic nerve. Semin Neurol. 2009;29(1):29-35.
13. Yu-Wai-Man P, Griffiths P. Steroids for traumatic optic neuropathy. Cochrane Database Syst Rev. 2007;(4):CD006032.
14. Yu Wai Man P, Griffiths PG. Surgery for traumatic optic neuropathy. Cochrane Database Syst Rev. 2005;(4):CD005024.
15. Nayak SR, Kirtane MV, Ingle MV. Fracture line in post head injury optic nerve damage. J Laryngol Otol. 1991;105(3):203-4.
16. Hathiram BT, Khattar VS, Rode S. Traumatic optic neuropathy. Otorhinolaryngology Clinics: An International Journal. 2011;3(3):188-96.
17. Edwards P, Arango M, Balica L, et al. Final results of MRC CRASH, a randomised placebo-controlled trial of intravenous corticosteroid in adults with head injury-outcomes at 6 months. Lancet. 2005;365(9475):1957-9.
18. Ropposch T, Steger B, Meço C, et al. The effect of steroids in combination with optic nerve decompression surgery in traumatic optic neuropathy. Laryngoscope. 2013;123(5):1082-6.
19. Nayak SR, Kirtane MV, Ingle MV. Transethmoid decompression of the optic nerve in head injuries: an update. J Laryngol Otol. 1991;105(3):205-6.

CHAPTER 16

Endoscopic Dacryocystorhinostomy

Milind Navalakhe

HISTORY

In the past three decades endoscopic dacryocystorhinostomy (DCR) has gained popularity due to the growing interest in endonasal endoscopic procedures among otorhinolaryngologists. Improved visualization and a wide range of instruments available have enabled the routine use of this procedure. Dacryocystorhinostomy was described by Killian in 1889.

The first surgery reported in literature was done by Caldwell, an ENT surgeon in 1893.[1] He performed a rhinostomy and removed part of inferior turbinate following the nasolacrimal duct to the lacrimal sac. His surgery however did not gain any popularity due to lack of advancement in instrumentation and considerable skill required for this procedure. In 1904, Toti first described the external approach and this was modified by Dupuy-Dutemps and Bourget. This led to the temporary shift of this surgery under the purview of ophthalmologists.[2]

West modified Caldwell's technique with a window resection over the lacrimal sac. Almost 100 years after the first description, Steadman and Mc Donagh and Meiring published early results using endoscopic approach. Massaro et al. published the report on use of LASER to aid endoscopic DCR in 1990. LASER fibers can be advanced through the canaliculi with simultaneous lacrimal endoscopic visualization.

The technical advancements in instrumentation and optics have once more brought this surgery into mainstream otorhinolaryngology practice.

ANATOMY

See Figure 16.1.

Lacrimal Gland

Lacrimal gland is situated superolaterally in the orbit. It is a serous acinus type of gland. It has two parts—a large orbital (upper) part and a smaller palpebral (lower) part about one-third the size of the orbital part. Both these parts are continuous posterolaterally around the levator aponeurosis.

Many small accessory lacrimal glands or Krause's glands are seen in or around the fornix, they are more numerous in the upper lid (about 42) than in the lower (about 6–8).

Lacrimal Ducts

About 6–12 lacrimal ducts open into the superior fornix from the palpebral part of the lacrimal gland. Ducts from accessory lacrimal glands unite to form a larger duct which opens into the fornix. Upper and lower puncta lie near the posterior border of the free margin of the lid about 6 mm from the inner canthus.

Lacrimal Sac

The lacrimal sac lies in the lacrimal fossa formed by the lacrimal bone, the frontal process of maxilla and the lacrimal fascia. It is about 12–15 mm long vertically and 6–8 mm wide. The upper portion of the fundus extends slightly above the

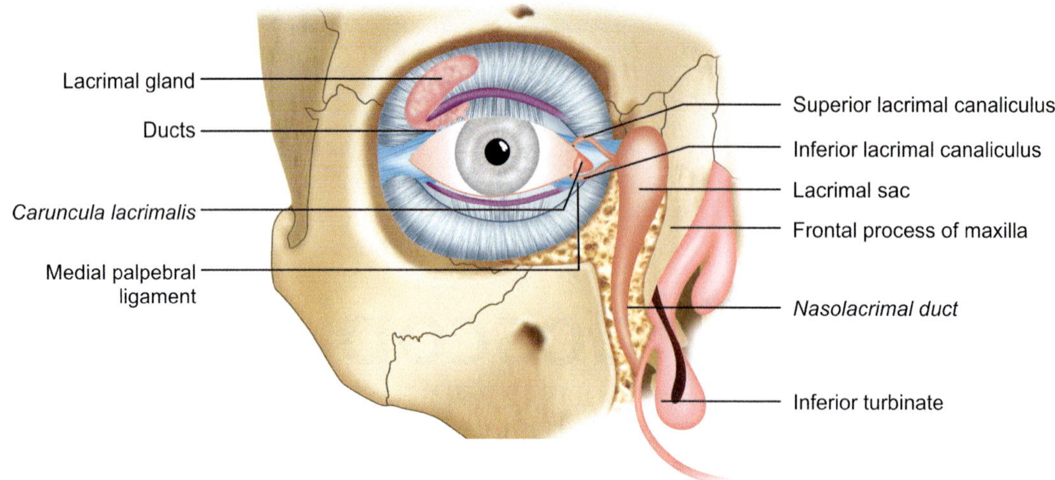

Fig. 16.1: Anatomy

level of the inner tarsal ligament. The common canaliculus opens into the lateral wall near its upper end. Lacrimal fascia forms the roof and lateral wall to the lacrimal fossa. Fascia separates the sac from the median palpebral ligament in front and the lacrimal part of orbicularis oculi behind. The lower-half of the lacrimal sac is related medially to the anterior part of middle meatus and upper-half is related to the anterior ethmoidal sinuses. The relation of anterior ethmoidal cells to lacrimal fossa is variable. The anterior ethmoidal cells may extend till the lacrimal fossa in more than 50% of patients. Mucosa of lacrimal sac is continuous with that of the conjunctiva through lacrimal canaliculi and with the nasal mucosa through nasolacrimal duct. The sac has a fibroelastic wall surrounded by fibers of the orbicularis oculi muscle.[3]

Valves (Fig. 16.2)

There are many valves involved in the lacrimal transport.[4] They are small mucosal folds within the lumen of the lacrimal system which vary between individuals. It is suggested that they help prevent intercompartment regurgitation of tears in retrograde direction.

- *Valve of Bochdalek:* This is the first valve of the lacrimal drainage system and is located at the lacrimal punctum
- *Valve of Foltz:* This valve is just after the punctum where the vertical canaliculus starts
- *Valve of Rosenmüller:* This valve is at the common canaliculus where it opens in the lacrimal sac. The valve is situated superiorly at this site. This is one of the most important valves in the lacrimal system
- *Valve of Huschke:* This is also at the common canaliculus before its opening into the lacrimal sac, situated inferiorly
- *Valve of median palpebral ligament:* The median palpebral ligament gives an impression on the lacrimal sac creating a mucosal valve
- *Valve of Taillefer:* This valve is within the wall of the nasolacrimal duct. The area from valve of Beraud/Krause to this valve is more prone to obstruction
- *Valve of Beraud or Krause:* This valve is near the lower end of the lacrimal sac
- *Valve of Hasner, Cruveilhier or Bianchi:* This is one of the most important valves of the lacrimal system situated at the lower end of the nasolacrimal duct, at its opening into the nasal cavity.

Dimensions

See Figure 16.3.

ENDOSCOPIC ANATOMY (FIG. 16.4)

Endoscopically, the area 5–8 mm anterior to the uncinate process is the area of the lacrimal sac. Nasolacrimal duct

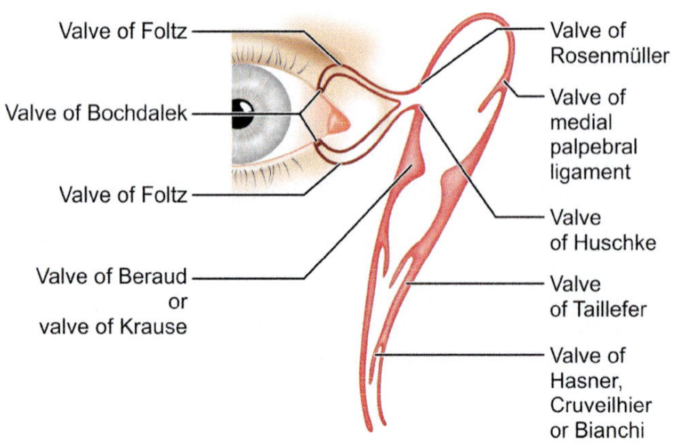

Fig. 16.2: Valves

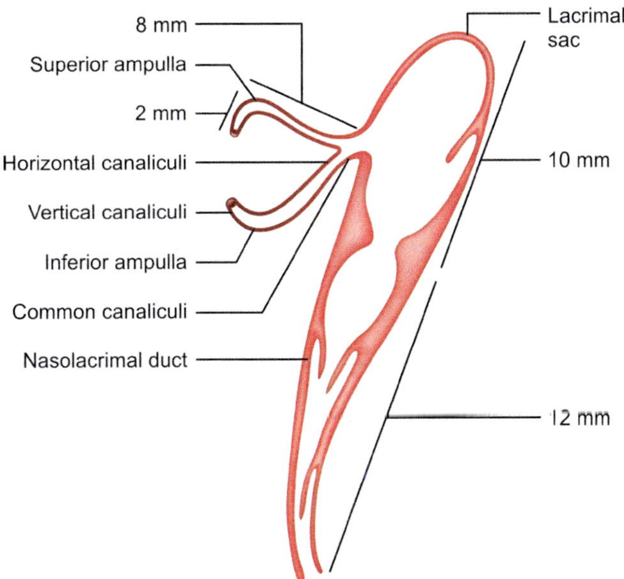

Fig. 16.3: Dimensions

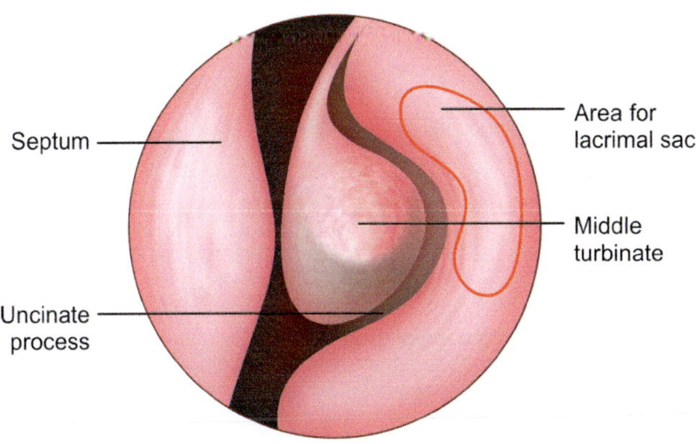

Fig. 16.4: Endoscopic anatomy

opens in the inferior meatus under the inferior turbinate. The distance between the uncinate process and the lacrimal sac is variable.[5]

PHYSIOLOGY OF LACRIMATION

Ocular tear film layer consists of three components:
1. Inner deep mucous layer
2. Middle watery layer
3. Outer surface oily layer.

Conduction of the tear film:
- Absorption through the conjunctiva
- Evaporation from the surface
- Flow into nasolacrimal duct, which is an active process.

Blink reflex helps in tear transport. It carries tears from the conjunctival surface to puncta. Contraction of orbicularis oculi pulls median palpebral ligament and anterior sac wall. This produces suction pump action that pulls tears into the sac through puncta and canaliculus. This distends the lacrimal sac. The elasticity of the sac wall initiates action of contraction of its contents. Propulsion action of sac wall on its contents pushes the tears downward aided by gravity into the nasolacrimal duct.

Neural Supply

Secretomotor fibers are supplied by the facial nerve. The greater superficial petrosal nerve is the branch of the facial nerve arising at the geniculate ganglion. The greater superficial petrosal nerve then unites with the deep petrosal nerve to forms the vidian nerve. After synapse in pterygopalatine ganglion the lacrimal branch is given which supplies the lacrimal gland. The sensory supply to the lacrimal gland is by the ophthalmic division of trigeminal nerve (V1). The afferent nerve for the blink reflex is the trigeminal nerve and the efferent is the facial nerve.

CLINICAL FEATURES OF DACRYOCYSTITIS

- Epiphora (Management of a patient with epiphora is described in Flow chart 16.1)
- Purulent discharge from lacrimal puncta
- Rarely, cutaneous fistula.

Preoperative Evaluation of the Patient

A complete history and thorough ENT and ophthalmological evaluation is essential before the surgery is planned. The most important tools in preoperative evaluation include sac syringing (Flow chart 16.2) and a diagnostic nasal endoscopy.

DIAGNOSTIC NASAL ENDOSCOPY

This is essential to rule out any associated nasal pathology. In case of patients with deviated nasal septum which limits endoscopic access to the sac on the side of surgery, the surgeon must first perform a septoplasty prior to endoscopic DCR.

A space occupying lesion blocking the nasolacrimal duct opening in also ruled out.

Contraindications of endoscopic DCR:
- Punctal block
- Canalicular block
- Common canalicular block

Flow chart 16.1: Management of a patient with epiphora

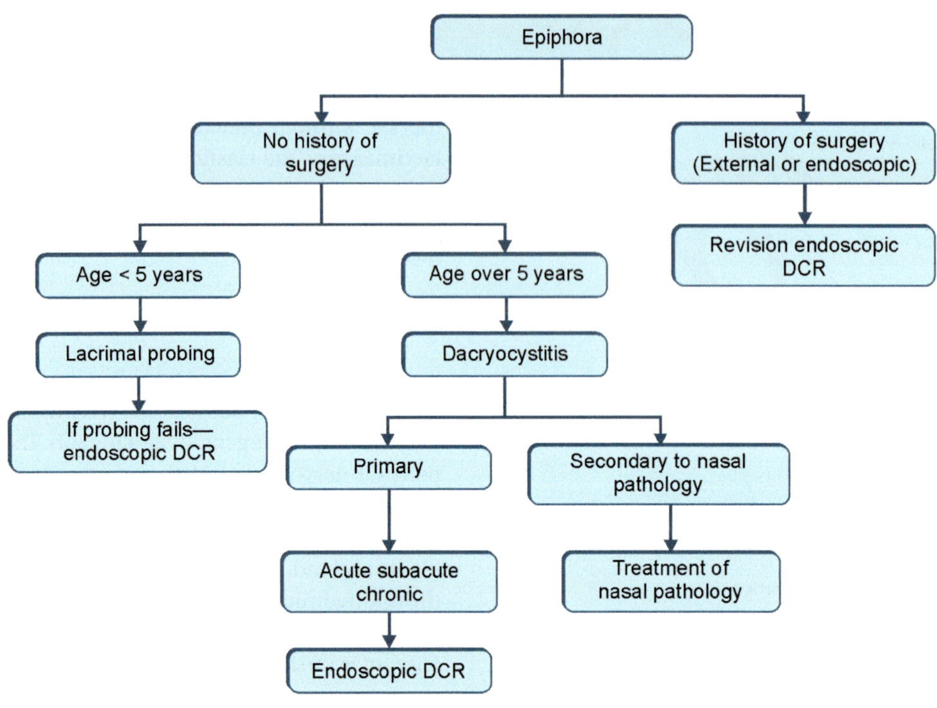

Abbreviation: DCR, dacryocystorhinostomy

Flow chart 16.2: Preoperative evaluation of a patient with dacryocystitis

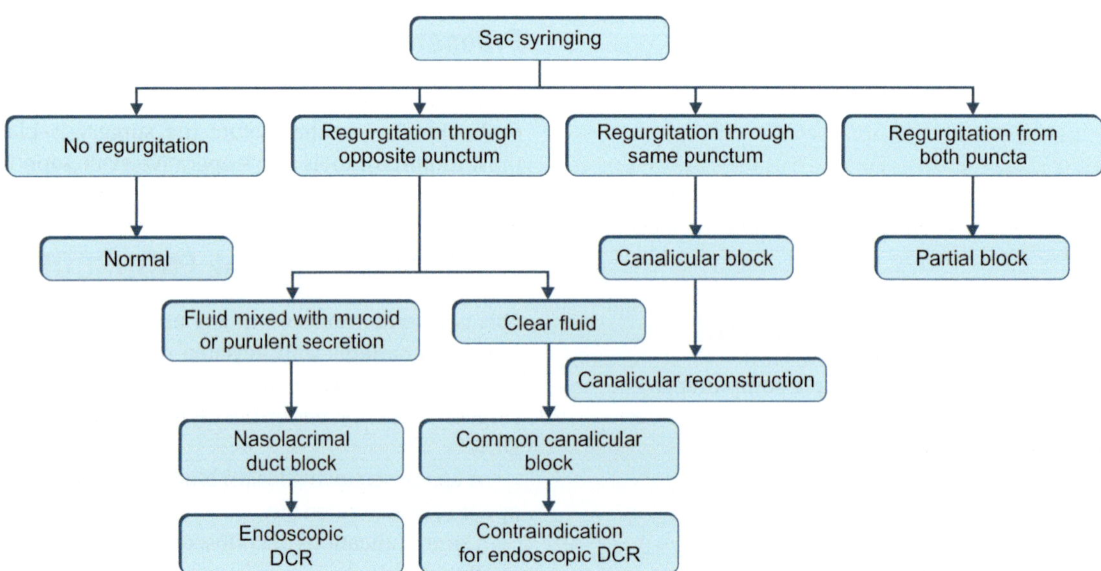

- Lacrimal sac tumors
- External compression of the nasolacrimal duct
- Nasal pathology causing dacryocystitis.

PREOPERATIVE PATIENT PREPARATION

Patient is explained the procedure, pros and cons of surgery and anesthesia and written informed valid consent is taken.

The procedure may be done under general anesthesia or local anesthesia.

It is extremely important the nose is packed with 4% lignocaine with adrenaline moistened cottonoids prior to the surgery for adequate decongestion and better visualization.

ANESTHESIA

Adult endoscopic DCR can be done under local anesthesia with sedation. The infiltration used is 2% lignocaine with 1:2,00,000 adrenaline. This solution is injected endoscopically anterior to uncinate process on the lateral wall. Externally the area of lacrimal sac is infiltrated with the same solution. The block is given 10 minutes prior to surgery.

Pediatric patients are always operated under general anesthesia.

General anesthesia is also required for adult patients who are anxious/uncooperative and prefer it to local anesthesia.

STEPS OF SURGERY

- Adequate decongestion of nasal cavity is done with 4% lignocaine with 1:2,00,000 adrenaline
- A diagnostic nasal endoscopy is done
- Any associated nasal pathology is ruled out or dealt with appropriately, for example, septoplasty for deviated nasal septum
- The middle turbinate and uncinate processes are identified. The area anterior to the uncinate process is the region of the lacrimal sac
- The infiltration is given in this region with 2% lignocaine with 1:2,00,00 adrenaline
- An incision is made with a unipolar cautery forceps or an insulated ball probe or with a sickle knife. A square shaped mucosal flap is elevated with a Freer periosteum elevator and is reflected backward on middle turbinate
- The anterior lacrimal crest is identified. A 1-mm Kerrison bone punch is used to remove the bone covering the lacrimal sac. The frontal process of maxilla and lacrimal bone are removed for exposing the lacrimal sac. Complete removal of bone will ensure adequate exposure of the lacrimal sac. All bone chips must be removed
- Using a no. 12 blade, a sharp incision is made over the sac in inferior to superior direction, taking care not to damage the lateral wall of the sac

- The medial wall of the sac is then excised using a 45° angled scissors. Care must be taken that the tissue is cut sharply, and not pulled. Alternatively, the mucosal flap is split into upper- and lower-half and is used to cover the raw area created by bone removal. This can help in preventing granulations in these areas postoperatively
- Once the lumen is visualized, sac syringing is done using diluted methylene blue to check the adequacy of the lumen created
- A silicon stent is then placed. There are two schools of thought regarding use of stent, some surgeons prefer to keep a stent *in situ* for 4 months, other do not use the stents. In our experience, we have used silicon stents routinely for all our patients. Stent is a must in cases of revision surgeries and post-traumatic cases
- The metallic end of the silicone stent is first inserted from the lower punctum and once it reaches the nose via the common canalicular opening, it is held with a straight Blakesley forceps and pulled out. While doing this the silicone end attached to the metallic part of the stent must be supported by an Adson's forceps to prevent the stent from sliping out.
- Similarly, the upper punctum is dilated and the opposite end of the metallic part of the silicone stent is inserted. When it comes out through the same common canalicular opening, it will confirm there is no false passage created. This end is also pulled out of the nose in a similar fashion.
- To prevent the over tightening of the stent between the two puncta, lacrimal probe is placed under the stent. Over tightening of the stent causes irritation and foreign body sensation in the eye.
- Another silicone tubing of 1.5 mm inner diameter and 3–4 cm in length is threaded over the nasal end of the stent all the way till it reaches the inside of the lumen of the lacrimal sac. This ensures one large opening in the sac.
- Once the silicone tubing is in place, the two ends of the stent are tied to form a knot. With the assistant making the knot, the surgeon slides it down with a knot slider. The 8 to 10 similar knots are taken. This ensures that after 4 months, even if some knots slip, there will still be the other knots holding the stent in place.
- The lacrimal probe is removed and it is ensured that the loop of the stent around the medial canthus is neither too loose nor too tight.
- If required nasal packing can be done to achieve adequate hemostasis
- If the patient has a fistula, a fistulectomy has to be performed externally.

CHALLENGES FACED IN SURGERY

- Bleeding
- Difficulty in getting the first punch for bone removal

- Small fibrosed contracted sac
- Deviated nasal septum
- Stenosed puncta
- Thick bone
- Accidentally opening the orbit or the ethmoids
- Diverticulae.

STEPS TO ENHANCE SUCCESS RATES IN ENDOSCOPIC DACRYOCYSTORHINOSTOMY

- Surgeon must do the sac syringing before surgery
- Deviated nasal septum must be corrected with septoplasty
- Preserve mucosal flaps
- Adequate removal of bone
- Complete exposure of lacrimal sac
- Follow-up diagnostic nasal endoscopy for cleaning of crusts and prevention of adhesion formation and granuloma formation
- If stent is not used then regular sac syringing weekly for 4 weeks.

PACK REMOVAL AND TREATMENT

Patient has nasal pack postoperatively which can be removed after 24 hours.

Adequate oral broadspectrum antibiotics, analgesic, anti-inflammatory, antihistaminic medication should be given postoperatively for 1 week. Patient is given lubricant eyedrops. Nose should be cleaned and any crusts after pack removal should be removed. Liquid paraffin nose drops are given for lubrication. This helps to remove crusts and keep operated area clean. It is essential for the patient to perform regular nasal douching for 3 months postoperatively.

STENT REMOVAL AND RESULTS

Stent removal is done 4 months after surgery, by cutting the stent at medial canthus and removing stent from the nose. By this time the track is well formed and lined with epithelium. While removing the stent one should be gentle to nasal mucosa to avoid creating a raw surface. Sac syringing is done on removal of stent to check the patency.

ADVANTAGES OF ENDOSCOPIC DACRYOCYSTORHINOSTOMY

- Bilateral DCR can be done in the same sitting

- Both nasal and lacrimal pathology can be handled at the same time
- Patient does not have an external scar
- There is lesser morbidity and lesser duration of hospital stay
- There are lesser chances of bleeding
- No eye padding is required postoperatively
- The sac is opened under endoscopic vision
- Decreased risk of postoperative adhesions
- No risk of injury to medial canthus leading to stricture formation
- Recent studies have shown that the success rate is higher following endoscopic approach
- Normal pumping mechanism of the lacrimal system is unaltered
- Revision surgery is easier
- Lacrimal abscess can be drained and an endoscopic DCR can be done in the same sitting
- Patient can be followed up with nasal endoscopy to look for any mucosal overgrowth or granulomas at the site of the stent and adhesions.

COMPLICATIONS

Complications of Surgery

Intraoperative

- *Bleeding:* Bleeding can be due to damage angular vein or generalized bleeding from the mucosa. There are various ways to control the bleeding:
  - Adequate preparation of the nasal mucosa with topical decongestants. No focus of infection should be present.
  - Stop all anticoagulant therapy at least 72 hours prior to surgery
  - Evaluate the patient for any coagulopathy
  - Blood pressure should be assessed and monitored preoperatively. Adequate control is imperative.
  - Use of local adrenaline packing can significantly decrease the bleeding.
- *Injury to the lamina papyracea:* Careful identification of the thin papery bone, lamina papyracea must be done to avoid any damage to it. The orbital periosteum is seen even after the lamina papyracea is broken. Hence, careful identification helps to prevent fat prolapse into the nose
- *Opening the orbit:* With the usage of powered instruments, orbital complications can be extremely serious
- *False passage:* False passage can be created when the probing is forceful and in a wrong direction. There are chances of creating false passage during stent insertion.

Postoperative

- Swelling of the eye may be due to subcutaneous emphysema may occur after surgery which is treated with gentle eye massage and local ice application
- *Bleeding:* Intraorbital hemorrhage can occur due to damage to the orbital vessels
- *Sump syndrome:* Collection of pus in the remnant sac after surgery. It may regurgitate on pressure. This can be avoided with adequate bony removal
- *Corneal abrasion:* It can occur due to prolonged exposure of the cornea during surgery. It can be avoided by adequate lubrication to the eye
- Synechia formation
- Failure of surgery remains the worst complication.

Complications of Stent (Silicone)

- Stretching of puncta
- Granuloma
- Allergic conjunctivitis with stent in place
- Adhesions at medial canthus
- *Extrusion of the silicone stent:* It can prolapse out of the punctum and into the eye or it may be pulled out by a child causing foreign body sensation and irritation
- Foreign body sensation, if the stent is loose or tight.

CONCLUSION

The endoscopic DCR has many advantages over external DCR. The endoscopic approach without a scar makes, it a better choice for patients. The exposure of the sac is much better endoscopically. Both the sides can be operated simultaneously if the patient has bilateral pathology. The opening made in the sac is much larger. The medial canthal ligament is not handled as well as the sac which preserves the anatomy and physiology of the sac resulting in better outcomes of the surgery.

REFERENCES

1. Massegur H, Trias E, Adema' JM. Endoscopic dacryocystorhinostomy: modified technique. Otolaryngol Head Neck Surg. 2004;130(1):39-46.
2. Harish V, Benger RS. Origins of lacrimal surgery, and evolution of dacryocystorhinostomy to the present. Clin Experiment Ophthalmol. 2014;42(3):284-7.
3. Jones LT. An anatomical approach to problems of the eyelids and lacrimal apparatus. Arch Ophthalmol. 1961;66:111-24.
4. Gustav A, et al. Endoscopic Transnasal Dacryocystorhinostomy (chapter 34). In: Microendoscopic Surgery of the Paranasal Sinuses and Skull base: Springer; 2000.pp.415-24.
5. Wormald PJ, Kew J, Van Hasselt A. Intranasal anatomy of the nasolacrimal sac in endoscopy dacryocystorhinostomy. Otolaryngol Head Neck Surg. 2000;123(3):307-10.

CHAPTER 17

Endoscopic Management of Epistaxis

Sujata Muranjan

INTRODUCTION

Epistaxis is one of the most common emergencies in ear, nose, and throat (ENT). It is a distressing symptom causing considerable patient anxiety. It therefore needs effective and prompt control with minimal morbidity. Whether spontaneous or otherwise, epistaxis is experienced by up to 60% of people in their lifetime with only 6% requiring medical attention.[1] Although most cases resolve with first aid measures, some are complex and may require specialist intervention. This is especially so in the elderly population with their associated morbidity who often require more intensive treatment and subsequent admission. The majority of hospital admissions for epistaxis are therefore seen in the age group of 60–70 years, but there is a bimodal age incidence, with an earlier peak in childhood.[2]

In ancient Greece, sheep's wool lubricated with oil was used by Hippocrates on pugilistic noses to control nasal bleeds. Over the years the understanding of this condition has improved and its management has undergone considerable refinement. Sophisticated nasal packs, nasal endoscopes with excellent optics and illumination and refined techniques of arterial angiography and embolization are now included in the armamentarium for controlling moderate to severe epistaxis.

ANATOMY

The nose plays an important role in warming, humidifying and conditioning the inspired air. It has a rich blood supply from branches of both the external and the internal carotid arteries.

The anterior part, the roof and the part of the lateral nasal wall above the middle turbinate are supplied by branches of the anterior and posterior ethmoidal arteries which are branches of the internal carotid artery. The rest of the nasal cavity is supplied by branches of the external carotid artery through the sphenopalatine artery, the main artery of the nose, and the greater palatine artery. Both these are branches of the internal maxillary artery, the terminal branch of the external carotid artery (Fig. 17.1).

The nasal septum has a blood supply similar to that of the lateral nasal wall. In addition to this, the anterior most part is supplied by the superior labial artery a branch of the facial artery and branches of the alar artery. All these belong to the external carotid artery system. An area of anastomosis exists between all these arteries on the anteroinferior part of the nasal septum. This is the "Little's area". Bleeding from this site causes anterior epistaxis. Posterior bleeding occurs primarily from the branches of the sphenopalatine artery (SPA) chiefly the posterior septal artery[3] which runs just above the roof of the choana and onto the posterior part of the nasal septum.

The anterior ethmoidal artery branches off from the ophthalmic artery within the orbit. It then runs in the bony orbitocranial canal in relation to the roof of the ethmoid sinus just posterior to the area of the frontal recess (Figs 17.2 and 17.3). The vertical skull base turns to become more horizontal at this level. The artery enters the cranial cavity and then

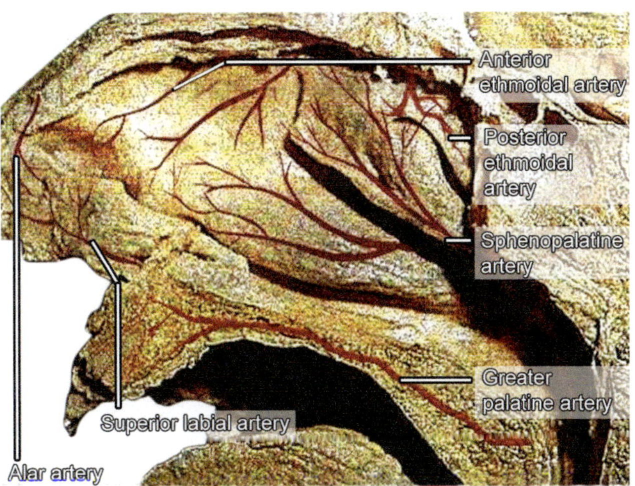

Fig. 17.1: Blood supply of the lateral nasal wall

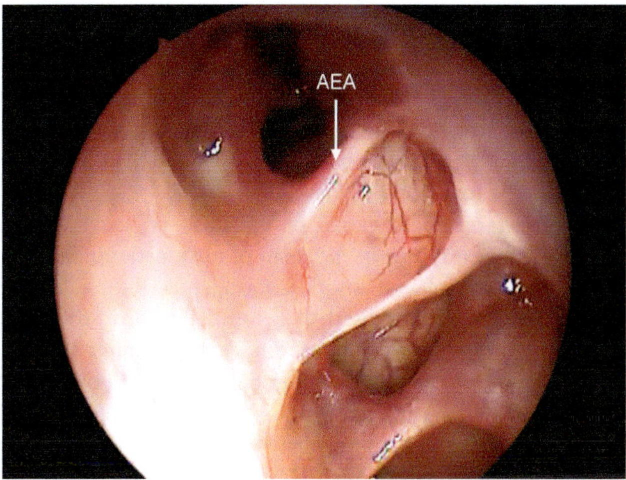

Fig. 17.2: Endoscopic view of the anterior ethmoidal artery (AEA) marked by arrow

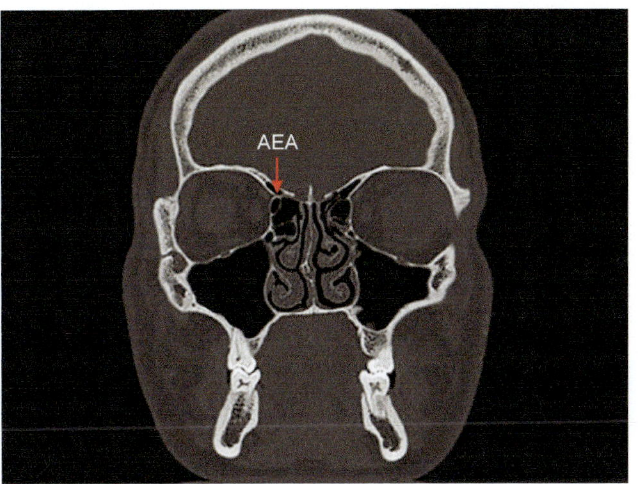

Fig. 17.3: Computed tomography coronal section showing the anterior ethmoidal artery (AEA) marked by the red arrow

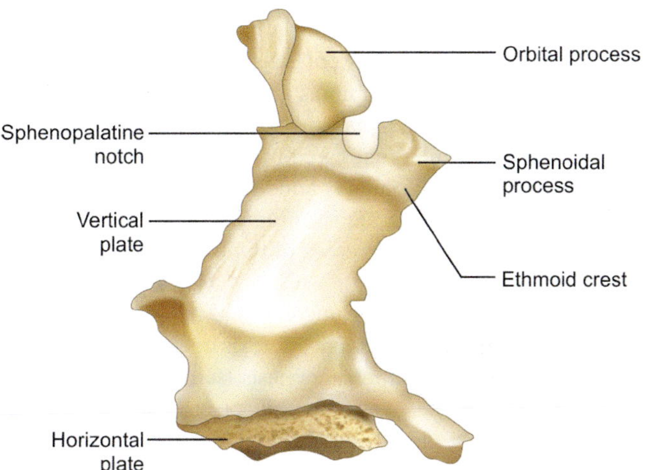

Fig. 17.4: Palatine bone with the sphenopalatine notch

descends through a foramen in the cribriform plate to re-enter the nasal cavity. Bleeding from the anterior ethmoidal artery is rare in cases of spontaneous epistaxis. It is however prone to trauma during endoscopic sinus surgery. The traumatized artery can retract into the orbit and continue to bleed therein giving rise to an orbital hematoma. It is imperative to diagnose and manage this promptly to prevent blindness.

Anatomy of the sphenopalatine foramen and artery is somewhat complex. The perpendicular plate of the palatine bone has an anterior process, the orbital process and a posterior one, the sphenoidal process. A notch termed the sphenopalatine notch exists between the two (Fig. 17.4). This is closed off superiorly by the sphenoid bone to form the sphenopalatine foramen. The sphenopalatine artery exits from the pterygopalatine fossa through this foramen to enter the nasal cavity. This sphenopalatine foramen is located just above the ethmoid crest on the palatine bone to which is attached the middle turbinate. Lee reported that the SPA will divide into 2–4 branches before exiting the sphenopalatine foramen. The majority of cases (70%) will have only two branches.[4] In 12% of cases the septal branch of the SPA will emerge from a separate foramen.[5] It is essential to locate this septal branch and ligate it following endoscopic ligation of the SPA.

CAUSES OF EPISTAXIS

There exist a number of etiological factors that can cause epistaxis (Table 17.1). These can be classified into idiopathic, local or systemic.

Very often epistaxis is idiopathic where no discernible cause can be found.

A common local cause of epistaxis is nasal trauma which could be minor in the form of nose picking or major following maxillofacial injuries. Iatrogenic trauma leading to epistaxis is encountered in a hospital setting following procedures like nasogastric tube insertion or after nasal or sinus surgery. An occasional foreign body, particularly in a child, may cause unilateral blood stained nasal discharge. Of the congenital causes, Osler's disease or hereditary hemorrhagic telangiectasia is a rare condition in which multiple telangiectatic lesions are present in the nasal mucosa. These can bleed and give rise to spontaneous epistaxis. Inflammatory conditions like acute rhinosinusitis or infective sinonasal polyposis can occasionally cause epistaxis. Structural anomalies like septal spurs, deviations or septal perforations can cause crusting and subsequent bleeding. Hemangiomas of the nasal septum, juvenile nasopharyngeal angiofibromas and inverted papillomas are some benign neoplasms causing epistaxis whereas malignant tumors like squamous cell carcinoma, adenocarcinomas and granulomas like lymphomas and Wegener's granulomatosis are other local causes. Environmental factors occasionally causing epistaxis are extremes of temperature, dry climates and high altitudes.

In the systemic group, uncontrolled hypertension is one of the most common causes of epistaxis frequently warranting hospitalization on an emergency basis. Hematological diseases with coagulopathies like Hemophilia, Christmas disease and diseases causing platelet dysfunction like thrombocytopenia and von Willebrand's disease have the propensity to cause profuse nasal bleeding. Epistaxis may also be encountered in patients on anticoagulant drugs like heparin, warfarin or antiplatelet agents like aspirin or clopidogrel. Patients with systemic diseases leading to renal and hepatic failure like uremia or cirrhosis of liver can also present with epistaxis.

PATHOPHYSIOLOGY

The rich blood supply of the nasal mucosa makes it prone to bleeding even with minor trauma. The blood vessels within the nasal mucosa run superficially and are therefore comparatively unprotected. In most cases, it is damage to the mucosa and vessel wall that results in bleeding. Occasionally spontaneous rupture of these blood vessels may occur during forceful Valsalva's maneuver, e.g. during heavy weightlifting. In elderly patients the ruptured atherosclerotic blood vessels

TABLE 17.1: Causes of epistaxis
Idiopathic
Local causes
Congenital: Osler's disease or Hereditary hemorrhagic telangiectasia
Traumatic: Nasal picking, maxillofacial injuries, iatrogenic trauma
Inflammatory: Acute rhinosinusitis, infective sinonasal polyposis
Structural anomalies: Septal spurs, deviations or septal perforations
Neoplastic: *Benign:* Hemangioma, juvenile nasopharyngeal angiofibroma, *inverted papillomas* *Malignant:* Squamous cell carcinoma, adenocarcinoma
Granulomas: Tuberculosis, fungus, sarcoid, lymphoma, Wegener's granulomatosis
Environmental
Systemic
Hypertension
Hematological diseases: Hemophilia, Christmas disease, Thrombocytopenia, von Willebrand's disease
Drugs: Heparin, warfarin, aspirin or clopidogrel
Uremia
Cirrhosis

fail to undergo contraction and can therefore lead to profuse and prolonged epistaxis. The areas of nasal mucosa which frequently bleed are Little's area, septal mucosa, lateral nasal wall and nasopharynx. Bleeding can also occur from existing nasal pathologies.

MANAGEMENT

A stepwise approach (Flow chart 17.1) to epistaxis management is advocated. This should follow an order of assessment and initial management or first aid followed by direct therapy, tamponade and finally vascular intervention if the need arises.

While assessing a patient with a recent history of epistaxis it is important to enquire about the amount of blood loss. This could be of a mild, moderate or severe nature. One needs to know if the bleeding occurred spontaneously or following trauma and if it was unilateral or bilateral. Enquiry has to be made about history of similar such episodes in the past. Eliciting history of medical diseases in particular hypertension and cardiac illness is relevant since many of these patients may be on blood thinning medications like aspirin and clopidogrel which can compound the problem and make control of the nasal bleed difficult.

Flow chart 17.1: Stepwise management of epistaxis

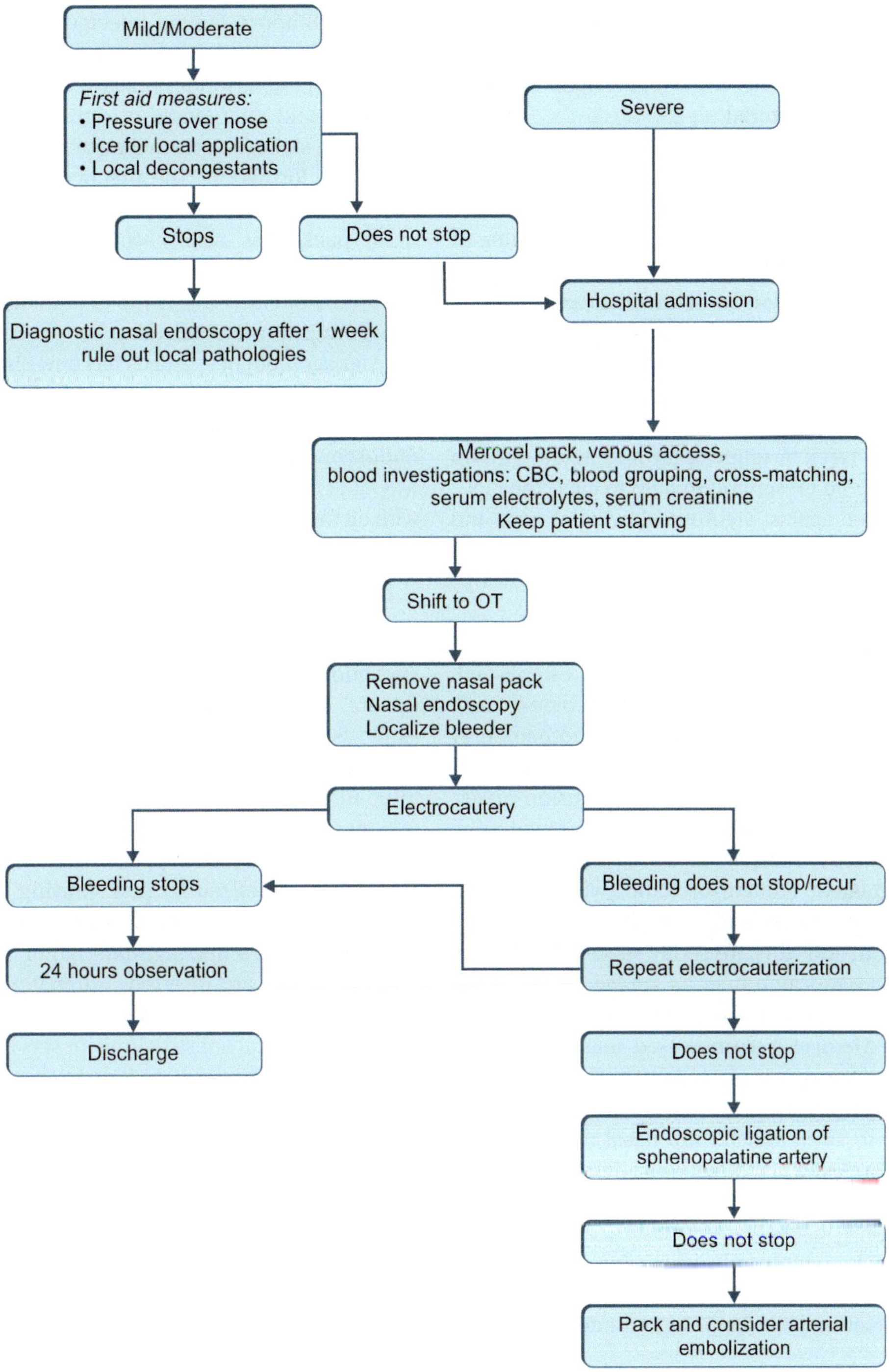

Mild/Moderate

First aid measures:
• Pressure over nose
• Ice for local application
• Local decongestants

Stops

Does not stop

Severe

Diagnostic nasal endoscopy after 1 week rule out local pathologies

Hospital admission

Merocel pack, venous access, blood investigations: CBC, blood grouping, cross-matching, serum electrolytes, serum creatinine Keep patient starving

Shift to OT

Remove nasal pack
Nasal endoscopy
Localize bleeder

Electrocautery

Bleeding stops

Bleeding does not stop/recur

24 hours observation

Repeat electrocauterization

Discharge

Does not stop

Endoscopic ligation of sphenopalatine artery

Does not stop

Pack and consider arterial embolization

Vital parameters particularly the pulse and blood pressure need to be recorded. Presence of pallor has to be assessed. These details give an idea of the approximate blood loss which helps decide whether intravenous fluids or blood products need to be administered.

If the vital parameters are stable and the epistaxis is mild, first aid measures such as digital pressure over the lower soft cartilaginous part of the nose along with ice application and instillation of local decongestants such as oxymetazoline or xylometazoline may be tried. The patient is asked to sit up and lean forward and clear any clots from the pharynx by spitting out any collection in the throat. Thus swallowing the blood can be prevented.

In mild cases of epistaxis, if the bleeding stops completely with the above treatment the patient may be asked to continue decongestants for a week. A saline spray and liquid paraffin nose drops may also be prescribed to help to clear the clots. The patient is advised against vigorous blowing of nose and is asked to follow-up for a diagnostic nasal endoscopy after a week. It is mandatory to perform a diagnostic nasal endoscopy to rule out a local pathology.

Moderate to severe epistaxis warrants hospital admission. A venous access has to be first established. Blood is also collected and sent for a complete blood count and determination of blood group and the blood bank may be requested to keep adequate units of whole blood or packed cells ready in case the need for transfusion arises. Studies have shown that routine clotting studies need to be performed only if there is a suspected clotting diathesis or the patient is anticoagulated.[6] Fluid resuscitation when indicated has to be initiated. An anterior rhinoscopy is performed in the emergency room and clots are gently sucked out. A local anesthetic such as lignocaine may be sprayed in the nose and after its action sets in, in a few minutes, temporary packs may be inserted. Merocel is compressed foam made of a polyvinyl alcohol polymer. It is convenient and easy to insert within a casualty setting. Water or normal saline is instilled over it causing it to swell and fill the nasal cavity thereby applying pressure over the bleeding points. It may also allow clotting factors to localize and reach a critical level facilitating coagulation.[3] Merocel packs are effective in 85% of cases. These packs help in temporarily stemming the bleeding which allows time to stabilize the patient. During this time the blood pressure if elevated can be brought under reasonable control.

The old practice of inserting lubricated ribbon gauzes is now practically given up. Not only is their insertion traumatic with the propensity to cause unwanted mucosal abrasions, but so is their removal which can also called bleeding. The subsequent mucosal trauma and necrosis can lead to a vicious circle of rebleeding and repacking. Packs which are left *in situ* for over 48 hours can get infected and cause rhinosinusitis. They can cause hypoxia[7] especially in elderly age group by depressing the nasopulmonary reflex. In addition to causing epiphora and dacryocystitis, tight nasal packs can lead to vestibular stenosis, columellar or alar necrosis and delayed synechiae formation. The practice of insertion of posterior nasal packs either in the form of balloon catheters or formal nasal packs has also become more or less redundant. Posterior nasal packs including balloon tamponade will fail in 26–52% of cases[8,9] and the next management step will be either surgery or embolization.

Management of epistaxis has now changed over the years with a move away from traditional approaches of prolonged admissions and reliance of extensive nasal packing. Endoscope-guided management of epistaxis has paved a new way of actively managing this condition. Thus nasal packing with all the associated complications can now be avoided.

ENDOSCOPIC ELECTROCAUTERIZATION

When the general condition is stabilized and adequate starvation is confirmed, the patient is shifted to the operation theatre. The procedure is carried out under local anesthesia as far as possible. General anesthesia is avoided to prevent fluctuations in the blood pressure which can occur during intubation and extubation. Sedation is also avoided since the patient needs to be awake to prevent aspiration of blood.

The temporary nasal packs are removed gently. The nasal cavity is anesthetized by first spraying it with a solution of 4% Lignocaine. Cottonoids® soaked with a solution of 4% lignocaine with a decongestant either adrenaline or oxy or xylometazoline are inserted. Adrenaline as a decongestant is avoided in case of a hypertensive patient. After adequate action of the local anesthetic agent sets in, under endoscopic guidance both the nasal cavities are systematically examined to localize the bleeder. The Little's area is examined first followed by examination of the entire nasal septum. This is followed by inspection of the choana and the nasopharynx. The endoscope is then withdrawn and the middle meatus is inspected paying close attention to the area of exit of the SPA near posterior end of the middle turbinate. On identification of the bleeding point, the blood is aspirated with an insulated suction and the bleeding point is touched with the side of the suction and cauterized with the help of a monopolar cautery thereby sealing off the blood vessel (Figs 17.5 and 17.6).

Endoscopic cauterization has several advantages. In addition to confirming the bleeding site, other nasal pathologies if present can be identified simultaneously. There is no trauma to the surrounding mucosa, the complications of

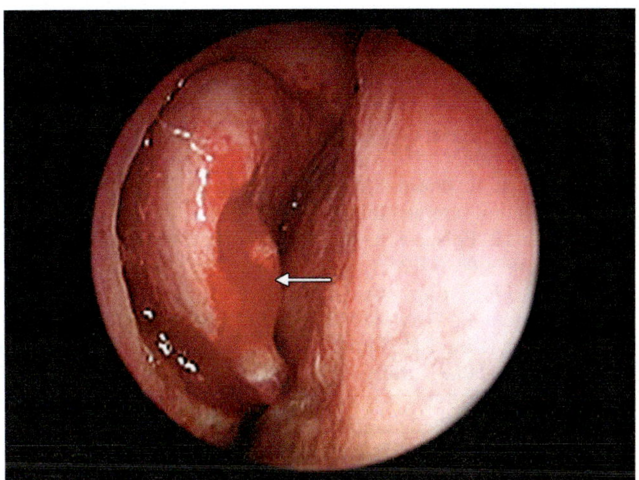

Fig. 17.5: Bleeding from the middle turbinate localized with diagnostic nasal endoscopy

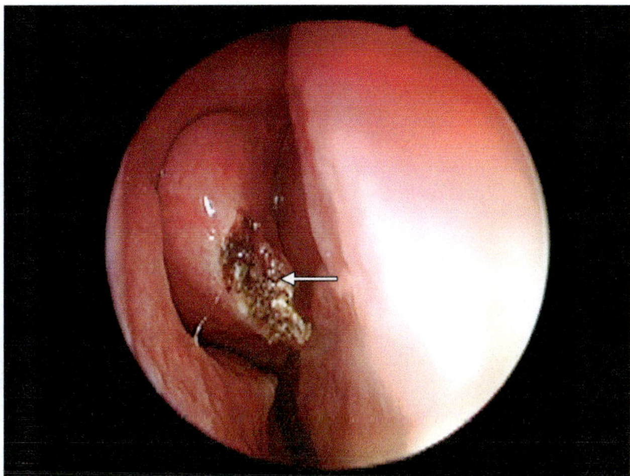

Fig. 17.6: Bleeding points on the middle turbinate cauterized

nasal packing are avoided and the duration of the hospital stay is also shorter.

ENDOSCOPIC LIGATION OF SPHENOPALATINE ARTERY

In cases refractory to attempts of endoscopic electrocauterization, recurrent intermittent posterior epistaxis, as well as intractable posterior epistaxis, endoscopic ligation of the SPA is reserved as an option. The procedure of SPA ligation was first described in 1992 by Budrovich and Saetti[10] and majority of large studies report success rates of around 90%.[11] This has in fact been shown to be the most effective and cost-efficient definitive treatment for posterior epistaxis.[12]

The procedure which was initially done under general anesthesia has now been described under local anesthesia[13] keeping in mind the co-morbid conditions of the group of patients requiring this procedure. A greater palatine foramen block may be combined with local anesthetic infiltration into the lateral wall of the middle meatus near the posterior end of the middle turbinate prior to the procedure.

The procedure of pterygopalatine fossa infiltration through the greater palatine foramen has been described by PJ Wormald.[14] The foramen is identified by transoral palpation of the hard palate in line with the third molar tooth. A 25G needle is bent to an angle of 45 degrees approximately 2.5 cm from its tip and is used to inject 2 mL of 2% lignocaine with adrenaline 1:80,000 solution into the foramen. Immediate blanching of the hemipalate confirms accurate placement of the needle and subsequent vasoconstriction. Thakkar and Sharan have also advocated infiltration of a high volume injection of saline

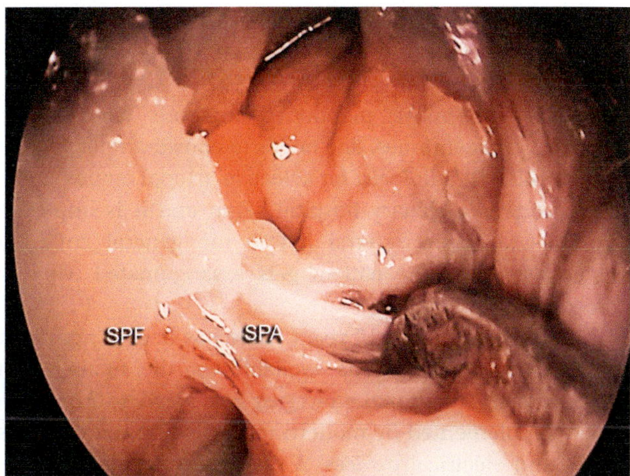

Fig. 17.7: Endoscopic view showing the sphenopalatine artery (SPA) exiting from the sphenopalatine foramen (SPF)

(3 mL) at the same site to pressure tamponade the vessel.[15] Under endoscopic guidance 2 mL of the same local anesthetic solution is injected with a 25G spinal needle in the lateral nasal wall in the middle meatus just in front of the posterior end of the middle turbinate. An incision is made in the lateral wall 1 cm anterior to the posterior attachment of the middle turbinate. A mucosal flap is raised and the ethmoidal crest is identified alongwith the SPA as it exits the sphenopalatine foramen (Fig. 17.7). The artery is ligated using metal clips or is alternatively cauterized with a bipolar cautery (Fig. 17.8). The mucosal flap is then replaced. Some authors advocate bilateral SPA ligation with or without anterior ethmoidal artery ligation for the treatment of intractable epistaxis that

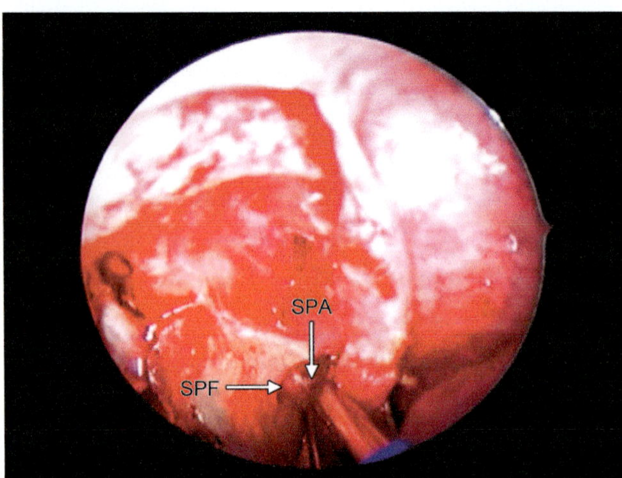

Fig. 17.8: Sphenopalatine artery cauterized with bipolar cautery

has failed conventional nasal packing.[16] Complications are minor and include increased nasal crusting and palatal numbness.[17]

If all the above mentioned methods fail and the epistaxis still continues, one needs to consider referral to an interventional radiologist for selective arterial embolization. This requires a tertiary hospital setup and it is important to make a timely referral before the general condition deteriorates and the patient gets exsanguinated with the bleeding.

Thus over the past 10 years, there has been a significant expansion in the options available for the management of epistaxis. Traditional strategies like nasal packing have been supplemented by modern technology using the latest optic and electrical devices. A stepwise management plan has to be followed while treating these patients. The treating surgeon should aim toward reducing patient morbidity as well as hospital stay. Newer options of endoscopic electrocauterization which limit patient morbidity and complications must be considered. Endoscopic ligation/cauterization of SPA is a feasible option for recurrent and intractable posterior epistaxis. All these procedures have now been standardized and are not only safe, but also successful and effective management options for the treatment of this commonly occurring ENT emergency.

REFERENCES

1. Petruson B, Rudin R. The frequency of epistaxis in a male population sample. Rhinology. 1975;13:129-33.
2. Juselius H. Epistaxis. A clinical study of 1,724 patients. J Laryngol Otol. 1974;88:317-27.
3. Pope LE, Hobbs CG. Epistaxis: an update on current management. Postgrad Med J. 2005;81:309-14.
4. Lee HY, Kim HU, Kim SS, et al. Surgical anatomy of the sphenopalatine artery in lateral nasal wall. Laryngoscope. 2002;112:1813-8.
5. Wareing MJ, Padgham ND. Osteologic classification of the sphenopalatine foramen. Laryngoscope. 1998;108:125-7.
6. Thaha MA, Nilssen EL, Holland S, et al. Routine coagulation screening in the management of emergency admission for epistaxis—is it necessary? J Laryngol Otol. 2000;114:38-403.
7. Elwany S, Kamel T, Mekhamer A. Pneumatic nasal catheters: Advantages and drawbacks. J Laryngol Otol. 1986;100:641-7.
8. Schaitkin B, Strauss M, Hounck JR. Epistaxis: medical versus surgical therapy, a comparison of efficacy, complications and economic considerations. Laryngoscope. 1987;97:1392-5.
9. Shaw CB, Wax MK, Wetmore SJ. Epistaxis: a comparison of treatment. Otolaryngol Head Neck Surg. 1993;109:60-5.
10. Budrovich R, Saetti R. Microscopic and endoscopic ligature of the sphenopalatine artery. Laryngoscope. 1992;102:1391-4.
11. Feusi B, Holzman D, Steuer J. Posterior epistaxis: systematic review of the effectiveness of surgical therapies. Rhinology. 2005;43:300-04.
12. Douglas R, Wormald PJ. Update on epistaxis. Curr Opin Otolaryngol Head Neck Surg. 2007;15:180-3.
13. Jonas N, Viani L, Walsh M. Sphenopalatine artery ligation under local anesthesia: A report of two cases and review of the literature. Local Reg Anesth. 2010;3:1-4.
14. Wormald PJ, Athanasiadis T, Rees G, et al. An evaluation of effect of pterygopalatine fossa injection with local anaesthetic and adrenalin in the control of nasal bleeding during endoscopic sinus surgery. Am J Rhinol. 2005;19:288-92.
15. Thakar A, Sharan CJ. Endoscopic sphenopalatine artery ligation for refractory posterior epistaxis. Indian J Otolaryngol Head Neck Surg. 2005;57(4):301-3.
16. Asanau A, Timoshenko AP, Vercherin P, et al. Sphenopalatine and anterior ethmoidal artery ligation for severe epistaxis. Ann Otol Rhinol Laryngol. 2009;118(9):639-44.
17. Snyderman CH, Goldman SA, Carrau RL, et al. Endoscopic sphenopalatine artery ligation is an effective method of treatment of posterior epistaxis. Am J Rhinol. 1999;13:137-40.

CHAPTER 18

Juvenile Nasopharyngeal Angiofibroma

Renuka Bradoo, Milind V Kirtane, Anagha Joshi

INTRODUCTION

Juvenile nasopharyngeal angiofibroma (JNA) is a highly vascular, histologically benign yet locally aggressive head and neck tumor. It is a slow growing tumor which originates from the posterior nasal and nasopharyngeal region in adolescent males. It has been variously described as juvenile fibroma, angioma, angiofibroma, fibroangioma and bleeding fibroma of adolescence. Its management continues to be a challenge because of its vascularity and its propensity to grow through narrow bony crevices along the base skull with intracranial and intraorbital extension. This often makes complete excision of the tumor difficult, resulting in the often reported recurrences.

The first description of JNA probably dates to the fourth century BC when Hippocrates first observed nasal polyps. It was only in 1847 that Chelius described JNA as "a tumor which commonly occurred in a person about the time of puberty". Friedberg first used the term angiofibroma in 1940.[1] The first successful excision of a probable JNA is credited to Liston in 1841 at University College Hospital in London.

EPIDEMIOLOGY

Juvenile nasopharyngeal angiofibroma (JNA) accounts for 0.05–0.5% of all head and neck tumors.[2,3] The most common age group is 10–18 years, with an average age of around 14 years.[4] The youngest case reported in literature was a newborn infant.[5] Fu et al. have reported a case of JNA in a 79-year-old man.[6] JNA occurs almost exclusively in males and rarely occurs in females. The highest incidence of 16% in female patients was reported by Handousa in Egypt.[7] Chromosomal studies are advised in these patients.

ETIOPATHOGENESIS

In spite of the numerous theories proposed to explain the origin of JNA, the exact histogenesis of the tumor remains debatable. The tumor is most commonly believed to arise at the site where the sphenoidal process of the palatine bone articulates with the base of the sphenoid and the horizontal ala of the vomer.[8] This area forms the superior border of the sphenopalatine foramen and lies just above the posterior end of the middle turbinate.

Speculations on the tissue's origin were first made in the 19th century by Nelaton,[9] Verneuil,[10] and Tillaux,[11] who defined angiofibromas as fibrous neoplasms arising from periosteum or embryonic fibrocartilage of the skull base. Authors such as Martin et al.[12] and Dane[13] focused on a hormonal imbalance as the cause of these tumors. In 1942, Brunner,[14] described endothelium-lined vascular spaces in the fascia basalis and proposed that angiofibromas originated from this tissue. Similarities to nasal erectile tissue were noted by Osborn.[15] Schiff[16] suggested that angiofibroma was ectopic vascular tissue that grew as a result of alterations in pituitary activity. Maurice and Milad,[17] interpreted angiofibromas as hamartomas resulting from misplaced genital erectile tissue. In addition to these two main theories of either fibrous or vascular origin, many other hypotheses have been proposed. One such theory proposes that these tumors originate from non-chromaffin paraganglionic cells present at the terminal end of the maxillary artery.[18]

The last decade has seen numerous studies being conducted in an attempt to understand the underlying deranged molecular mechanisms which lead to the formation of this tumor, most commonly in adolescent boys. Immunocytochemical techniques have shown androgen receptors in both vascular and stromal elements of the tumor. In contrast, few progesterone receptors and no estrogen receptors have been found.

The role of factors such as transforming growth factor (TGF-β1) and vascular endothelial growth factor (VEGF) has been studied.[19] Nagaii et al. found that transforming growth factor (TGF) β1 and IGF-II show statistically increased expression in these tumors than in controls suggesting that they may be growth regulators of nasopharyngeal angiofibromas. It is thought that the over expression of IGF-II might be associated with a tendency to recurrence and poorer prognosis.[20] Mutations in the adenomatous polyposis coli (APC) gene on chromosome 5q might be involved in the pathogenesis of sporadic juvenile angiofibromas. Platelet derived growth factor (PDGF-B) can contribute, at least in part to neovascularization and fibrosis.[21]

Recent evidence suggests that angiofibromas are extra-colonic manifestations of familial adenomatous polyposis.[22,23] JNA has been reported to occur more commonly among patients with familial adenomatous polyposis (FAP), suggesting that it is a true neoplasm with alterations of the APC/β-catenin pathway.[24]

Schick et al. studied sex chromosome structure in JNA. They found a significant loss of chromosome Y in combination with a gain of chromosome X.[25]

Even as an extensive research to discover the etiological factor(s) in this tumor continues, a widely accepted theory of origin is yet to be established.

PATHOLOGY

On gross examination the tumor is a soft to firm, lobulated, non-encapsulated mass which is pinkish red in color. It has a broad, sessile base in the posterior part of the nasal cavity and the nasopharynx. The consistency and friability of the tumor depends on the relative percentage of vascular to fibrous tissue within it, which may vary in individual tumors. It is generally noted, that the fibrous component and nodularity increases with increase in age of the patient.

Microscopically, the tumor is composed of thin walled vessels of varying caliber interspersed in a mature connective tissue stroma. The vessels typically have a single endothelial cell lining without a muscularis layer (Fig. 18.1). This explains the propensity of the tumor to bleed profusely as the vessels do not constrict on being cut. The tumor cells show features of both fibroblasts and smooth muscle cells and are termed as myofibroblasts.

MODE OF SPREAD

The tumor usually originates where the palatine bone articulates with the body of the sphenoid to form the sphenopalatine foramen. It has a propensity to grow through narrow bony crevices along the base skull widening fissures and foramina without destroying the underlying bone. Large tumors are frequently bilobed or dumbbell-shaped, with one portion of the tumor filling the nasopharynx and the other portion extending through the pterygopalatine fossa into the infra temporal fossa (Fig. 18.2).

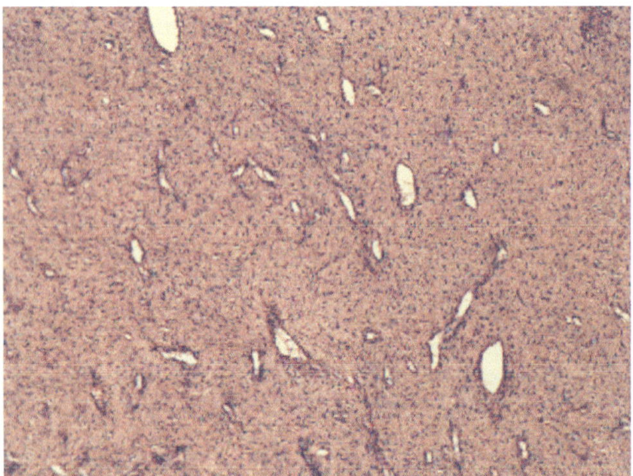

Fig. 18.1: Histological section (H & E, original magnification × 100) showing vascular channels of varying caliber amidst dense fibrocollagenous stroma

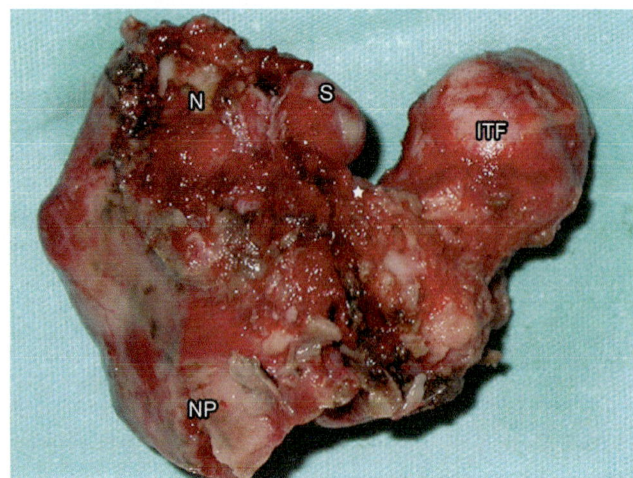

Fig. 18.2: Postoperative tumor specimen showing tumor extensions (N-nasal; NP-nasopharyngeal; S-intrasphenoid; ITF-infratemporal; *-site of sphenopalatine foramen)

The tumor extends medially into the nasal cavity. It then extends anteriorly for a variable distance but more often extends posteriorly under the nasopharyngeal mucous membrane into the nasopharynx. A large nasopharyngeal component may also block the posterior choana of the opposite nostril and push the soft palate downwards.

Superior growth takes place into the sphenoid sinus by erosion of its floor. Here it tends to remain in the submucosal plane. The cavernous sinus may become invaded if the tumor erodes the lateral wall of the sinus.

Lateral spread involves the pterygopalatine fossa causing anterior bowing of the posterior wall of the maxillary sinus. Extension into the maxillary sinus itself is infrequent. It can continue to grow laterally into the infratemporal fossa. The tumor may directly erode the greater wing of sphenoid or widen and pass through the foramen ovale to enter the cranial cavity lateral to the cavernous sinus.

From the pterygopalatine fossa it can pass through the inferior orbital fissure to enter the orbit. When the orbital apex is involved the tumor may extend through the superior orbital fissure to involve the cavernous sinus. Intracranial spread is usually extradural and can occur through the superior orbital fissure, lateral wall of the sphenoid sinus or the greater wing of the sphenoid.

Extranasopharyngeal angiofibroma is extremely rare and generally occurs in older patients and females where it tends to be less vascular and aggressive. There have been reports of angiofibromas on the nasal septum, middle turbinate, hard palate and alveolar ridge.[26-29]

Spontaneous regression of the tumor remains a debatable issue and has been reported in residual tumors.[30,31]

CLASSIFICATION

There are numerous classifications described in literature. However, the Andrew-Fisch classification[32] and Radkowski (revised Sessions) classification[33] are particularly useful in planning management protocols and predicting prognosis.

Andrew-Fisch Classification (1989)

Stage I: Tumor limited to the nasopharynx and nasal cavity. Bone destruction is negligible or limited to the sphenopalatine foramen.

Stage II: Tumor involving the pterygopalatine fossa or the maxillary, ethmoid or sphenoid sinus with bone destruction.

Stage IIIa: Tumor involving the infratemporal fossa or orbital region without intracranial involvement

Stage IIIb: Tumor involving the infratemporal fossa or orbital region with intracranial, extradural (parasellar) involvement.

Stage IVa: Intracranial, intradural tumor without infiltration of cavernous sinus, pituitary fossa or optic chiasma.

Stage IVb: Intracranial intradural tumor with infiltration of cavernous sinus, pituitary fossa or optic chiasma.

Radkowski Classification

Stage Ia: Tumor limited to posterior nares and/or nasopharyngeal vault.

Stage Ib: Extension into one or more paranasal sinuses.

Stage IIa: Minimal lateral extension into the pterygopalatine fossa.

Stage IIb: Full occupation of the pterygopalatine fossa with or without superior erosion of orbital bones.

Stage IIc: Extension into the infra temporal fossa or extension posterior to pterygoid plates.

Stage IIIa: Erosion of the base skull (middle cranial fossa/base of pterygoids).

Stage IIIb: Erosion of skull base with extensive intracranial extension with or without extension into the cavernous sinus.

BLOOD SUPPLY

The tumor is always supplied by the ipsilateral maxillary artery, but as it grows, it develops blood supply from other adjacent structures and blood vessels, including branches of the internal carotid artery (ICA). Other major feeding vessels are the maxillary artery of the opposite side and the ascending pharyngeal artery. There may also be a feeding artery from the vidian canal. ICA supply is seen in tumors involving the basisphenoid and sphenoid sinus, in tumors with an intracranial component or in recurrent tumors where the external carotid artery has been ligated during the first surgery.

CLINICAL FEATURES

Unilateral nasal obstruction and epistaxis in a young male patient are the hallmarks of this disease. The epistaxis is profuse, recurrent in nature and usually from one nostril. The patient may present with anemia. The degree of nasal obstruction depends on the size of the tumor. A large nasopharyngeal extension can cause snoring, mouth breathing, adenoid facies, rhinolalia clausa and signs of eustachian tube dysfunction, such as blocking of ears, otalgia and a conductive hearing loss. The patient may also have a sense of heaviness on one side of the face though headache is not very common.

A small tumor extension into the pterygopalatine fossa or infratemporal fossa does not cause any specific symptoms. However, a large mass may present with a bulge in the cheek and proptosis if the orbit is involved (Fig. 18.3).

Intracranial involvement is also usually asymptomatic and is detected only on radiological investigations. However, a case of meningitis, diabetes insipidus, proptosis and ptosis has been noted by the authors (Bradoo, Joshi) due to involvement of the meninges, compression of the pituitary gland and involvement of the orbit and cavernous sinus. Symptoms suggestive of direct neural involvement such as blindness are very rare. The authors have noted two such cases.

DIAGNOSIS

A preliminary diagnosis can usually be made on the basis of the history and clinical examination of the patient. A nasal endoscopy helps confirm the diagnosis (Fig. 18.4).

Plain X-rays of the paranasal sinuses show anterior bowing of the posterior wall of the maxillary sinus (Holman-Miller sign) and increase in the maxilla-coronoid distance (Handousa sign). However, they do not have any place in today's diagnostic armamentarium. A CT scan of the paranasal sinuses with contrast is the gold standard for the diagnosis of JNA. The enhancement and mode of spread of the tumor is characteristic. Both axial and coronal cuts with bony and soft tissue windows are necessary to evaluate the tumor in detail. Sagittal reconstructions may further help in understanding the three-dimensional spread of the tumor along the base skull (Figs 18.5A to C).

An MRI study reveals a lobulated tumor of variable signal intensity on T2 weighted images, often appearing relatively hypointense because of its fibrous tissue content. This differentiates it from the high intensity signal of sinus secretions. Prominent vascularity is seen as flow voids within the tumor, with intense enhancement on both CT and MR images. An MRI is essential in case of an intracranial extension

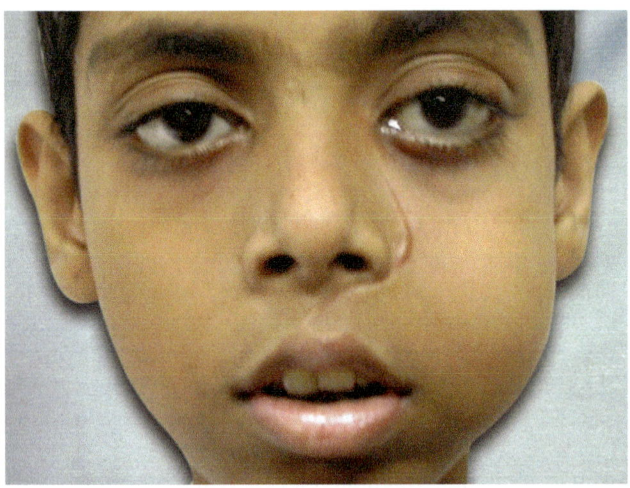

Fig. 18.3: Patient of JNA presenting with a bulge on the cheek and a facial scar from previous surgery

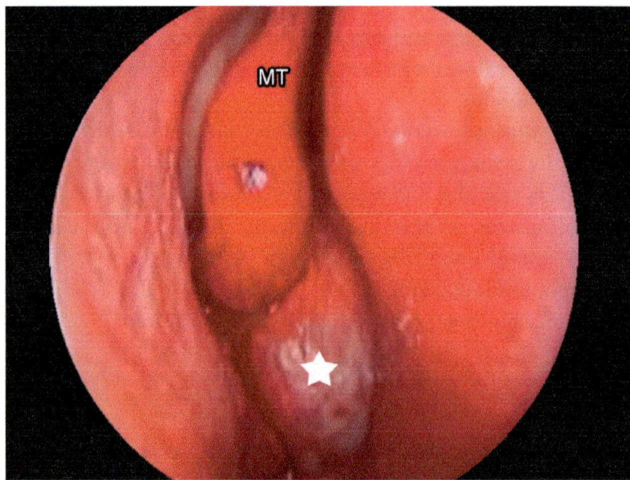

Fig. 18.4: Endoscopic picture of the tumor (*) in the right nasal cavity medial to the middle turbinate (MT)

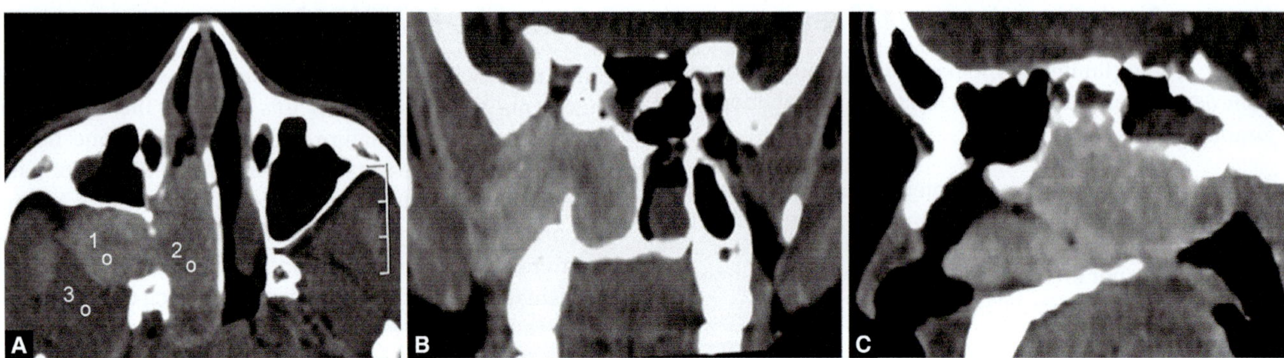

Figs 18.5A to C: Contrast-enhanced axial (A), coronal (B), sagittal (C) CT scans showing characteristic mode of spread of tumor

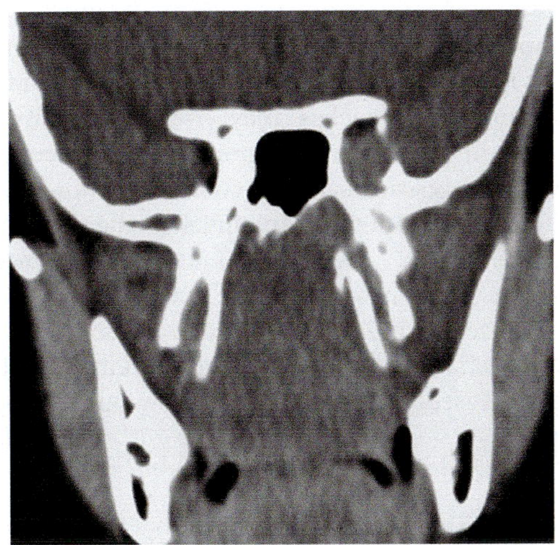

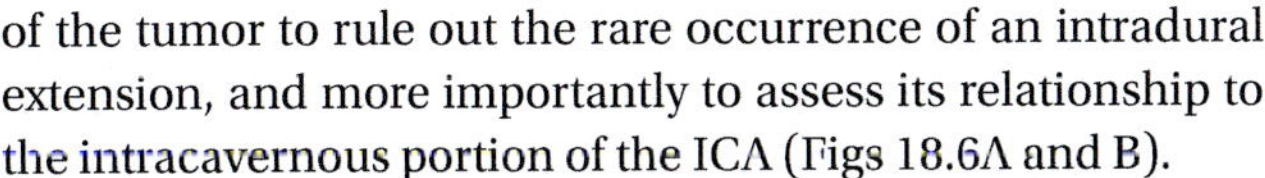

Fig. 18.6A: CT scan showing involvement of the cavernous sinus

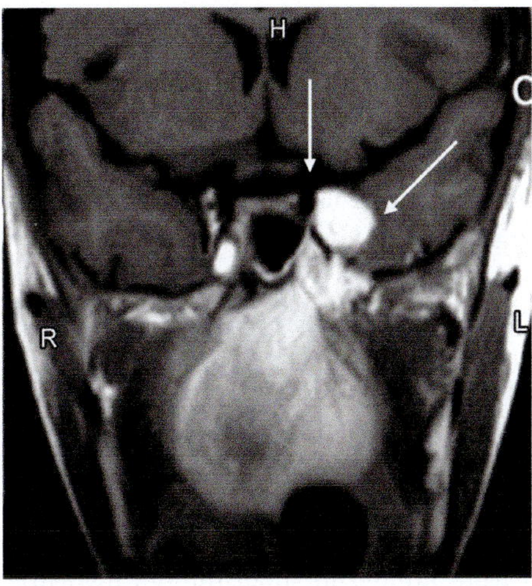

Fig. 18.6B: MRI scan showing relationship of the tumor to internal carotid artery (ICA) within the cavernous sinus and the extradural nature of the tumor

of the tumor to rule out the rare occurrence of an intradural extension, and more importantly to assess its relationship to the intracavernous portion of the ICA (Figs 18.6A and B).

The MRI may also help to better delineate the tumor in case of extensive involvement of the infratemporal fossa and orbit.

An MR angiography is useful in intracavernous extensions of the tumor. It helps to diagnose compression or encasement of the ICA by the tumor.

Although MR angiography has the advantage of being a non-invasive procedure, it cannot replace digital subtraction angiography (DSA) which is necessary to delineate feeder vessels and to selectively, embolize them. Angiography demonstrates an intense tumor blush with arterial supply via branches of the internal maxillary, ascending pharyngeal, and palatine arteries. The anastomotic connections between the internal and external carotid arteries are frequently enlarged and this has to be taken into account when performing preoperative embolization.

The characteristic CT and angiographic appearances usually obviate the need for a biopsy. Due to the risk of hemorrhage, a biopsy is advisable only in those cases where the histopathological diagnosis seems doubtful, e.g. in the rare event of a female patient of JNA. The evaluation of the patient is not complete without an otoscopy, tuning fork tests, evaluation of the central nervous system (CNS) and an ophthalmological examination.

TREATMENT

The management of JNA has always been a formidable challenge. Various modes of management such as surgery, hormone therapy, radiotherapy using either external beam radiation or gamma knife, cryotherapy and electrocoagulation have been tried. However, surgery remains the mainstay and treatment of choice for JNA.

Surgical Management

Various open surgical approaches such as transpalatal, lateral rhinotomy, Weber Fergusson, midfacial degloving, maxillary swing, facial translocation, transhyoid and transmandibular have been used to resect the tumor. The description of so many surgical approaches in literature bears testimony to the fact that no single approach has been found ideal for the management of all stages of the tumor.

The basic underlying surgical principles for removal of this tumor are: wide exposure of the tumor, subperiosteal dissection, and en bloc removal.

Open Surgical Approaches

Three of the most preferred open approaches are the Weber Fergusson, transpalatal and the midfacial degloving approach.

The transpalatal approach[34] offers good exposure of the nasopharynx and the posterior nasal cavity. The advantage of this approach is absence of an external scar, however, large lateral extensions are difficult to access. One of the complications of this approach is a palatal perforation.

The Weber Fergusson incision is an extension of the lateral rhinotomy approach. The advantage is that it offers a good exposure of the lateral limit of the tumor. Its major disadvantage is a disfiguring facial scar. It also offers only a unilateral approach to the tumor. Anesthesia of the cheek is a frequent occurrence with this approach.

The midfacial degloving approach[35,36] gives a wide bilateral exposure to the nasal cavity, nasopharynx and the infratemporal fossa. This approach is one of the only open approaches that offers a very wide exposure of the tumor bed without leaving a facial scar. It can occasionally cause vestibular stenosis.

Endoscopic Approach

Endoscopic excision of JNA was first described by Kamel.[37] With better imaging studies, safer and selectively targeted embolization, better optics and increasing surgical experience, endoscopic excision of angiofibromas is now an accepted modality of treatment (Figs 18.7A and B). Initial endoscopic attempts were limited to small tumors involving the nose, nasopharynx with minimal involvement of infratemporal fossa. However, a number of tertiary referral centers across the world are now reporting endoscopic excision of much larger tumors.

The authors' (Bradoo, Joshi) experience of endoscopic excision in 91 cases includes successful removal of tumors with intraorbital and intracranial extensions with or without cavernous sinus involvement.

Embolization of the tumor is a prerequisite to endoscopic excision. This significantly decreases the blood loss and makes for better visualization with the endoscope. Newer techniques of embolization make use of microcatheters and very fine polyvinyl alcohol (PVA) particles (150–250 µm). This ensures a more distal and selective embolization of the tumor bed thus reducing the risk of complications (Figs 18.8A and B). There is no clear consensus on the interval between embolization and surgery and it varies from 24 to 72 hours. The authors prefer a minimum period of 48 hours.

Although the long-term outcomes are yet to be analyzed, there is increasing evidence that endoscopic/endoscope-assisted open approaches may overcome many of the limitations of conventional approaches. Endoscopy allows meticulous subperiosteal dissection of tumor extensions under direct vision thus minimizing the possibility of recurrence. Blood loss is minimum requiring fewer transfusions. Tight nasal packs are not necessary and hence postoperative morbidity is significantly decreased. There is no facial disfigurement. It lessens the duration of hospital stay and endoscopic monitoring on follow-up of the patient is possible.

Radiotherapy

Radiotherapy arrests the growth of the tumor, and this stabilization may take two to three years. Although reduction in size of the tumor is seen, residual tumor persists. Certain centers[38] advocate radiation therapy as a primary modality of treatment. The authors believe that this is too radical an approach for benign tumors in young patients; especially where an accepted alternative mode of treatment is available. The long-term complications of radiotherapy may be far worse than the disease itself, viz. growth retardation, panhypopituitarism, temporal lobe necrosis, cataracts, radiation keratopathy, skin, thyroid and nasopharyngeal malignancies and sarcomatous transformation of the tumor. Radiation treatment should therefore be reserved for unresectable, residual or recurrent tumors. A dose of 3600–4000 cGy in 14–16 fractions is given over 3–6 weeks. Modern techniques such as intensity modulated radiation therapy (IMRT) should increase the efficacy and safety of this treatment. Targeted radiation with a Gamma knife can be

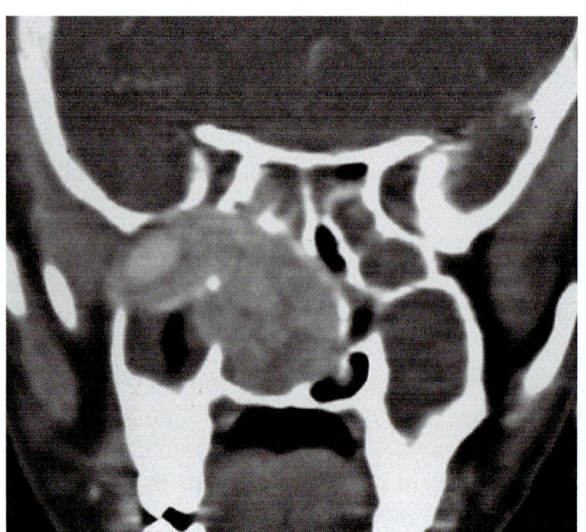

Fig. 18.7A: Preoperative CT scan of patient showing tumor with its extensions

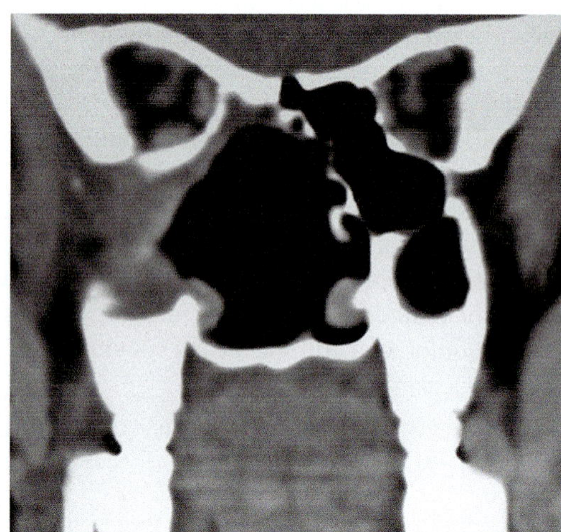

Fig. 18.7B: Postoperative CT scan of same patient after endoscopic excision showing complete removal of tumor

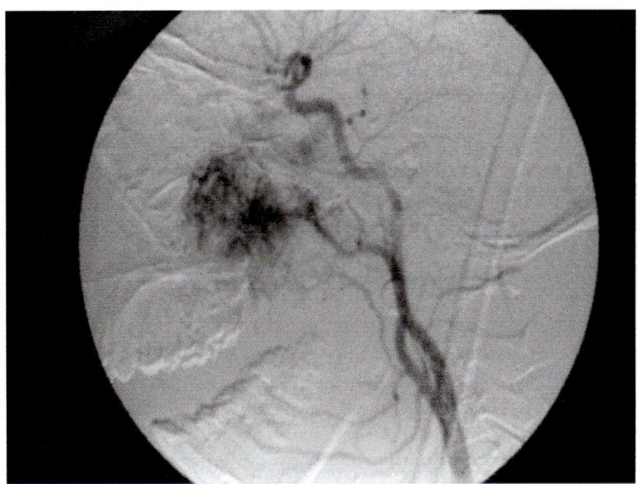

Fig. 18.8A: *Digital subtraction angiography:* Pre-embolization tumor blush

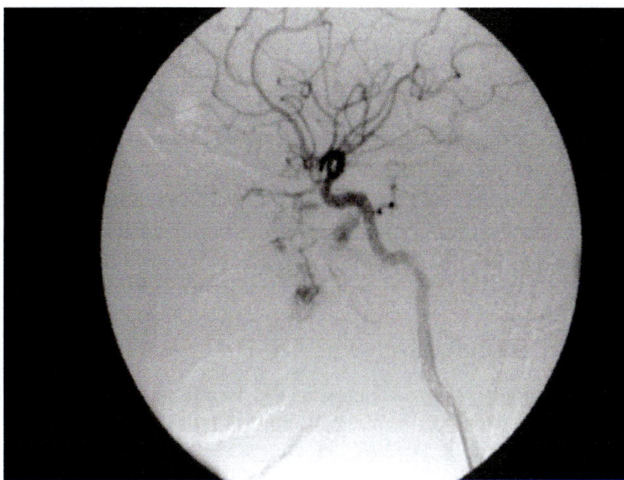

Fig. 18.8B: *Post-embolization film:* Absence of tumor blush

given for residual intracranial tumors. Long-term results on this therapy are awaited.

Medical Treatment

There is no established medical line of treatment available which has conclusively proved effective against JNA, although hormonal therapy has been empirically used. Response of the tumor to both androgens and estrogens has been demonstrated and may be useful in decreasing the vascularity of tumor just prior to surgery. They have also been used as adjunctive therapy in recurrent and inoperable tumors.[39,40] In the light of suggested androgen dependence of JNA, anti-androgen drugs like cyproterone acetate have been used as it has a dual anti-androgenic effect of target organ inhibition and suppression of plasma testosterone. Hormone therapy should be restricted only to tumors not resectable by surgery, as administration of these drugs, particularly during puberty, can significantly interfere with psychophysical development of the patient.

The authors believe that cryotherapy, electrocoagulation, embolization alone and injection of sclerosing agents, though described in literature, do not play a significant role in the management of JNA.

COMPLICATIONS

Severe hemorrhage, intracranial involvement and recurrence are the most common complications of JNA. Facial disfigurement due to swelling in the cheek or temporal region, proptosis and diplopia are also commonly seen. Much rarer complications include panhypopituitarism, meningitis, blindness and superior orbital fissure syndrome.

Surgery of the tumor is also not without risks. Minor sequelae include palatal perforation, paresthesias of the face, vestibular stenosis, nasal synechie and epiphora. More serious complications include severe hemorrhage from the tumor itself, the cavernous sinus or rarely the ICA, cranial nerve injuries and dural tears with cerebrospinal fluid (CSF) leaks. These complications are rare and more likely to occur in non-embolized, extensive tumors (Stage IV).

PROGNOSIS

Recent advances in technology such as better imaging techniques, use of the endoscope, and selective embolization of the tumor have played a significant role in improving the prognosis of these tumors.

There are various factors which directly "impact" the long-term prognosis in these patients. A primary tumor has a far better prognosis than a previously operated one. Recurrence rates of 55% in extensive tumors,[41,42] 25% in moderate site tumors[43] and 15% in small tumors[44] have been quoted. However, in the authors' experience, mere size of the tumor is not the only prognostic factor. The regions involved also play a major role in deciding the prognosis. Certain sites like the superior orbital fissure and the cavernous sinus are more difficult to approach and there is greater chance of recurrence if these areas are involved. A large intracranial component would naturally worsen the prognosis. Very friable tumors and those with a significant residual post-embolization blush are also difficult to manage. A previous history of early recurrence with rapid regrowth of the tumor suggests an aggressive lesion.

Certain surgical factors also affect prognosis. A relatively bloodless surgery, where all the extensions of the tumor have been dissected under direct vision and delivered en bloc, has a good prognosis with a low chance of recurrence. Good preoperative planning to decide on a customized treatment plan in every individual case also goes a long way in improving the prognosis.

Finally, the key to the decisive management of this enigmatic tumor may lie with understanding its molecular biology and etiopathogenesis.

REFERENCES

1. Friedberg SA. Nasopharyngeal Fibroma. Arch Otolaryngol. 1940;31:313-26.
2. Sivanandan R, Fee WE. Benign and malignant tumours of the nasopharynx. In: Cummings CW, Flint FW, Harker LA, et al. (Eds). Cummings otolaryngology head and neck Surgery, 4th edition. New York: Elsevier, Mosby; 2005. pp. l669-972.
3. Batsaki's JG. Tumours of the Head and Neck: Clinical and Pathological Considerations, 2nd edition. Baltimore: Williams & Wilkins; 1979. pp. 296-300.
4. Bensch H, Ewing J. Neoplastic diseases, 4th edition. Philadelphia: WB Saunders and Company; 1941.
5. Chaikovski VK. Angifibroma of the nose in a 14-day-old infant girl. Zh Ushn Nos Gorl Bolezn. 1967;27:103-4.
6. Fu YS, Perzin KH. Non epithelial tumours of the nasal cavity, paranasal sinuses, and nasopharynx; a clinicopathologic study. I: General features and vascular tumours. Cancer. 1974;33:1275-88.
7. Handousa F, Farid H, Elwi AM. Nasopharyngeal fibroma: a clinico-pathological study of seventy cases. J Laryngol Otol. 1954;68:647-66.
8. Neel HB, Whicker JH, Devine KD, et al. Juvenile Angiofibroma: review of 120 cases. Am J Surg. 1973;126:547-76.
9. Nelatori M. Polype fibreux de la base du crane: considerations generales. Gaz Hop. 1853; 26:22.
10. Verneuil V. Seances de la Societe de Chirurgie de Paris pendant l'annee. 1860. Bull Soc Chir. 1861.
11. Tillaux P. Traite danatomie topographique avec applications a la chirugie, edition 2. Paris: P Asselin. 1878.pp.348-9.
12. Martin H, Ehrlich HE, Abels JC. Juvenile nasopharyngeal angiofibroma. Ann Surg. 1948;127:513-36.
13. Dane WH. Juvenile nasopharyngeal fibroma in state of regression. Ann Otol Rhinol Laryngol. 1954;63:997-1014.
14. Brunner H. Nasopharyngeal angiofibroma. Ann Otol Rhinol Laryngol. 1942;51:29-65.
15. Osborn DA. The so called juvenile angiofibroma of the nasopharynx. J Laryngol Otol. 1959;73:295-316.
16. Schiff M. Juvenile nasopharyngeal angiofibroma: a theory of pathogenesis. Laryngoscope. 1959;69:981-1016.
17. Maurice M, Milad M. Pathogenesis of juvenile nasopharyngeal fibroma. J Laryngol Otol. 1981;95:1121-6.
18. Girgis ICH, Fahmy SA. Nasopharyngeal fibroma: its histopathological nature. J Laryngol Otol. 1973;87:1107-23.
19. Ferrara N, Houck K, Jakeman L, et al. Molecular and biological properties of the vascular endothelial growth factor family of proteins. Endocr Rev. 1992;13:18-32.
20. Coutinho-Camilfo CM, Brentani MM, Butugan O, et al. Relaxation of imprinting of IGF II gene in juvenile nasopharyngeal angiofibromas. Diagn Mol Pathol. 2003;12:57-62.
21. Nagai MA, Butugan O, Logullo A, et al. Expression of growth factors, proto oncogenes and p-53 in nasopharyngeal angiofibromas. Laryngoscope. 1996;106:190-5.
22. Ferouz AS, Mohr RM, Paul P. Juvenile nasopharyngeal angiofibroma and familial adenomatous polyposis: an association? Otolaryngol Head Neck Surg. 1995;113:435-9.
23. Giardiello FM, Hamilton SR, Krush AJ, et al. Nasopharyngeal angiofibroma in patients with familial adenomatous polyposis. Gastroenterology. 1993;105:1550-2.
24. Abraham SC, Montgomery EA, Giardiello FM, et al. Frequent β-catenin mutations in Juvenile Nasopharyngeal Angiofibromas. Am J Pathol. 2001;158:1073-8.
25. Schick B, Rippel C, Brunner C, et al. Numerical sex chromosome aberrations in juvenile angiofibromas: genetic evidence for an androgen dependant tumour? Oncol Rep. 2003;10:1251-5.
26. Capodiferro S, Favia G, Lacaita MG, et al. Juvenile angiofibroma: report of a case with primary intraoral presentation. Oral Oncol Extra. 2005;41:1-6.
27. Antoniades K, Antoniades DZ, Antoniades V. Juvenile angiofibroma: report of a case with intraoral presentation. Oral Surg Oral Med Oral Pathol Oral Radiol Endod. 2002;94(2):228-32.
28. Handa KK, Kumar A, Singh MK, et al. Extranasopharyngeal angiofibroma arising from nasal septum. Int J Pediatr Otorhinolaryngol. 2001;58;163-6.
29. Huang RY, Damrose EJ, Blackwell Ke, et al. Extranasopharyngeal angiofibroma. Int J Pediatr Otorhinolaryngol. 2000;56(1):59-64.
30. Neel HB, Whicker JH, Devine KD, et al. Juvenile Angiofibroma: Review of 120 Cases. Am J Surg. 1973;126:547-58.
31. Stansbie JM, Phelps PD. Involution of residual juvenile nasopharyngeal angiofibroma (a case report). J Laryngol Otol. 1986;100:599-603.
32. Andrews JC, Fisch U, Valvanis A, et al. The surgical management of extensive nasopharyngeal angiofibromas with the infratemporal fossa approach. Laryngoscope. 1989;99:429-37.
33. Radkowski D, Mcgill T, Healy GB, et al. Angiofibroma: changes in staging and treatment. Arch Otolaryngol Head Neck Surg. 1996;122:122-9.
34. Wilson CP. Observations on the surgery of the nasopharynx. Ann Otol Rhinol Laryngol. 1957;66:5-40.
35. Casson PR, Bonaro PC, Converse JM. The midfacial degloving procedure. Plast Reconstr Surg. 1974;53(1):102-3.
36. Conley J, Price JC. Sublabial approach to the nasal and nasopharyngeal cavities. Am J Surg. 1979;138:615-8.
37. Kamel RH. Transnasal endoscopic surgery in juvenile nasopharyngeal angiofibroma. J Laryngol Otol. 1996;110(10):962-8.
38. Briant TDR, Fitzpatrick P, Book H. The radiologic treatment of Juvenile nasopharyngeal angiofibroma. Ann Otol Rhinol Laryngol. 1970;79:1108-12.
39. Martin H, Ehrlich HE, Abels JC. Juvenile nasopharyngeal fibroma. Ann Surg. 1948;127:513-36.
40. Patterson C. Juvenile nasopharyngeal angiofibroma. Otolaryngol Clin North Am. 1973;6:839-60.
41. Economou TS, Abemayor E, Ward PH. Juvenile nasopharyngeal angiofibroma: an update of the UCLA experience, 1960-1985. Laryngoscope. 1988;98:170-5.
42. McCombe A, Lund VJ, Howard DJ. Recurrence in juvenile angiofibroma. Rhinology. 1990;28:97-102.
43. Roger G, Tran Ba Huy P, Froelich P, et al. Exclusively endoscopic removal of Juvenile Nasopharyngeal Angiofibroma. Arch Otolaryngol Head Neck Surg. 2002;128:928-35.
44. Scholtz AW, Appenroth E, Jolly KK, et al. Juvenile Nasopharyngeal Angiofibroma: Management and Therapy. Laryngoscope. 2001; 111:681-7.

CHAPTER 19

Pituitary Tumors

Nishit J Shah, Chandrashekhar E Deopujari, Gauri M Kapre

INTRODUCTION

The pituitary has been called the master gland of the body because of its central role in directing the activity of other glands.[1] The average size of the pituitary gland is 14 mm (transverse) × 8 mm (sagittal) × 6 mm (vertical).[2] It has important anatomic relations with the hypothalamus, optic nerves, cavernous sinus, carotid artery, and cranial nerves. The anterior, intermediate, and posterior lobes of the pituitary gland function as three separate endocrine organs, each characterized by distinct cell populations which secrete specific hormones. The anterior lobe secretes thyroid stimulating hormone, corticotropin, luteinizing hormone, follicle stimulating hormone, growth hormone, and prolactin. The posterior lobe releases oxytocin and antidiuretic hormone. The intermediate lobe is rudimentary in human beings but it is known to produce melanocyte stimulating hormone.

Pituitary tumors constitute around 10–15% of all intracranial neoplasms.[3] Adenomas are the most common benign epithelial tumors of the pituitary gland, malignant cell infiltration being relatively rare.[4] Characteristically, they are slow growing and mostly arise from the adenohypophysis.

These pituitary adenomas can be classified in three ways:
1. According to histology
2. According to size
3. According to function.

Histological Classification

There are two cell types encountered in the pituitary; the chromophobic cells and the chromophilic cells which may be basophilic or eosinophilic. Depending on the cell of origin the tumor will have specific secretory functions. Eosinophilic cells secrete growth hormone (GH) and prolactin, while basophilic cells secrete adrenocorticotropic hormone (ACTH), thyroid-stimulating hormone (TSH), follicle-stimulating hormone (FSH), luteinizing hormone (LH) and melanocyte-stimulating hormones (MSH). By immunohistochemical staining the secretory cells in an adenoma can be identified and the hormone produced by this adenoma can be predicted.

Classification by Size

According to the size of the adenoma they are classified as either micro-or macroadenomas.[5] Macroadenomas are more common (Fig. 19.1):
- Microadenoma   < 10 mm
- Macroadenoma   > 10 mm
- Giant adenoma extends far beyond sellar and parasellar regions.

Microadenomas are usually secretory (functional) tumors but having little impact on the visual system whereas macroadenomas cause sellar enlargement and pressure symptoms.

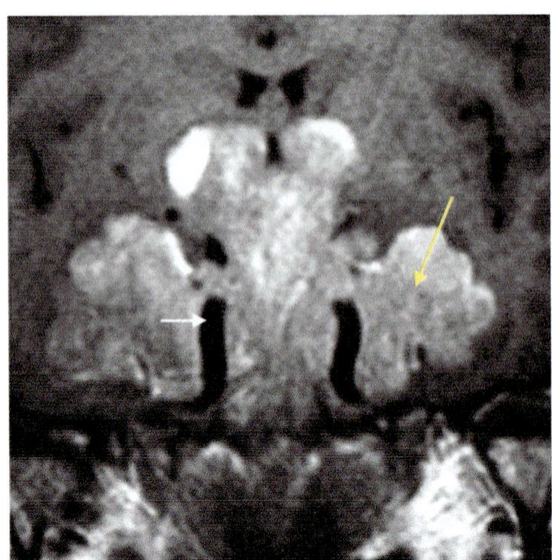

Fig. 19.1: Macroadenoma of pituitary. White arrow indicates the internal carotid artery and the yellow arrow shows the tumor extension lateral to it. It would be impossible to remove such massive parasellar extension by endoscopic approach

In the authors' series of 671 pituitary tumors (operated by the endoscopic trans-sphenoid route during a 10 years period from 2001–2010), 576 (85.84%) were macroadenomas and 95 (14.16%) were microadenomas.

Wilson[6] has given a grading system for pituitary tumors based on extrasellar extension
- *Stage 0:* No suprasellar extension
- *Stage A:* Extension into suprasellar cistern only
- *Stage B:* Extension into anterior recess of third ventricle
- *Stage C:* Obliteration of anterior recess and deformation of floor of third ventricle
- *Stage D:* Intradural extension into the anterior, middle or posterior cranial fossa
- *Stage E:* Extradural invasion into the cavernous sinus.

Classification as Per Function

Depending upon their ability to secrete hormones, pituitary tumors can also be subdivided as functioning or non-functioning adenomas. Functioning or secretory adenomas are further subdivided on the basis of the hormone they produce as:
- Prolactinomas
- GH secreting adenomas
- ACTH secreting adenomas
- TSH secreting adenomas
- Gonadotropinomas.

Nonfunctioning adenomas are said to be the most common followed by prolactinomas, GH secreting adenomas and ACTH secreting tumors.[7]

In our series, we documented 440 (65.57%) nonfunctioning tumors and 231 (34.42%) functioning tumors. Amongst the functioning tumors; 94 (40.69%) were prolactinomas, 77 (33.33%) were GH secreting tumors, 55 (23.8%) were ACTH secreting tumors, 3 (1.2%) were TSH secreting tumors and 2 (0.86%) were gonadotropinomas.

Other differential diagnosis for sellar tumors include:
- Rathke's pouch cyst
- Craniopharyngioma
- Chordoma
- Glioma
- Plasmacytoma
- Epidermoid/Dermoid cyst
- Granuloma
- Metastatic tumors.

EPIDEMIOLOGY

Pituitary tumors represent around 10–12% of all intracranial neoplasms. An overall population incidence of 0.6–2.8/100,000 has been reported with a slight female preponderance. Not infrequently, they are found as incidentalomas.[7]

CLINICAL FEATURES

A patient with a pituitary adenoma may present with symptoms associated with hormonal imbalance or due to the mass effect caused by the tumor.

Endocrine Effects

a. *Prolactinomas:* They are more common in women. These tumors typically present with amenorrhea, infertility and sometimes associated galactorrhea. In men there may be no specific symptoms other than decreased libido or potency and hence the tumors are usually of the macroadenoma variety at the time of presentation.[8] A very large adenoma may replace the entire normal adenohypophysis and patient may present with symptoms of panhypopituitarism.

b. *GH secreting tumors:* Depending on whether the hormonal imbalance starts before or after complete skeletal growth, patients present with either features of gigantism or of acromegaly. Thickening of the skin over the lip, coarse facial features with enlarged jaw, frontal skull bossing, macroglossia, enlarged hands and feet, hyperhidrosis, etc. is noted.[9] The effects of GH are insidious and thus diagnosis may be delayed. GH is an insulin antagonist and hence some patients may present with features of diabetes mellitus (DM).

c. *ACTH secreting tumors:* Patients with these tumors present with features of Cushing's syndrome such as obesity, moon face, buffalo hump, hirsutism, muscle weakness, cutaneous striae, etc. Due to the other metabolic actions of glucocorticoids, patients may suffer from hypertension or diabetes mellitus. It is noteworthy that most of these tumors are microadenomas and may often be missed on imaging and hence the onset of symptoms is quite insidious and a considerable amount of time may elapse before a pituitary adenoma can be diagnosed.[10]

d. *TSH secreting tumors:* These are relatively rare and patients will present with features of thyrotoxicosis like palpitations, weight loss, excessive sweating, etc.

e. *Gonadotropinomas:* These tumors usually present with irregular menses in women and low testosterone levels and decreased libido in men. They are usually macroadenomas at the time of presentation.

MASS EFFECT OF TUMOR

Most of the macroadenomas are nonsecretory and hence do not cause hormonal disturbances and therefore remain undiagnosed till they attain a size large enough to cause compression of the surrounding vital structures and cause subsequent symptoms.[11] The clinical features depend on the size of the tumor and the direction in which it spreads. For example, a tumor growing laterally may encroach upon the cavernous sinuses. Such tumors may remain asymptomatic or may present as palsy of the third cranial nerve. Inferiorly growing tumors occupy the sphenoid sinuses. Patient may be asymptomatic or may present with headache. However, the most common direction of growth remains superiorly, as that is the path of least resistance being limited only by the membranous diaphragm sellae. Here the optic chiasma lies is close relation with the tumor, particularly the inferomedial fibers of both the optic nerves, causing visual loss in bilateral upper outer quadrants.[12] Usually, such defects may not be noticed by the patient and may be detected only on visual perimetry. When the stalk of the pituitary is compressed the secretion of vasopressin is affected which manifests as diabetes insipidus with patients suffering from electrolyte imbalance, altered serum osmolality, etc.

Occasionally, a very large tumor may cause compression of the surrounding normal pituitary gland and subsequent features of hypopituitarism. This is especially true for non-secreting tumors.[13]

INVESTIGATIONS

Hormonal assay will help to determine whether a tumor is functioning or nonfunctioning. This will aid in determining further management, e.g. prolactinomas are very well managed medically with bromocriptine and surgery may easily be avoided in cases which to respond to medical therapy.

In case of secretory tumors, a fall in the levels of the particular secreted hormone in the postoperative period may give an indication about adequacy of excision. Postoperative period hormonal assays also prove invaluable for guiding hormone replacement therapies required for maintaining endocrine balance.

For accurate estimation of ACTH levels, 24 hours urinary free cortisol is determined. Raised plasma cortisol with loss of diurnal variation indicates Cushing's disease.[3] Dexamethasone suppression tests aid further confirmation. Inferior petrosal sinus sampling is also a reliable indicator. Comparison of the measurement of the hormone in a blood drawn from the inferior petrosal sinus versus that from a peripheral vessel will give an indicator of increased hormone production at the level of the pituitary. A comparative gradient between levels drawn from both side sinuses will give a more localizing indication about the site of lesion.[14]

Growth hormone values on a random sample may not be reliable as it has a very short half-life. Hence clinical features coupled with radiology provide a better clue.

Sometimes when the entire normal gland has been replaced or compressed by tumor, features of panhypopituitarism may be noted.

Blood glucose levels and impaired glucose tolerance test (GTT) are observed in GH as well as ACTH secreting tumors as both these hormones inhibit insulin.

Radiological Investigations

Magnetic resonance imaging (MRI) forms the mainstay in diagnosing pituitary tumors. Size and site of the tumor, along with details of spread to the cavernous sinuses, ICA, optic nerves can be accurately described on MRI.[15] Extent of the tumor into the suprasellar or parasellar region must be noted. Depending on the signal intensity on T1- and T2-weighted imaging, cystic and solid components of the tumor can be noted (Figs 19.2 and 19.3).

Small functioning microadenomas especially ACTH secreting tumors are often missed on imaging.[10] But the normal anterior pituitary is usually visible with gadolinium enhanced T1-weighted image, allowing the microadenoma to be delineated. Areas of focal calcification must be noted as this is highly indicative of a craniopharyngioma. During the postoperative period, serial imaging can lead to early detection of a recurrence if any.

However, from an ENT surgeon's point of view, it is also important to ask for a preoperative CT scan of the paranasal sinuses to provide anatomical details about bony landmarks. CT scan is required (a) to find out other anatomical variations that may obstruct approach to the sphenoid sinus (b) to know

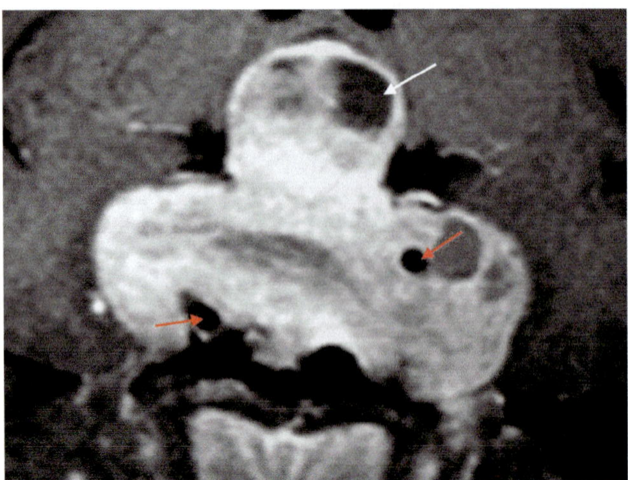

Fig. 19.2: A macroadenoma with a large suprasellar component with cystic degeneration within it (white arrow). The carotids have been displaced laterally (red arrows)

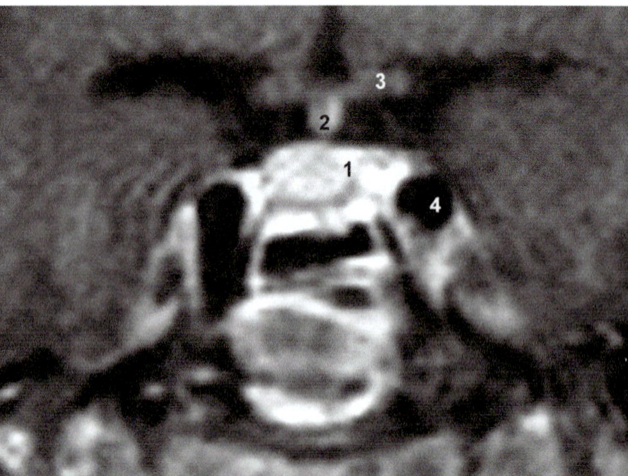

Fig. 19.3: A pituitary microadenoma displacing the normal gland laterally (1), pituitary stalk is seen superiorly (2) along with the optic chiasm (3) and the carotids laterally (4)

the extent of sphenoid sinus pneumatization (c) to look for variations in the attachments of the intra- and inter-sphenoid septae (d) to know the size of the sella, and (e) to ascertain sellar erosion and extent of tumor extension into the sphenoid sinus (Fig. 19.4).

Perimetry

Perimetry is important to assess visual impairment if any. Small defects in the form of superotemporal field defects may not be noticed by the patient himself, and will only be detected on perimetry.

▍ MANAGEMENT (FLOW CHART 19.1)

Medical Management

Hormonal suppression therapy is an option in the treatment of functioning adenomas. For example, prolactinomas can be managed with dopamine agonists like bromocriptine, cabergoline, etc. which reversibly block the prolactin receptors preventing action of the excess circulating hormone.[16] Treatment may be required to be carried on for a prolonged period and very often surgery may be reserved only for patients who do not respond to therapy. The drug may even be withdrawn in cases where there is stabilization of hormone levels and no evidence of tumor.[17]

For GH producing tumors, somatostatin analogs like octreotide, lanreotide are used. However, these drugs have significant side effects and are also very expensive. Pegvisomant is a newly developed GH receptor antagonist which shows some promise.[18]

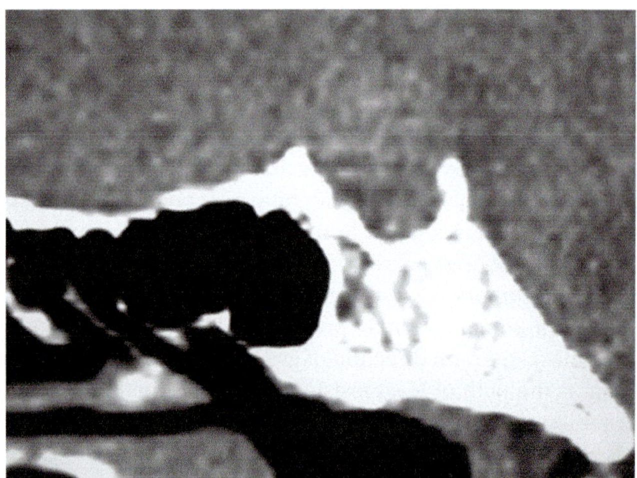

Fig. 19.4: Conchal type of sphenoid pneumatization which makes endoscopic trans-sphenoidal approach difficult. It is advisable to use navigation images in such cases

Tumor regression with medical line of management in case of ACTH and TSH secreting tumors has not been noted and drug therapy is directed to counter the peripheral effects of the circulating hormone (with metyrapone and neomercazole respectively) and in order to prepare the patient for surgery.

Radiotherapy

Radiotherapy is very rarely employed and its use is mainly restricted to control growth of tumors which could not be completely excised surgically or where tumor recurrence

Flow chart 19.1: Management choices for pituitary adenomas

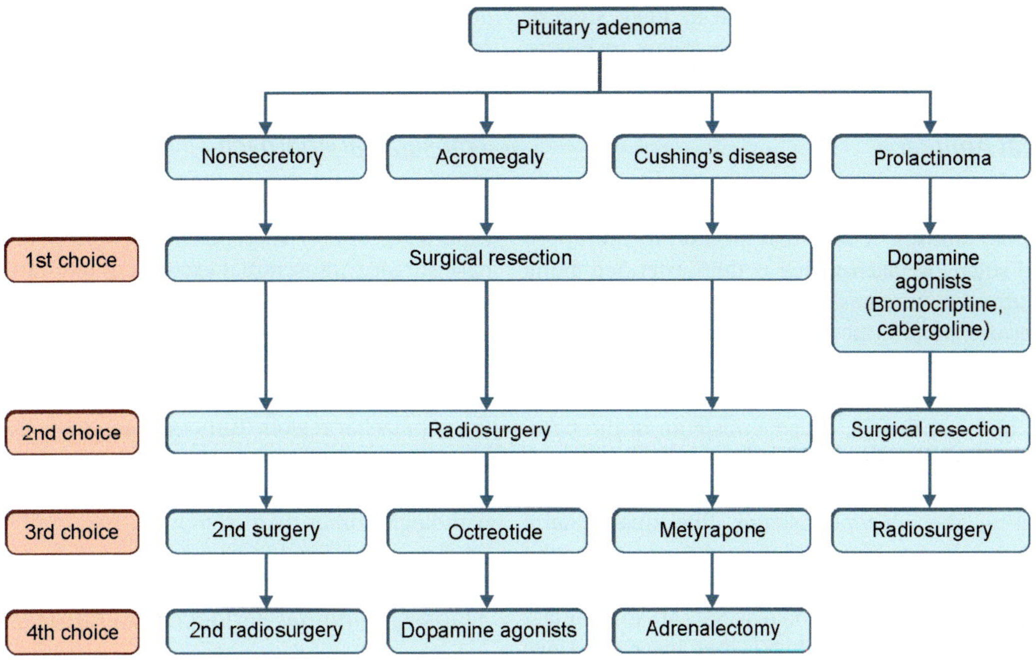

is an imminent possibility. Objectives of radiotherapy are control of tumor growth, normalization of hormone secretion and preservation of neurological function by the avoidance of surgery.[19] Radiotherapy has been described in the treatment of corticotropin producing tumors in patients who have undergone adrenalectomy to prevent Nelson's syndrome.[20] Adverse effects of radiation therapy include long-term hypopituitarism, risk of optic neuropathy and also secondary primary developing in the irradiated field.

Gamma Knife

Gamma knife radiosurgery is a radiation therapy technique using cobalt. Narrow ionizing beam radiations are used to destroy a predetermined volume of tumor. This avoids any surgical intervention and thus the consequent adverse effects of surgery. Stereotactic radiosurgery is characterized by a highly precise definition of the target. Due to this feature, radiosurgery is reserved for small lesions which are well defined on imaging.

Most studies recommend a maximum dose of 8 Gy to minimize the risk of optic neuropathy. A minimum distance of 2–5 mm between the tumor and the optic apparatus is advisable.[21] However, for actively functioning tumors, where a larger dose may be required to bring about hormonal control, doses up to 10 Gy are permissible.[21]

The main drawback of gamma knife surgery is delayed remission. This implies that radiosurgery will be efficacious in patients with tumors that have a low secretory activity or those in whom antisecretory drugs are at least partially active. Radiation induced hypopituitarism is the most frequent side effect seen in 20–40% cases.[22,23] The incidence of hypopituitarism is less with stereotactic surgery than with fractionated radiotherapy. However, special attention needs to be exercized to minimize the radiation exposure to the pituitary stalk and the normal pituitary gland to avoid these effects.[24]

Surgical Management

Nowadays, surgical treatment is the primary choice for almost all primary tumors of the pituitary. The history of evolution of pituitary surgery is intrinsically linked with the history of skull base surgery. It was as early as 1907 when Schloffer performed the first transethmoidal-transsphenoidal pituitary surgery. In 1910, Cushing developed the trans-septal transsphenoidal approach. Hardy (1969) modified the trans-septal approaches by combining them with the operating microscope. Jankowski et al (1992) have been credited with the first endoscopic transnasal transethmoidal pituitary tumor removal. Sethi in 1995 adopted the endoscopic trans-septal transsphenoidal approach. Endoscopic transnasal transsphenoidal approach has remained the mainstay of surgical approaches since being popularized by HD Jho and Carrau et al in 1996. Surgical control rates in most series with long-term follow-up ranges between 50 and 90%.[25]

Trans-septal Approach

The trans-septal route provides a direct midline approach to the sphenoid sinuses. A sublabial incision in the upper gingivolabial sulcus is taken which is then extended along the periosteum of the premaxilla. This gives exposure of the piriform aperture, anterior nasal spine and the anterior end of the nasal septum. The mucoperichondrium is elevated completely off the quadrilateral cartilage on one side to reach the rostrum of the sphenoid. Mucoperiosteum of the nasal floor is also lifted off. Nasal mucosa is elevated off the septum far enough on both sides to allow the cartilage to be displaced without tearing the mucoperiosteum. The quadrilateral cartilage is then separated from the floor of the nose and the posterior bony septum. The bony septum is then excised till the anterior wall of the sphenoid is reached. An appropriate sized Hardy's self retaining speculum is then inserted to give a stable view. The surgeon shifts to the operating microscope at this stage to carry out further steps of the procedure.

The advantages of the trans-septal approach are that it is a stable, relatively avascular, midline approach without any facial scarring. However, the surgeon gets a very narrow, limited field of vision. Risk of rhinological complications like septal perforations, collapse of the nasal tip, denervation of upper incisors, etc. are involved in this approach.[26]

Transethmoidal Approach

For this approach, an incision is made starting from the medial end of the eyebrow, curving downwards to the upper end of the piriform aperture of the nose. After elevating the skin and soft tissue off the underlying bone, the lacrimal bone is exposed. A window is made through it to gain access to the nasal cavity via the medial wall of the orbit. The ethmoid sinus complex has to be opened up. It may be necessary to remove the posterior end of the middle turbinate and posterior part of the lamina papyracea to ease access. The posterior bony septum is then excised to expose the anterior wall of both the sphenoid sinuses and the pituitary fossa is approached through this. A self-retaining speculum is applied and the operating microscope is used for a magnified vision.

The vision is through the ethmoids while the instrumentation can be carried out through the nasal cavity which eases approach. This route provides a good lateral exposure but superior exposure is limited.[27,28] As the anterior half of the nasal cavity is untouched, deformities of the septum and nasal tip, etc. are avoided. However, a facial scar will be seen. Bleeding may be more in this approach as compared to other routes. Scarring at the frontal recess and frontal sinus ostium with consequent frontal sinusitis or frontal mucocele formation are also known complications.

Transcranial Approach

With the increasing technological backup and growing experience of ENT surgeons in the field of endoscopic skull base surgery, transcranial excision of pituitary tumors is not the first line treatment anymore. All tumors that are amenable to endoscopic transsphenoidal excision must be attempted to be removed by this route. Transcranial approach may be needed for tumors that are too large and extending far into the suprasellar region. Tumors which have the classic "hour glass" shape with a waist at the diaphragm, may be difficult to remove endoscopically.[29] In revision surgeries, especially for pathologies other than adenomas, transcranial surgery may be considered (Fig. 19.5).

Trans-sphenoidal Endoscopic Approach

This is the standard approach to all pituitary tumors today world over and has been discussed in details here.

The areas one needs to focus on are supra and parasellar extent, encasement of the internal carotid artery (ICA), cystic or hemorrhagic areas, anterior extension, positioning of the normal gland and the probability of a differential diagnosis. Lateral extension of tumor will require a wider exposure including opening of the posterior ethmoids. It is not advisable to chase tumor lateral to, or encasing the ICA and only experienced surgeons should attempt removal of tumor from there or the cavernous sinus (Fig. 19.1). Also anterior

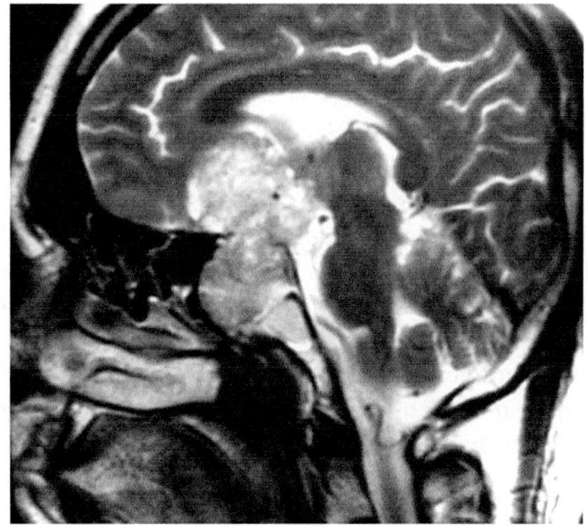

Fig. 19.5: "Hour glass"-shaped suprasellar component of a pituitary macroadenoma. A contraindication for endoscopic approach

extension requires planum exposure above the superior intercavernous sinus and skills in drilling, coagulation and reconstruction.

EQUIPMENT

One must have the necessary equipment before attempting skull base surgery, as that will dictate the ease of surgery and also whether one can handle all the potential complications. Amongst those that we think are essential are:

- Excellent quality endoscopes: at least 0° and 45°
- HD camera (or minimum; 3 chip) with compatible monitor
- Pneumatic drill with appropriate handpiece and burs
- Bipolar rotatable cautery forceps (optionally with suction)
- Material for hemostasis including Surgicel®, Fibrillar®, Floseal® or Surgiflo® these are registered trademark names of commonly used market products
- Complete set of instruments including curettes, keyhole suctions, fine scissors and forceps
- Set-up for navigation surgery (Fig. 19.6).

ANESTHESIA AND POSITION

The patient is operated under general anesthesia. A lumbar drain is inserted in patients with large tumors where significant reconstruction is likely to be required. Draping and preparation is done for the nose and right thigh (in case fascia lata graft may be required). The patient is supine with the head elevated about 30° and slightly turned to face the surgeon. The nurse will be at the head end of the table and the monitor and assistant on the left side opposite the main surgeons. A second monitor may be provided for viewing for the assistant and nurse. The nose is packed with patties soaked in a solution of 4% xylocaine with adrenaline (Fig. 19.7).

SURGICAL TECHNIQUE

We describe the technique as followed in our institute. We use a binostril, two surgeon technique for all cases. Following a diagnostic endoscopy, the first step is to gently laterally fracture the inferior turbinates, taking care not to damage the mucosa. Patties are then inserted between the middle turbinate and the septum to allow gentle lateralization of the middle turbinates and expose the superior turbinate. The superior turbinates are similarly lateralized to then expose the sphenoid ostium. One must remember to stay in the inferior half of the turbinates to find the ostium which usually lies just posterior to the superior turbinate. This is done on both sides. A common mistake is to go too high, towards the cribriform plate and that can cause mucosal damage and make further vision difficult as well as potentially increasing the risk of a CSF leak. In case of a large concha bullosa, it may be necessary to do a conchoplasty, by removing the lateral lamella, to allow lateralization of the turbinate.

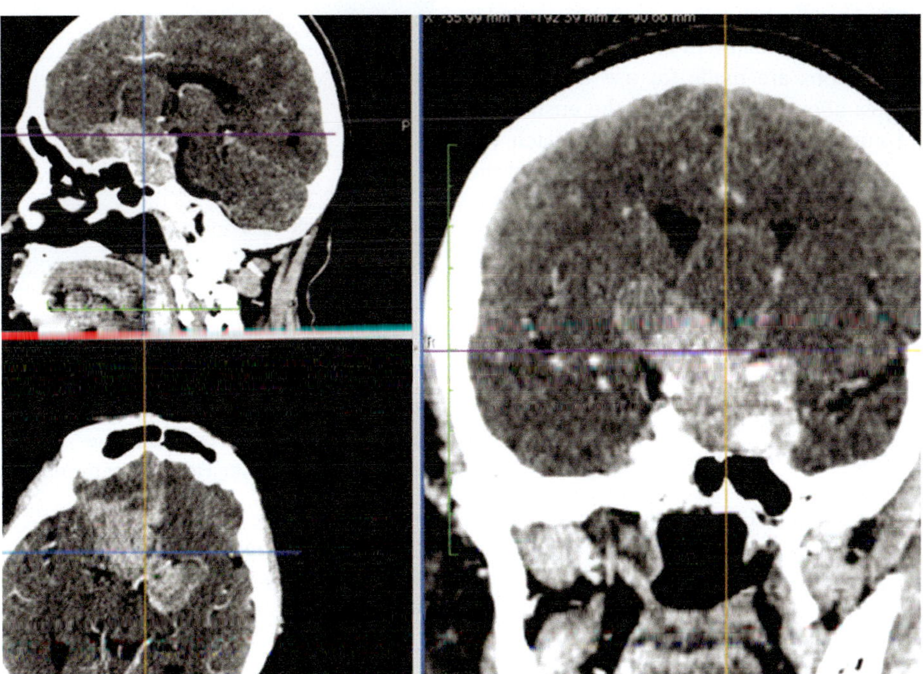

Fig. 19.6: Intraoperative navigation image showing the probe in the upper part of the tumor

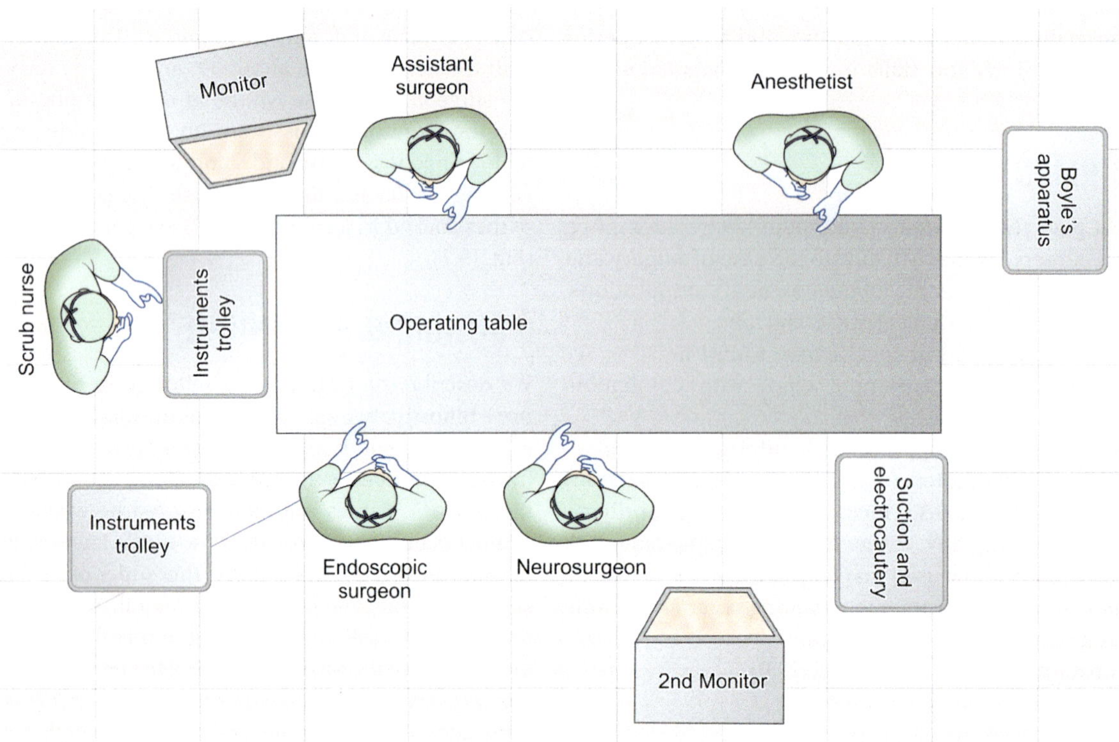

Fig. 19.7: Operating room set-up

The first incision actually takes into consideration the final reconstruction. Usually we use a pedicled vascular septal flap (Hadad flap)[30] for closure in case of CSF fistulae, and so the initial incisions are made for use of this flap. The incision starts just above and medial to the eustachian tube opening and curves above the choana to reach the inferior septum and come anteriorly to end just short of the mucocutaneous junction. The second part of the incision starts at the upper part of the sphenoid ostium and comes forward on the nasal septum at the same level as the upper aspect of the sphenoid ostium until the anterior end of the middle turbinate, where it curves upwards and continues anteriorly till the mucocutaneous junction. A vertical limb then joins the superior and inferior incisions. A small lateral extension is made till the root of the superior turbinate. The incisions are customized in length and width for the patient and the expected defect.

The mucoperichondrium is then elevated off the septum proceeding posteriorly to elevate the mucoperiosteum off the anterior face of the sphenoid septum so that it is now attached laterally based on the posterior septal artery, a branch of the sphenopalatine artery (Fig. 19.8). This flap is then tucked away into the nasopharynx, protected by a piece of polyvinyl

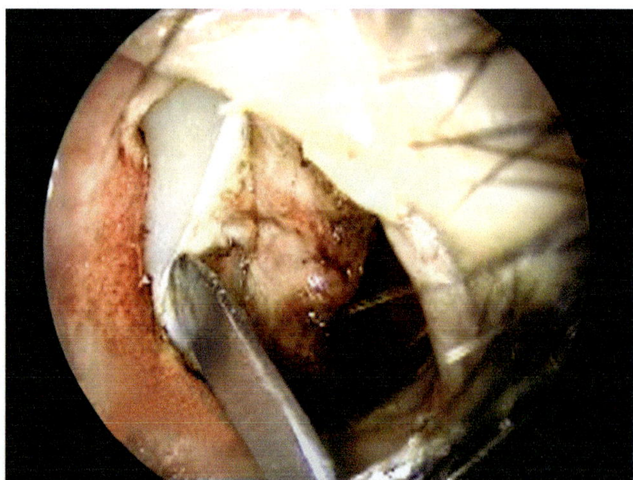

Fig. 19.8: Elevation of the nasoseptal flap

alcohol sponge. On the other side, we take a reverse flap. A vertical incision is taken from the sphenoid ostium down towards the choana. Like the other side, an upper and lower incision are taken which then come anteriorly along the nasal septum, but only till the anterior end of the middle turbinate.

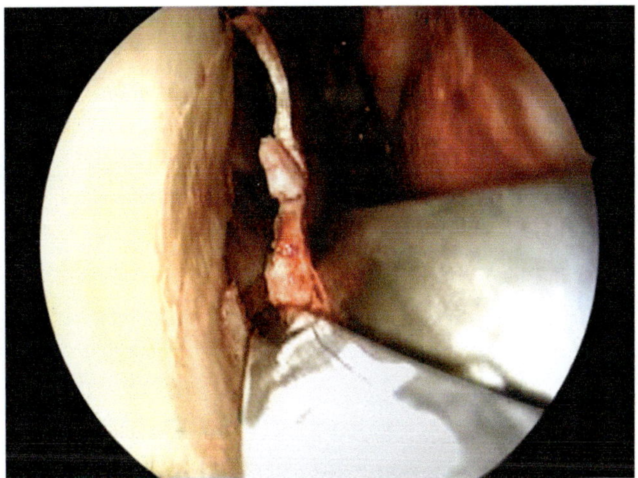

Fig. 19.9: Posterior septectomy

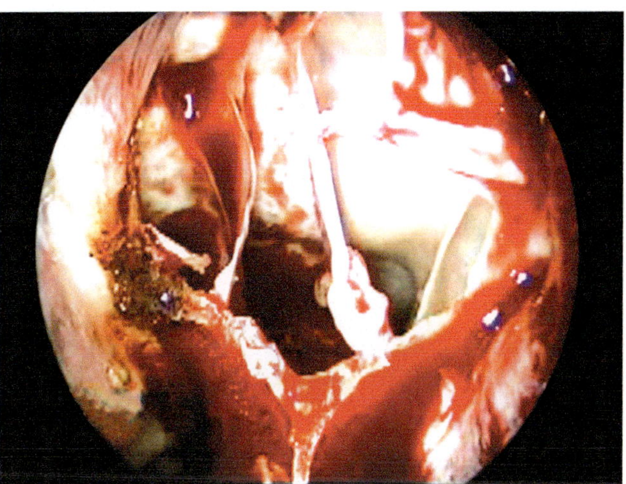

Fig. 19.10: Wide exposure of the sphenoids following removal of the rostrum

This mucoperichondrial flap is then elevated based anteriorly till the bony-cartilage junction. A posterior septectomy is then done by removing the exposed bony septum (between the upper and lower incisions), preferably as a single bony piece or at least one large piece that may aid in sellar reconstruction (Fig. 19.9).

The reverse flap is then brought out through the septectomy onto the opposite side and sutured to the cut anterior mucosal edge to cover the exposed cartilage from taking of the septal flap. If the likelihood of intra-operative CSF leak is minimal, we then do not take this flap initially, but instead start with a "rescue" or "reserve" flap. Here only the superior and inferior incisions are taken till the anterior end of the middle turbinate, and the mucoperiosteum reflected inferiorly to expose the bony septum and the anterior sphenoid wall. Surgery then continues as described earlier with a posterior septectomy. In the event of a CSF leak, the same incisions are extended anteriorly to complete the formal septal flap. The advantage is that morbidity due to septal exposure is reduced, whilst still affording the option of a septal flap. The disadvantage is the slightly reduced working space and exposure, which however can easily be overcome with a little experience.

The next step is to open the sphenoid sinuses by removing the rostrum and the anterior wall, again if possible keeping the bony piece intact (Fig. 19.10). Superior exposure of the anterior sphenoid wall above the ostium, is generally not required unless there is a large suprasellar tumor, that requires exposure superior onto the sphenoid planum. Inferiorly, the exposure is usually till the floor of the sinus to afford adequate space under the sellar floor. Laterally, exposure is till the superior turbinate. If there is a significant parasellar extension that requires exposure of the cavernous sinus, then the inferior half of the superior turbinate is resected and the posterior ethmoids opened to view the orbital apex. This step considerably enhances exposure and increases ease of surgery and may occasionally be done even for smaller tumors in case of restricted operative space. The intersphenoid septum is removed to enable a clear view of the above mentioned structures. One must keep in mind that the septum usually deviates to attach to the ICA or the optic nerve, thus care must be taken especially near the attachment. A preoperative CT scan is very useful if there are multiple septae or the presence of sphenoethmoidal (Onodi) cells, as MRI does not demonstrate bone very well. If the sphenoid is not well pneumatized or if there is a conchal type of pneumatization, navigation is essential, as the bone needs to be drilled to expose the sella, which should be done only under navigation control. Thus, conchal pneumatization of the sphenoid, although not favorable for transsphenoidal approach, is no longer a contraindication.[31]

The mucosa is removed over and around the sella and the floor of the sphenoid sinus (to prepare the bed for the septal flap). At this stage, the neurosurgeon joins the ENT surgeon for tumor removal. The ENT surgeon holds the endoscope in his left hand and irrigates the field with the right hand. The neurosurgeon has a suction tip in his left hand and another instrument (curette, forceps, scissor, suction, etc.) in his right hand. Thus in the right nostril are the endoscope, irrigation cannula and suction, while in the patient's left nostril is the main instrument held by the neurosurgeons right hand. Both are on the right side of the patient, with the endoscopist being closer to the head end allowing free hand and elbow movement for the neurosurgeon.

Before the sella is opened, one should have a panoramic view of the entire area to include the tuberculum sella anteriorly and above the sella, the optic nerve canals supero-laterally, the bulge of the internal carotid artery (ICA) in its

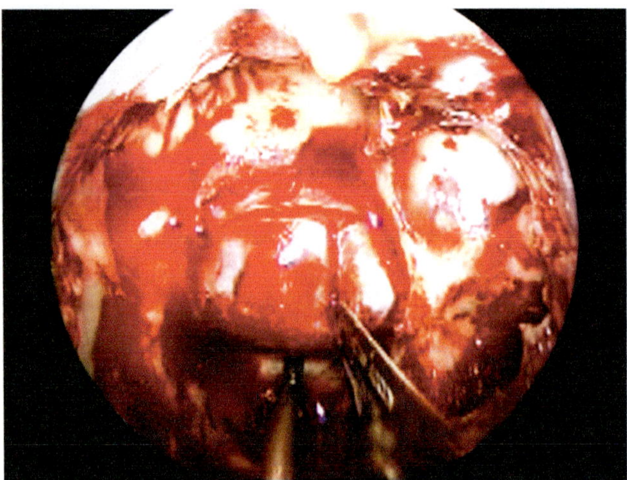

Fig. 19.11: Dural incision

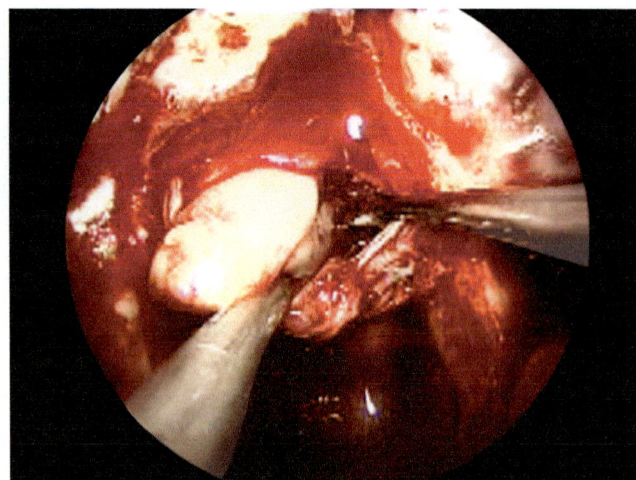

Fig. 19.12: Tumor being removed

cavernous segment just below the optics, the vertical segment of the ICA inferolaterally and a touch more posterior and the floor of the sella inferiorly. The sella is opened as widely as possible with a diamond burr, the lateral limits being the cavernous sinus, superiorly and inferiorly being the inter-cavernous sinuses. Though it is not essential to have the "4 blue sign" in every case, an attempt must be made to have maximum exposure. This allows for safer tumor removal under vision. The dural incision may be taken in a number of ways, we generally use a cruciate or an "I" incision (Fig. 19.11).

Tumor removal may be done extracapsular to ensure complete tumor excision, but it does require a higher level of experience and skill and will increase the risk of a CSF leak. Intracapsular tumor dissection is easier, but leaves the potential for residual tumor. We use both techniques depending on the size of the tumor and pathology. The sellar part of the tumor is the first to be removed starting inferiorly and continuing laterally (Fig. 19.12). Depending on the approach, one may use fine dissection instruments, scissors and suction for extracapsular and curettes, forceps and suction for intra-capsular surgery. Once the inferior and lateral parts are cleared, one can address the suprasellar part. It is prudent to do this part last, as occasionally the diaphragm or suprasellar cistern can collapse into the field obscuring the view, as well as trapping pockets of tumor that may then be challenging to clear. Complete tumor removal is ascertained by complete descent of the diaphragm sellae. With the endoscope in the sella, one should be able to visualize the complete diaphragm, the medial walls of the cavernous sinus, and the inferior wall ensuring there is no residual tumor. Rarely an angled scope (45°) may be used, like in giant pituitary tumors (Fig. 19.13).

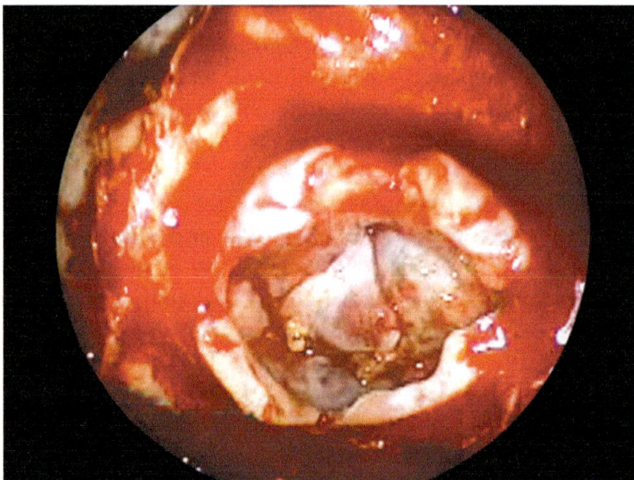

Fig. 19.13: Diaphragm descended after complete tumor removal

Once complete tumor is excised, bleeding usually stops, but hemostasis must be achieved completely. Warm saline irrigations are given, any bleeders are cauterized, and use of hemostatic material used judiciously to avoid over-packing in the sella. Nasal packing is done only if there is bleeding from the nasal mucosa. If packs have been kept, they are usually removed in 24–48 hours.

If there is a CSF leak, then the defect needs to be meticulously repaired. Reconstruction of the defect may be done in a number of ways. It is probably best to use the pedicled septal flap that was prepared at the start of the surgery, or to convert the reserve flap into a formal pedicled septal flap (Figs 19.14A and B). This gives the maximum security and ensures the best possible repair for the defect.

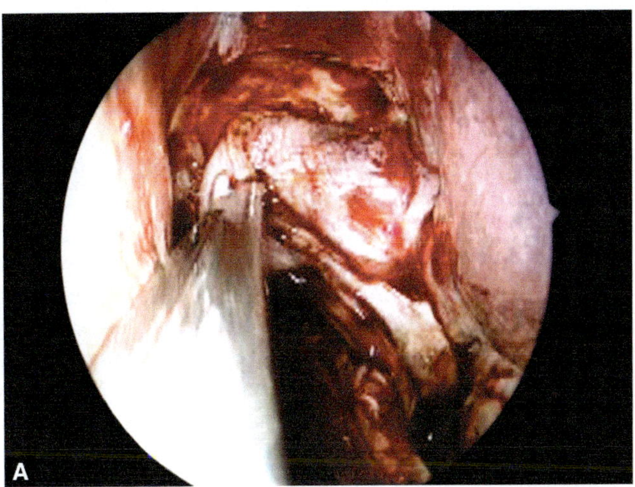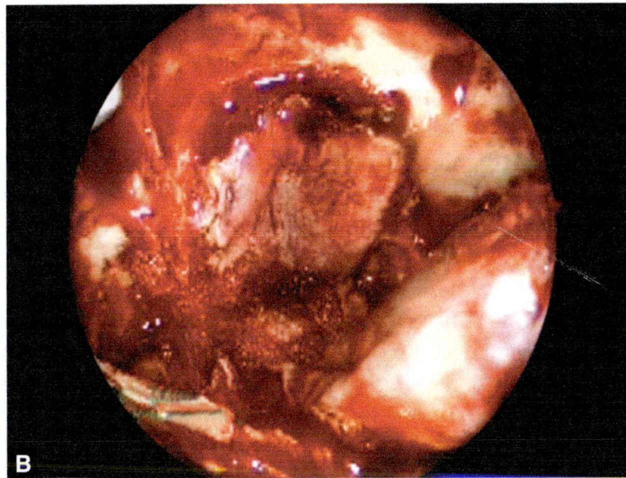

Figs 19.14A and B: Positioning of the septal flap for reconstruction of the defect

If however, one is not familiar with the flap or if a flap is not possible (e.g. revision surgery), then other methods need to be employed. Most commonly, we use fascia lata and fat from the thigh, along with tissue glue. This could be used as single or multiple layers depending on the size of the defect. Occasionally, we use bone or cartilage from the septum, or bone from the anterior sphenoid wall or the intersphenoid septum to strengthen the sella wall. This is done when the force of CSF with pulsations is high. Following reconstruction for CSF fistulae, nasal packs are inserted and kept for 4–5 days. A lumbar drain may be additionally utilized to keep the CSF pressure low.

Postoperatively, the patient must undergo nasal cleaning to keep the nose free of crusts and prevent the formation of synechiae. Usually, we see the patient in the first and second week, and more often only if required. The patient will be advised to use a saline spray to help keep the nose clean.

The main advantage of endoscopic skull base surgery is that we get a good visualization of the field where we are operating. The scope takes the surgeon right at the focus of action in the surgery. Moving the scope around in the operative field serves as a quick reckoner for the relative position of our instruments and surrounding anatomical structures. There is very minimal trauma to the normal soft tissue and bone, unlike in an external approach where there is significant tissue handling with consequent trauma. An external incision is avoided. Endoscopic skull base surgery ensures a better access, a decreased overall incidence of complications, improved surgical outcome and rapid patient recovery. All of this leads to a shortened hospital stay with less expenditure for the patient. The bacterial colonization of a normal nasal cavity is very minimal and hence infectious complications after an endoscopic skull base surgery are rare.

Prophylactic pre-operative antibiotics coupled with skull base reconstruction with a vascularized pedicle flap further lower the chances of an ascending infection.

The main disadvantage of this technique is that part of the space available for instrumentation is occupied by the endoscope and maneuvering instruments in restricted space is a skill which needs to be learnt. However, in our opinion, the binostril approach aids easy movements of the scope as well as the instruments and overcomes this disadvantage. Another drawback maybe the fact that the image obtained is a 2D image. However, moving the scope in and out of the field compensates for this and gives us depth perception while operating. Nowadays programs converting 2D images to 3D images are available but the precision may be lost in this and this technique still has some scope for improvement.

COMPLICATIONS

Intraoperative

- *Hemorrhage:* This may be from the tumor itself, intercavernous sinuses, cavernous sinuses or very rarely the internal carotid artery or its branches. Tumor bleeding can be managed by cauterization and local hemostatic patties. Having a pistol grip bipolar suction cautery in one's armamentarium is very beneficial for controlling most of the bleeding vessels during pituitary surgery. Intercavernous sinuses may not be effectively cauterized as the cautery may occasionally widen the rent in the sinus. Packing the area with oxidized cellulose (Surgicel®) and absorbable gelatin sponge will by and large control such bleeding. Bleeding from the cavernous sinuses however, may not be so easy to control and obscures surgical field making further tumor removal difficult. Packing the bleeding sinus and patiently proceeding with further careful dissection is needed. In such an event, commercial preparations of lyophilized human gelatin matrix (Floseal®, Surgiflo®) which contains fibrin elements, coagulation factors and protein C will ensure formation of a coagulum and achieve hemostasis. Visualization of surgical field is not impeded since the excess sealant material can easily be washed off. In the rare event of an ICA damage, the bleeding is catastrophic. Immediate packing to achieve pressure hemostasis is done while waiting for further definitive control. A large roller gauze pack may be used for tamponade. Definitive control will entail interventional radiological assistance with balloon/coil occlusion to block the artery.

- Bleeding from the nose is usually minor and from small mucosal vessels. Preoperative decongestant drops, intraoperative vasoconstrictor (xylocaine + adrenaline) patties usually tide over such bleeding. Generalized mucosal oozing may be managed by intermittently giving warm saline irrigations and this will keep the surgical field clean. A posterior septal branch of the sphenopalatine artery runs along the inferior part of the anterior wall of the sphenoid and may be damaged during sphenoidotomy. Bipolar cauterization of the offending vessel or carefully elevating the mucosa off the rostrum before widening the bone will prevent bleeding. When we have harvested a nasoseptal flap, caution must be exercised so as not to damage the vascular pedicle with the bipolar cautery.

- *CSF leak:* A CSF leak, if present is almost always detected intraoperatively. Specially in cases of large tumors or those with suprasellar extensions, and in cases of craniopharyngioma excision; chances of encountering a CSF leak are very high and the surgeon should be well prepared for such an eventuality. It might be advisable in such cases to harvest a nasoseptal flap at the very beginning of the surgery. Meticulous reconstruction of the sellar defect with fat, fascia and sometimes the bone of the rostrum or septum usually is enough to seal off all defects. A mucoperiosteal flap from the middle turbinate may also be used. Fibrin glue is used to further augment the repair.

Postoperative Complications

Many of the complications can be avoided by thorough and vigilant care during the postoperative period, especially the early postsurgical days. Patient is kept in the intensive care unit (ICU) where his neurological status is monitored. Watchful eye regarding fluid electrolyte balance, hormonal replacement, antibiotic cover, etc. is required.

- *Hemorrhage:* Though uncommon, a postoperative hemorrhage can lead to an acute surgical emergency and the patient will be needed to be re-explored under anesthesia immediately. One must always search thoroughly for an offending vessel and cauterise it. Branches from the sphenopalatine artery are found to be the culprits in most of such cases.

- Very rarely a postoperative hemorrhage may cause an intracranial bleed. A thorough neurological monitoring in the early postoperative period may be the only key to detect such an event in the absence of any external hemorrhage, the actual site of bleed being hidden by the skull base repair. Early intervention in the form of immediate re-exploration mostly by external approach is required.

- *CSF leak:* In the rare event that a CSF leak is detected in the postoperative period patient is taken in for a formal CSF repair similar to the above mentioned technique. Postoperative monitoring is therefore important, particularly having a high index of suspicion in patients complaining of persistent watery rhinorrhea. Sending nasal fluid for biochemistry and beta 2 transferrin levels can help in making a diagnosis.[32]

- *Meningitis:* In this age of highly efficacious broad spectrum antibiotics the event of a patient landing with meningitis is unlikely. In cases with CSF leakage, the risk of developing an ascending infection leading to meningitis becomes marginally higher.

- *Synechiae:* Synechia may be formed due to abrasion or laceration over the nasal mucosa. As most of the instrumentation goes on through the left nostril, incidence of adhesions on the left side is higher. These have usually been seen to form between the middle turbinate and nasal septum and do not compromize the airway. Good postoperative care with saline nasal washes usually avoids such a complication. Our protocol is to undertake postoperative nasal cleaning under vision for 2–3 weeks postoperative to prevent adhesions.

- *Sphenoidal mucocele:* Sometimes in very large sellar defects, the entire sphenoid sinus may be packed with fat and obliterated as a part of CSF leak closure. If the mucosa of the sphenoid sinus has not been thoroughly removed before obliterating the sinus with fat, a sphenoidal mucocoele will ensue. With sufficient widening of the sphenoid however, this is an unlikely complication.

Endocrine Complications

Depending on the extent of resection and the extent of the tumor itself, postsurgery hypopituitarism may follow. It may be transient or permanent, in which case long-term hormone replacement therapy will be needed. Diabetes insipidus is a very likely outcome postpituitary surgery, especially when the stalk of the gland has been traumatized.[33] Monitoring the serum sodium levels and looking for fluid electrolyte imbalance becomes vital during the postoperative period. Treatment is with Desmopressin (DDAVP) in the immediate postoperative days followed by maintenance with anti-diuretic hormone analogs (oral form/nasal spray) for persistent cases.

Recurrence

Recurrence of a tumor can be detected by careful monitoring of the patient after the surgery. Therefore, there is emphasis for regular follow-up postoperatively. Recurrence of a functioning adenoma can be detected by serial hormonal assays during follow-up visits. Nonfunctioning adenomas can only be detected by serial imaging studies (MRI) (Figs 19.15A and B).

OTHER LESIONS IN THE PITUITARY

Craniopharyngioma

Craniopharyngiomas are benign tumors arising in the sellar suprasellar region thought to arise from remnants of the craniopharyngeal duct in relation to the primitive gut. They typically have cystic as well as solid components.[34] There is a peak in incidence in childhood and adolescence and another in the sixth decade. But not uncommonly, tumors may remain undetected until they are large enough to press upon surrounding important structures and produce symptoms. Although they are histologically benign, they are considered as an aggressive form of tumor due to their tendency to become adherent to the surrounding structures making resection difficult. On MRI scanning calcification within a sellar lesion is typically indicative of a craniopharyngioma. It is often difficult to distinguish a craniopharyngioma from an adenoma in the pituitary. But more often than not, one can distinctly see the compressed pituitary at one end of the lesion in a craniopharyngioma whereas it may not be possible to identify a normal pituitary in case of an adenoma.

Rathke's Pouch Cyst

Rathke's cleft cyst is a cystic lesion found within the sella itself. It is considered to be derived from the remnants of Rathke's pouch, an invagination of the stomodeum. When such a remnant of the Rathke's pouch gets walled off and the secretions start building up inside, it forms a dilated cystic structure called the Rathke's cleft cyst. The epithelium lining

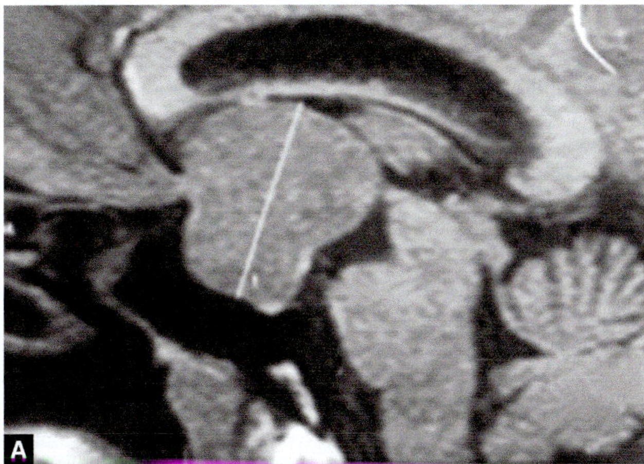
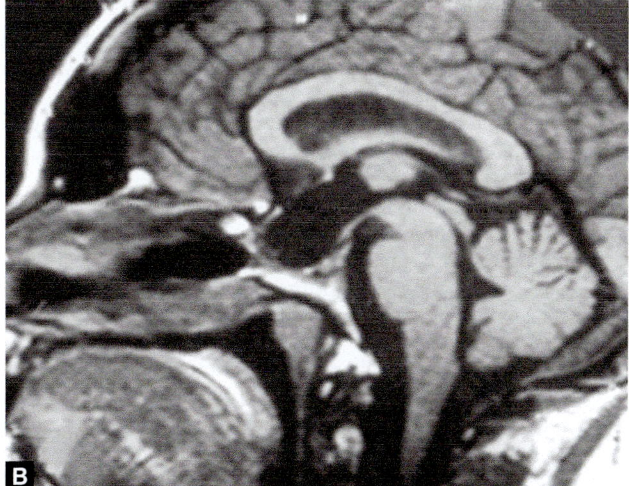

Figs 19.15A and B: Preoperative and postoperative MR images showing complete tumor removal

the cyst is ectodermal in origin and is either columnar or cuboidal.[35] The contents of the cyst are usually in the form of mucoid material which may be occasionally thick and opaque. That's why they are often referred as "machinery oil cysts". Such cysts may be found in 13–22% of normal pituitary glands.[36] If they attain significant size they produce signs and symptoms mimicking a pituitary adenoma. On MR imaging, however, a high intensity cystic component is typically noted which clinches the diagnosis.

Chordomas

They arise from remnants of the primitive notochord. They are slow growing tumors compressing upon critical surrounding structures. Radiographically, they appear as an expansile, osteolytic lesion with areas of calcifications associated with a soft tissue mass.

MALIGNANT TUMORS OF THE PITUITARY

Malignancies in the pituitary are rare (found in 0.2% of adenomas)[4] and are usually secretory (of the prolactin, ACTH secreting variety). Surgical debulking may be needed to be followed-up by radiotherapy in cases of incomplete resection. Infiltration from a nasopharyngeal carcinoma into the pituitary may be seen. Rarely, primary bone tumors, or metastases from bone tumors may be noted.

REFERENCES

1. Amar AP, Weiss MH. Pituitary anatomy and physiology. Neurosurg Clin N Am. 2003;14(1):11-23.
2. Kyo-Sung Ju, Hack-Gun Bae, Hyung-Ki Park, et al. Morphometric Study of the Korean Adult Pituitary Glands and the Diaphragma Sellae. J Korean Neurosurg Soc. 2010;47(1):42-7.
3. Buatti JM, Marcus RB. Pituitary adenomas: current methods of diagnosis and treatment. Oncology (Williston Park). 1997;11(6):791-6; discussion 798, 803-4.
4. Pernicone PJ, Scheithauer BW, Sebo TJ, et al. Pituitary carcinoma: a clinicopathologic study of 15 cases. Cancer. 1997;79(4):804-12.
5. Hardy J. Transphenoidal microsurgery of the normal and pathological pituitary. Clin Neurosurg. 1969;16:185-217.
6. Wilson CB. A decade of pituitary microsurgery. The Herbert Olivecrona lecture. J Neurosurg. 1984;61(5):814-33.
7. Yamada S. Epidemiology of pituitary tumors. In: Tharpar K, Kovacs K, Scheithauer BW, Lloyd RV (Eds). Diagnosis and management of pituitary tumors. Totowa: Humana Press, 2001:57-69.
8. Gillam MP, Molitch ME, Lombardi G, et al. Advances in the treatment of prolactinomas. Endocr Rev. 2006;27(5):485-534.
9. Melmed S. Acromegaly pathogenesis and treatment. J Clin Invest. 2009;119(11):3189-202.
10. Colombo N, Loli P, Vignati F, et al. MR of corticotropin-secreting pituitary microadenomas. AJNR. 1994;15(8):1591-5.
11. Kovacs K, Scheithauer BW, Horvath E, et al. The World Health Organization classification of adenohypophysial neoplasms. A proposed five-tier scheme. Cancer. 1996;78:502-10.
12. Cury ML, Fernandes JC, Machado HR, Elias LL, Moreira AC, Castro M. Nonfunctioning pituitary adenomas: clinical feature, laboratorial and imaging assessment, therapeutic management and outcome. Arq Bras Endocrinol Metabol. 2009;53(1):31-9.
13. Molitch ME, Thorner MO, Wilson C. Management of prolactinomas. J Clin Endocrinol Metab. 1997;82(4):996-1000.
14. Doppman JL, Oldfield E, Krudy AG, et al. Petrosal sinus sampling for Cushing syndrome: anatomical and technical considerations. Work in progress. Radiology. 1984;150:99-103.
15. Indrajit IK, Chidambaranathan N, Sundar K, Ahmed I. Value of dynamic MRI imaging in pituitary adenomas. Neuroradiol. 2001;11(4):185-90.
16. Beverly MK Biller, Colao Annamaria, Petersenn Stephan, et al. Prolactinomas, Cushing's disease and acromegaly: debating the role of medical therapy for secretory pituitary adenomas. BMC Endocr Disord. 2010;10:10.
17. Colao A, Di Sarno A, Cappabianca P, et al. Withdrawal of long-term cabergoline therapy for tumoral and nontumoral hyperprolactinemia. N Engl J Med. 2003;349(21):2023-33.
18. Auriemma RS, Galdiero M, Grasso LF, et al. Complete disappearance of a GH-secreting pituitary macroadenoma in a patient with acromegaly: effect of treatment with lanreotide Autogel and consequence of treatment withdrawal. Eur J Endocrinol. 2010;162(5):993-9.
19. Chanson P, Salenave S. Diagnosis and treatment of pituitary adenomas. Minerva Endocrinol. 2004;29(4):241-75.
20. Yoon JW, Jo SK, Cha DR, et al. A case of Rathke's Cleft Cyst inflammation presenting with diabetes insipidus. Korean J Intern Med. 2001;16(2):132-5.
21. Douglas G Castro, Soraya AJ Cecilio, Miguel M Canteras. Radiosurgery for pituitary adenomas: Evaluation of their efficacy and safety. Radiotion Onco. 2010;5:109.
22. Castinetti F, Brue T. Gamma Knife radiosurgery in pituitary adenomas: Why, who, and how to treat? Discov Med. 2010;10(51):107-11.
23. Castinetti F, Nagai M, Morange I, et al. Long-term results of stereotactic radiosurgery in secretory pituitary adenomas. J Clin Endocrinol Metab. 2009;94(9):3400-7.
24. Feigl GC, Bonelli CM, Berghold A, et al. Effects of gamma knife radiosurgery of pituitary adenomas on pituitary function. J Neurosurg. 2002;97(5 Suppl):415-21.
25. Sheehan J, Steiner L, Laws ER. Pituitary adenoma: Is gamma knife radiosurgery safe? Nat Clin Pract Endocrinol Metab. 2005;1(1):2-3.
26. Er U, Gürses L, Saka C, et al. Sublabial trans-septal approach to pituitary adenomas with special emphasis on rhinological complications. Turk Neurosurg. 2008;18(4):425-30.
27. van Cauwenberge P, Calliauw L. The transethmoidal-transsphenoidal route to the pituitary gland. Technique, advantages, limitations and possible complications. Acta Otorhinolaryngol Belg. 1983;37(6):883-91.
28. Das K, Spencer W, Nwagwu CI, et al. Approaches to the sellar and parasellar region: anatomic comparison of endonasal-transsphenoidal, sublabial-transsphenoidal, and transethmoidal approaches. Neurol Res. 2001;23(1):51-4.
29. Youssef AS, Agazzi S, van Loveren HR. Transcranial surgery for pituitary adenomas. Neurosurgery. 2005;57(1 Suppl):168-75.
30. Hadad G, Bassagasteguy L, Carrau RL, et al. A novel reconstructive technique after expanded endonasal approaches: vascular pedicle nasoseptal flap. Laryngoscope. 2006;116(10):1882-6.
31. Hamid O, El Fiky L, Hassan O, et al. Anatomic variations of the sphenoid sinus and their impact on transsphenoids Pituitary Surgery. Skull Base. 2008;18(1):9-15.
32. Irjala K, Suonpaa J, Laurent B. Identification of CSF leakage by immunofixation. Arch Otolaryngol. 1979;105:447-8.
33. Loh JA, Verbalis JG. Diabetes insipidus as a complication after pituitary surgery. Nat Clin Pract Endocrinol Metab. 2007;3(6):489-94.
34. Zada G, Laws ER. Surgical management of craniopharyngiomas in the pediatric population. Horm Res Paediatr. 2010;74(1):62-6.
35. Raghunath A, Sampath S, Devi BI, et al. Is there a need to diagnose Rathke's cleft cyst preoperatively? Neurol India. 2010;58(1):69-73.

Endoscopic Approach to Sinonasal and Anterior Skull-Base Tumors

Prathamesh S Pai

INTRODUCTION

Sinonasal tumors form a small proportion of head and neck tumors. Certain nasal symptoms such as nasal obstruction and epistaxis might force patients to seek medical attention but it is incumbent on the treating physician to rule out a malignancy when dealing with a unilateral nasal swelling. Computerized tomography (CT) scans and nasal endoscopes are ubiquitous and have improved our ability to diagnose and manage sinonasal tumors. For malignant sinonasal tumors, surgery with or without radiation remains the treatment of choice barring a few exceptions. Various surgical approaches have been described to manage sinonasal tumors. For subcranial diseases transfacial approaches (medial maxillectomy, total maxillectomy) are adequate while for intracranial extensions craniofacial approach is suitable. Modifications such as sublabial approaches (midfacial degloving, Le Fort) avoid facial scarring whilst the subcranial approaches (Raveh) reduce brain retraction and dural tears.

Since Professor Messerklinger described 'Functional Endoscopic Sinus Surgery"[1] the transnasal access has been pursued with the microscope and later the endoscope for removal of sinonasal tumors. Professor Aldo Stamm and Professor Wolfgang Draf developed the microendoscopic transnasal route[2] while the Pittsburgh group led by Professor Ricardo Carrou, Professor Carl Synderman and Professor Amin Kassam described a modular "Expanded Endonasal Approach" to access the entire ventral skull base.[3,4] Their modular design simplified understanding of the complex skull base anatomy and paved the way for increased interest in endonasal tumor resection.

PROGRESS

Three millennia ago Egyptians[5] used the transcribriform approach to remove the brain without vitiating the skin during body embalming. Anterior nares act as natural ports for accessing the nasal cavity as well as the paranasal sinuses and have been used for removal of polyps and benign tumors over the past 100 years of modern medicine. But in the last two decades significant technological advances have further broadened the scope of the transnasal route.

Superior imaging has enhanced our understanding of the skull base anatomy while magnified clearer vision, better illumination and improved instrumentation have vastly improved our access and resection capabilities. Powered instruments such as microdebrider aid in quick and safe soft tissue clearance. High speed drills allow us to remove bone with impunity adjacent to vital structures such as dura, optic nerve or internal carotid artery. Real time intraoperative navigation and intraoperative computed tomography (CT) or magnetic resonance imaging (MRI) scanners have improved our safety manifold. High definition endoscopy gives us fabulous vision and three-dimensional (3D) endoscopy, an emerging technology promises to improve it further.[6]

BIOLOGY OF TUMORS

The sinonasal tumors are unique with varying biology. Understanding their natural history is pertinent to treatment planning.

Amongst benign tumors inverted papilloma (IP) and angiofibroma are more common.

Inverted papillomas are known to arise from the lateral nasal wall and involve adjacent sinuses. They have a potential for malignant transformation to squamous cancer in 5% of cases.[7] In IP surgical clearance has to be meticulous along with drilling of its base to prevent local recurrence. The specimen also needs careful pathological evaluation to rule out squamous cell carcinoma differentiation which will merit adjuvant radiation therapy. Busquets JM and Hwang P in their meta-analysis of conventional and endoscopic resection of IP have shown lower recurrence pattern in the endoscopic series.[8]

Juvenile nasopharyngeal angiofibromas (JNA) occur in young adolescent males and are vascular tumors which arise from cell rests along the sphenopalatine foramen and spread into the nose, paranasal sinuses and the infratemporal fossa. The JNA can remodel the adjacent greater wing of sphenoid and the orbital apex expanding the inferior orbital fissure to spread intracranially alongside the cavernous sinus. The treatment of choice is complete excision with drilling of the sphenopalatine region which can be done either externally or through endoscopic approach. Endoscopic access should not be attempted unless the surgeon is well versed in advanced endonasal skull base resection and manipulation of tumors in the vicinity of the cavernous sinus. Large JNAs are best dealt with via an open approach.

Amongst malignant tumors adenocarcinoma, esthesion-euroblastoma, neuroendocrine tumor, adenoid cystic carcinoma and squamous cell carcinoma are more common. Due to varied histologies in the paranasal sinuses it is very important to get immunohistochemistry done for accurate diagnosis. This will go a long way towards appropriate treatment planning and prognostication.

Sinonasal adenocarcinomas (SNACs) show a variety of growth patterns. These lesions are classified as intestinal or non-intestinal, the latter subclassified as low grade or high grade.[9] Well-differentiated adenocarcinomas carry the best prognosis with survival rates exceeding 70%.

Esthesioneuroblastomas (ENB) are olfactory groove neuroendocrine tumors. These carry extremely good prognosis when limited to the nose (Kadish A) or up to the cribriform plate (Kadish B). Even the advanced ENB going intracranially (Kadish C) or those with metastatic disease (Kadish D) do relatively better than the squamous cell, sinonasal undifferentiated, small cell neuroendocrine and other high grade cancers. ENB should be treated aggressively with surgery and radiation therapy and those with advanced stages even with combination including chemotherapy. Meta-analysis of ENB reports from 1990 to 2000 by Dulgerov[10] showed better survival in Hyams' grades I and II (56%) than in grades III and IV (25%). Five percent patients manifest with cervical lymph nodes metastases. Survival was significantly better in those without neck node metastases (64% versus 29%). Survival according to treatment modalities was 65% for surgery plus radiotherapy, 51% for radiotherapy and chemotherapy, 48% for surgery, 47% for surgery plus radiotherapy and chemotherapy, and 37% for radiotherapy alone. Higher Hyams grade tumors and presence of cervical lymph node metastases emerged as poor prognostic factors. A combination of surgery and radiotherapy seems to be the optimum approach to treatment. The exact role of chemotherapy in treatment protocols is still unclear.

Neuroendocrine tumors are notorious in the paranasal sinuses. It is very difficult for the pathologist to differentiate between sinonasal undifferentiated carcinoma (SNUC), neuroendocrine carcinoma (NEC), and small cell carcinoma (SmCC). Immunohistochemistry is mandatory for diagnosis. The MD Anderson Cancer Centre report[11] showed local control rate at 5 years for SNUC 78.6%, NEC 72.6% and 66.7% in SmCC. The regional failure (RF) rate at 5 years was 15.6% in SNUC, 12.9% in NEC, and 44.4% in SmCC. The distant metastasis rate at 5 years was 25.4% in SNUC, 14.1% in NEC, and 75.0% in SmCC. Thus neuroendocrine tumors cannot be clubbed together but should be differentiated for better treatment planning.

Adenoid cystic carcinomas (ACC) are indolent tumors with locally advanced stage at presentation. Since the ACC have neurotropic spread it is important to evaluate with an MRI scan to rule out involvement of the adjacent nerves. In the MD Anderson Cancer Centre report[12] of 105 patients over 14 years, most patients presented in advanced stages T3/T4 (76.7%) and yet did not have neck node metastasis N0 (98%). The local recurrence rate was 30%, and the distant metastases rate was 38% mostly in the lungs. The 5-year overall survival and disease specific survival rates were 62.9% and 70.9% which highlights the fact that though local recurrences develop in a significant percentage of patients, survival from this disease exceeds that of other sinonasal malignancies. Almost 40% of patients with local control of disease might manifest with lung metastasis albeit many years later.

Squamous cell carcinoma (SCC) is a high-grade cancer with high propensity to neural spread as well as local invasion. A careful evaluation of the disease epicenter and extension should precede selection for the endonasal approach.

EVALUATION

Tumors in the anterior skull base often appear extensive and forbearing. We require characterization of the involved

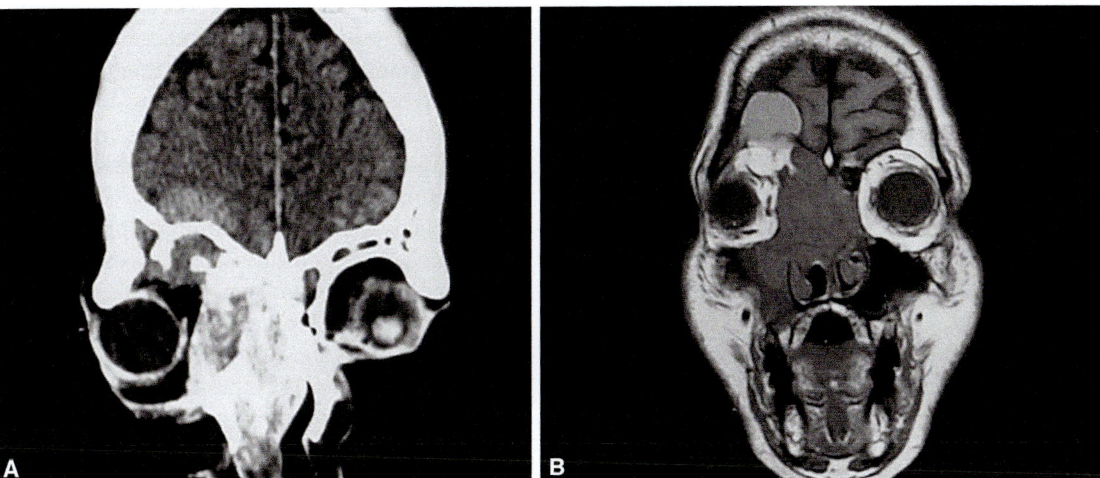

Figs 20.1A and B: CT and MR are essential for soft tissue delineation

structures, delineation of the orbit, dura and the cranial nerves. All this is possible with modern imaging. The new multi-detector CT scan machines are capable of better resolution up to 0.65 mm thickness as well as multiplanar reformatting. MRI scanners can delineate not only the anatomy but also characterize the lesions better. Sequencing in the MR can give us more information of the dural enhancement, characterize disease type and extent, and may well make the difference while contemplating extensive futile surgery. Hence it is mandatory to get CT scan and MRI for evaluating a paranasal sinus/anterior skull base tumor (Figs 20.1A and B).

With diagnostic nasal endoscopy we can evaluate the tumors with magnification and better illumination. Partial volume effect, a radiologic artefact which creates a false impression of tumor involvement of a structure can be verified with diagnostic nasal endoscopy. Structures seemingly involved by tumors on imaging can be delineated better giving a comprehensive evaluation of the disease extent. Thus imaging and endoscopy should be an integral part of paranasal and anterior skull base tumor evaluation.

TREATMENT

Most tumors in the paranasal sinuses and anterior skull base require combined modality treatment. Surgery forms an integral part of the combination along with radiation therapy. Surgery has traditionally been via the transfacial approaches such as lateral rhinotomy or the Weber Fergueson incision. Midfacial degloving approach allows us similar access to the midface with no facial scars. These approaches are well described and give us good access to the paranasal sinuses. For tumors reaching the skull base or with intracranial extension, traditional approach is a transfrontal craniotomy via either the bicoronal incision or the subcranial Raveh's approach combined with a transfacial access. This is called the craniofacial resection (CFR).

Conformal radiation therapy [3D or IMRT (intensity modulated radiation therapy)] is mandatory for the sinonasal region since the tumor is often in close proximity to vital structures. It also helps to contour the tumor bearing areas and protect the optic nerves and brain as much as possible.

Chemotherapy has an emerging role in the management of these tumors today:

1. Primary treatment modality in chemosensitive tumors, e.g. Ewing's sarcoma, embryonal rhabdomyosarcoma.
2. Induction chemotherapy in high grade tumors with a propensity for rapid growth and dissemination, e.g. small cell neuroendocrine tumors.
3. Neo-adjuvant chemotherapy in borderline resectable tumors.
4. Concurrent chemoradiation in grossly inoperable tumors in patients with good general condition.

WHY TRANSNASAL SURGICAL ACCESS?

Transnasal access is a natural trajectory. Experience in working in confined spaces, controlling hemorrhage and cerebrospinal fluid (CSF) leaks have led to application of endonasal route for benign tumors such as inverted papillomas[13] and juvenile nasopharyngeal angiofibromas. Sinonasal tumors lend themselves for endoscopic resection. Those tumors arising in the ethmoids grow locally within the nasal cavity and extend in all directions. These tumors tend to hang into the nasal cavity rather than infiltrate the surrounding structures. A complete resection of these tumors is possible with margins similar to conventional techniques.

In the past decade the transnasal access has grown further with forays made into the cranium. Professors Kassam, Carrou and Snyderman from Pittsburgh, USA have revolutionized the "Expanded Endonasal Approach".[3,4] This modular form of resection of the skull base has been made more appealing with in depth description of the steps of resection in the coronal and sagittal plane. The minimally invasive surgery is minimal only in its access but maximal in its capabilities. The ability to resect the skull base is more or less similar to the open techniques. Instrumentation in form of powered drills, microdebriders, angled scopes have given a tremendous fillip to this access. Neuronavigation has given more confidence in accessing these tumors which cross the skull base in vicinity of important structures such as the internal carotid artery, the optic nerves, ophthalmic, anterior and posterior communicating arteries, hypophysial vessels and the pituitary. Precise, magnified resection is possible today of all these structures which is required for a complete clearance of these tumors.

IS ENDONASAL ACCESS SUITABLE?

Disease control via complete tumor resection should be the prime objective. Endoscopic endonasal surgery is a new addition to the armamentarium and we need to evaluate its safety and efficacy.

The "en bloc" resection method is gold standard and there is no disputing its efficacy. But truly the actual ability to achieve "en bloc" resection in these tumors is doubtful. These tumors seldom come out intact and the posterior regions of these tumors are always removed piece meal. At the end of surgery we need to achieve negative margins. Whether you can achieve this via an "en bloc" surgery or via a piece meal resection is immaterial so long as you can get an oncologically safe clearance. This same logic has been proven in transoral laser microsurgery to be oncologically safe. Thus if there is a planned surgical method detailing exact structures to be removed and it is achieved via endonasal endoscopic resection then it would be as safe as conventional surgery.

In oncologic surgery, margins are essential for ensuring a safe resection. Sinonasal/anterior skull base tumor are bound by the orbit laterally, the brain superiorly, the optic nerves and internal carotid artery posterolaterally and the pituitary gland posteriorly. Surgical margins in these tumors would involve removing adjacent structures preserving the uninvolved vital structures with narrow margins. These margins are still possible. But when we deal with tumors extending to the sphenoid, the margins are even narrower. When the tumor extends intracranially the superior margin would be the dura which can be resected in a limited way till we reach the optic chiasma posteriorly. Brain involvement can never be cleared with margins. Hence in sinonasal/anterior skull base tumors the margins are close and usually "gross total resection" is possible at best. This cannot improve further by conventional techniques. Using the endoscopic access vital structures are visualized under magnification and illumination improving clearance of tumor. Frontal sinus, sphenoid and clivus are no longer blind areas and can be cleared optimally.

Tumors which arise around the ethmoids often do not involve the anterior facial skeleton or the nasal floor. In these tumors, access requires additional soft tissue and bone removal which can be time consuming and unnecessary for oncologic clearance. For suitable cases, the transnasal access is direct avoiding extensive bone and soft tissue dissection and reconstruction. Disassembly of the facial skeleton can be avoided. The tumor clearance can be tailor made to the tumor and margins similar to conventional surgery can be achieved. The uninvolved structures such as the nasolacrimal duct, frontal process of maxilla, inferior turbinate can be preserved without compromising on oncologic safety.

Morbidity of conventional surgery such as local infection, CSF leak and meningitis need to be reduced further. After adequate resection, the dural defect can be repaired endoscopically with layered closure ensuring reduced morbidity as seen in most series worldwide with CSF leak rates less than 4%.

Finally endoscopic resection should be undertaken only in those tumors feasible for complete excision via conventional methods to achieve similar control rates.

CONTRAINDICATIONS

The sinonasal and anterior skull base tumors require a 3D resection. The contraindications for a conventional surgical removal of tumors in this region are bilateral optic nerve involvement, internal carotid artery involvement, gross brain involvement and extensive dural enhancement.

Specifically for endonasal resection in addition to above the current contraindications are involvement of the anterior maxillary wall, the palate, outer table of the frontal bone and skin, extensive dural enhancement extending laterally and gross brain involvement. If we draw a meridian through the pupils, by and large the tumors with extension lateral to this meridian in the frontal sinus or dura are not amenable to an endonasal resection and require a conventional approach (Figs 20.2A and B).

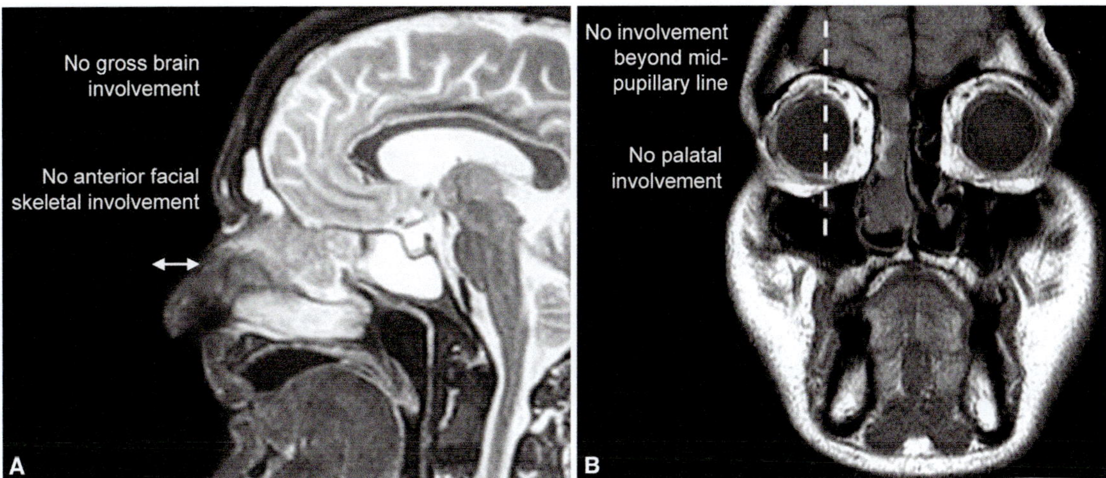

Figs 20.2A and B: Contraindications

Oncologic Results

The early 90s saw groups from Belgium, Austria, Germany and Italy remove select malignant tumors with encouraging results. Stammberger H, et al[14] from Graz, Austria published a report of 36 malignant paranasal sinus tumors resected endoscopically with the esthesioneuroblastomas having 100% survival with 37 months follow up. Goffart Y et al[15] from Belgium published a retrospective study of 78 cases from two centers in Belgium with 2-year and 5-year survival rates of 73.1% and 52.3% respectively. Nicolai P, Capabianca P, et al[16] from two centers in Italy reported on a 10 years follow up in 184 malignant tumors. The most frequent histotypes encountered were adenocarcinoma (37%), squamous cell carcinoma (13.6%), olfactory neuroblastoma (12%), mucosal melanoma (9.2%), and adenoid cystic carcinoma (7.1%). They reported a 5-year disease-specific survival of 91.4% for those resected exclusively endoscopically and 58.8% for those resected with cranioendoscopic techniques. The latest in these series of reports comes from the MD Anderson Cancer Center wherein Hanna E[17] reported 120 cases treated endoscopically, 93 (77.5%) exclusive endoscopic approach (EEA) and 27 (22.5%) treated with endoscopic assisted CFR. The 5 years local control rate was 85% with a medial follow-up of 37 months.

Preservation of Uninvolved Structures

In traditional surgery, the resection is standard irrespective of involvement of the structures. Medial maxillectomy involves removal of the frontal process of the maxilla, lacrimal bone, lamina papyracea, part of maxilla medial to the infraorbital foramen, the middle turbinate and the inferior turbinate along with the lacrimal sac and the nasolacrimal duct. Thus even though the nasolacrimal duct system is uninvolved, in a conventional medial maxillectomy we endup with marsupialization of the lacrimal sac and a potential for epiphora. What the endoscopic approach offers is ability to customize the resection to the tumor with the objective of removing the tumor base completely with margins as much as possible in that region. Since we can customize the resection to the tumor extent, uninvolved structures such as nasolacrimal duct, lacrimal sac can be spared.

Steps of Resection

Endonasal Endoscopic Resection

Subcranial disease: Today endoscopic medial maxillectomy, ethmoidectomy, frontoethmoidectomy, sphenoidectomy are all feasible. The resection is tailor made to the tumor with the objective of removing the tumor base completely with margins as much as possible in that region. The tumor is surveyed for feasibility of endonasal resection. The structures involved on imaging are determined and planned for sequential resection. The tumor is debulked centrally and the margins are achieved all around. In oncologic surgery the "next compartment" technique is followed for margins. For instance if the tumor is in the anterior ethmoids the margins achieved will be opening the frontal sinus superiorly and the posterior ethmoids posteriorly and lamina papyracea laterally. If the tumor involves the lateral nasal wall, the lateral margin would be achieved by removing the lamina papyracea and the maxillary sinus laterally and the frontal sinus superiorly and the sphenoid sinus posteriorly. The base is resected completely and as wide margins as suitable are achieved (Figs 20.3A and B).

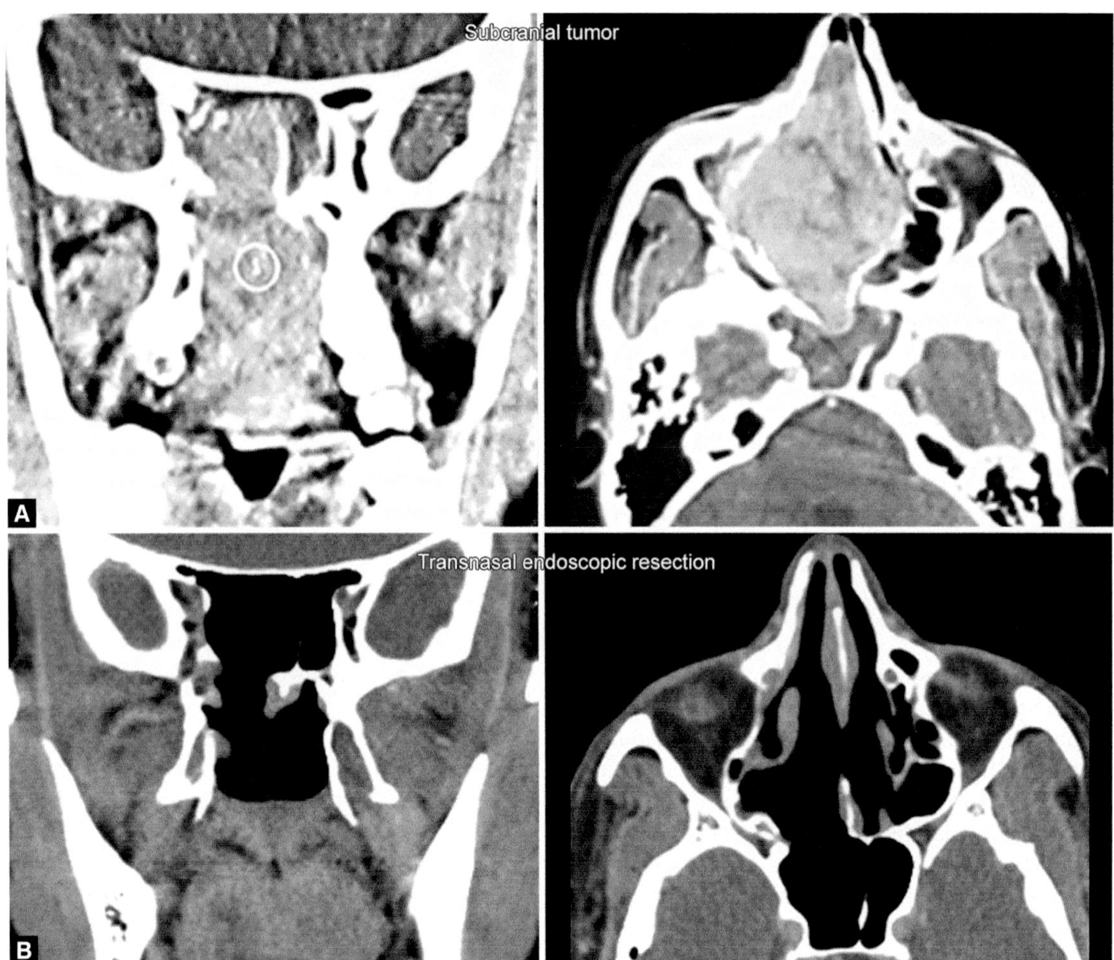

Figs 20.3A and B: Transnasal resection of subcranial tumor

Transcranial disease: For sinonasal tumors which have breached the anterior skull base and involve the dura the endoscopic endonasal trajectory is suitable to access and encompass the tumor with margins. Via the transnasal access a complete resection of the sinonasal component of the tumor is carried out. The base of the tumor is targeted next. To encompass the tumor all round exposure of normal dura is achieved. Bilateral complete ethmoidectomy with removal of the lamina papyracea exposes the supraorbital crest area. The Draf type III frontal sinus procedure combines both the frontal sinuses and gives access to the posterior wall of the frontal sinus which can be drilled to expose normal dura anterior to the tumor at the skull base. Wide sphenoidotomy is accomplished with removal of the rostrum of the sphenoid and floor followed by drilling of the intersphenoid septae. This gives good access to the optic chiasma and jugum sphenoidale anterior to it. Drilling the planum sphenoidale exposes the dura posterior to the cribriform region. Once the dura is exposed on all sides of the tumor at the cribriform, the ethmoidal vessels are coagulated with bipolar cautery. Keeping adequate margins, the dura is incised exposing the brain. After coagulating the tail of the sagittal sinus anteriorly the crista gala is exposed and separated from the dural envelope. Further dissection is with bipolar cautery separating the involved structures from the brain. Once the olfactory bulbs are reached they are cauterized with bipolar cautery and divided separating the tumor completely. Dural margins are assessed with frozen section and the dural defect repaired with fascia lata tissue and tissue glue. A nasal septal flap (Hadad-Carrou flap) if preserved can be used to provide a mucosal cover for the defect (Figs 20.4A and B).

Combined Approach

The endoscope is a useful tool in combination with conventional techniques. As mentioned before the endoscopic

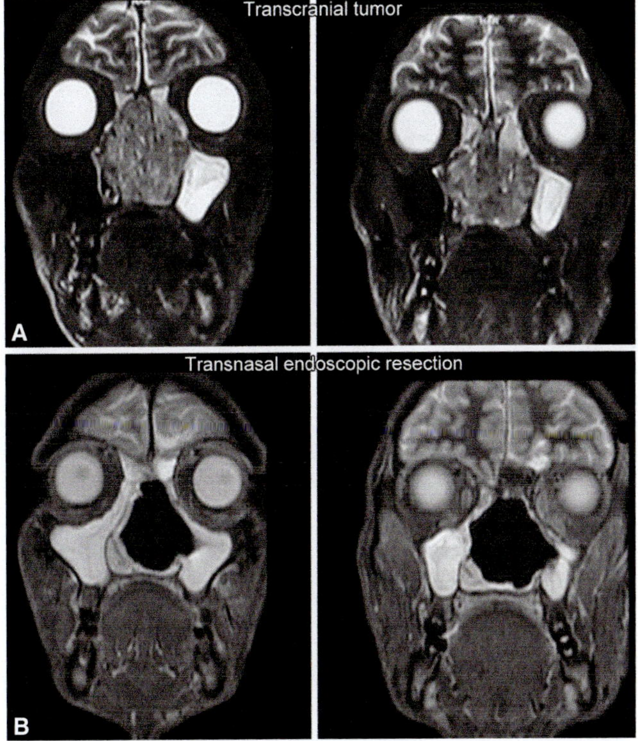

Figs 20.4A and B: Transnasal resection of a transcranial tumor

techniques allow better visualization with magnification and illumination. If the nasal component is amenable to endonasal resection then it is performed in conjunction with other procedures as required for an oncologically safe resection. Even after conventional medial maxillectomy it is good idea to use the endoscope to visualize the posterior ethmoids, frontal sinus and the sphenoid sinus. These areas in the far recesses of the skull are not well visualized conventionally.

Combined Endoscopic with Orbital Resection

When the sinonasal tumor involves the orbit, the sinonasal part of the tumor can be resected endonasally while the orbit can be resected conventionally.

Combined Endoscopic and Craniotomy Access (Cranioendoscopic Resection)

Intracranial extension of sinonasal tumors can be extensive. Tumors with dural involvement or enhancement laterally beyond the mid-pupillary line are not feasible for endonasal resection. When there is gross brain involvement not limited to midline it is not suitable for endonasal resection. In this situation if the nasal component is amenable for endoscopic resection then it is addressed transnasally along with a conventional cranial access for the intracranial component (Figs 20.5A to C).

DEBATE: ENDOSCOPIC SURGERY VERSUS CONVENTIONAL SURGERY

In my opinion there is no debate about the superiority of any single approach. Endoscopic approach is an addition to the existing armamentarium of the surgeon. Depending on the merits of each case the approach should be planned. When contemplating on the approach for resection of a sinonasal/anterior skull base tumor, you need to take into account the training of the surgeon and available resources. A surgeon should be trained in all aspects of conventional skull base surgery before venturing into endoscopic surgery. Endoscopic tumor resection is not an approach for the novice surgeon. The surgeon needs to gain experience in benign endoscopic surgery before venturing to tumor surgery. When dealing with malignant tumors the first chance is the best chance and a complete resection regardless of the approach is to be achieved. To manage malignant tumors the surgeon needs to be well versed in oncologic aspect of tumors and more importantly should have the maturity to stop and convert to a conventional approach in adverse situations.

AUTHOR'S EXPERIENCE

At the Tata Memorial Hospital from September 2002 to May 2012 we have performed 180 endonasal resections of benign (40) and malignant (140) lesions. Endonasal endoscopic resection was performed in 154 patients of which 3 needed to be converted to open procedures, one for control of hemorrhage while the other 2 were for oncologic safety. Endoscopic assisted craniofacial resection was performed in 15 patients while complete transnasal cranioendoscopic resection was performed in seven patients. Amongst the 140 malignant lesions, most common were adenocarcinomas 18% followed by esthesioneuroblastomas 13% and adenoid cystic carcinoma 9.5% amongst other varied histologies. CSF leak was seen in two patients. In one patient the skull base was repacked while in the other the patient recovered without any intervention. In two cases, a leak was suspected, but there was no conclusive evidence. Meningitis occurred in one patient which resolved on antibiotics without sequelae.

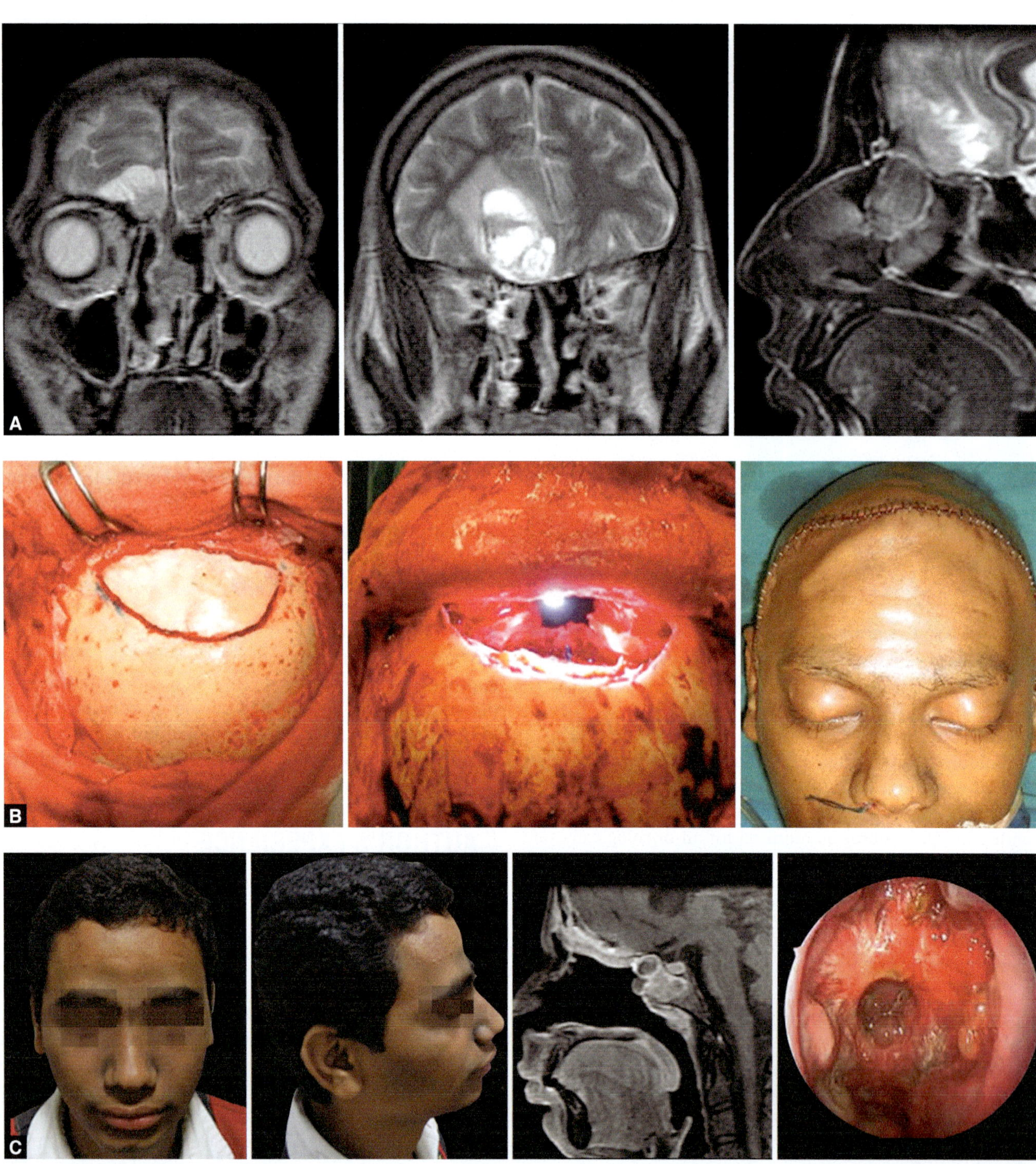

Figs 20.5A to C: Combined approach for transcranial tumor: (A) MR showing limited nasal tumor with transcranial spread; (B) Transcranial access via bicoronal flap and craniotomy and transnasal clearance; (C) Postoperative results showing excellent cosmesis, good cranionasal separation and well mucosalized nasal cavity

CONCLUSION

Minimal access surgery for sinonasal and anterior skull base tumors is now an established modality with proven safety. The endonasal access should be used whenever feasible either alone or in combination with external approaches with the sole aim of optimal resection. Prior to attempting endoscopic endonasal tumor surgery one should get adequate training with cadaver dissection and benign endoscopic surgery. Malignant tumors are best dealt with by surgeons in a multidisciplinary team with adequate knowledge of tumor biology and experience in conventional surgical techniques.

REFERENCES

1. Messerklinger W. Technics and possibilities of nasal endoscopy. HNO. 1972;20(5):133-5.
2. Stamm AC, Draf W, Stamm A. Micro-endoscopic Surgery of the Paranasal Sinuses and the Skull Base. Berlin: Springer; 2000.
3. Kassam A, Snyderman CH, Mintz A, et al. Expanded endonasal approach: the rostrocaudal axis. Part I. Crista galli to the sella turcica. Neurosurg Focus. 2005;19(1):E3.
4. Kassam A, Snyderman CH, Mintz A, et al. Expanded endonasal approach: the rostrocaudal axis. Part II. Posterior clinoids to the foramen magnum. Neurosurg Focus. 2005;19(1):E4.
5. Hoffman H, Hudgins PA. Head and skull base features of nine Egyptian mummies: evaluation with high-resolution CT and reformation techniques. AJR Am J Roentgenol. 2002;178(6):1367-76.
6. Fraser JF, Allen B, Anand VK, et al. Three-dimensional neurostereoendoscopy: subjective and objective comparison to 2D. Minim Invasive Neurosurg. 2009;52(1):25-31.
7. Mendenhall WM, Hinerman RW, Malyapa RS, et al. Inverted papilloma of the nasal cavity and paranasal sinuses. Am J Clin Oncol. 2007;30(5):560-3.
8. Busquets JM, Hwang PH. Endoscopic resection of sinonasal inverted papilloma: a meta-analysis. Otolaryngol Head Neck Surg. 2006;134(3):476-82.
9. Cordes B, Williams MD, Tirado Y, et al. Molecular and phenotypic analysis of poorly differentiated sinonasal neoplasms: an integrated approach for early diagnosis and classification. Hum Pathol. 2009;40(3):283-92.
10. Dulguerov P, Allal AS, Calcaterra TC. Esthesioneuroblastoma: a meta-analysis and review. Lancet Oncol. 2001;2(11):683-90.
11. Rosenthal DI, Barker JL, El-Naggar AK, et al. Sinonasal malignancies with neuroendocrine differentiation: patterns of failure according to histologic phenotype. Cancer. 2004;101(11):2567-73.
12. Lupinetti AD, Roberts DB, Williams MD, et al. Sinonasal adenoid cystic carcinoma: the M. D. Anderson Cancer Center experience. Cancer. 2007;110(12):2726-31.
13. Kamel RH. Transnasal endoscopic medial maxillectomy in inverted papilloma. Laryngoscope. 1995;105(8 Pt 1):847-53.
14. Stammberger H, Anderhuber W, Walch C, et al. Possibilities and limitations of endoscopic management of nasal and paranasal sinus malignancies. Acta Otorhinolaryngol Belg. 1999;53(3):199-205.
15. Goffart Y, Jorissen M, Daele J, et al. Minimally invasive endoscopic management of malignant sinonasal tumors. Acta Otorhinolaryngol Belg. 2000;54(2):221-32.
16. Nicolai P, Battaglia P, Bignami M, et al. Endoscopic surgery for malignant tumors of the sinonasal tract and adjacent skull base: a 10-year experience. Am J Rhinol. 2008;22(3):308-16.
17. Hanna E, DeMonte F, Ibrahim S, et al. Endoscopic resection of sinonasal cancers with and without craniotomy: oncologic results. Arch Otolaryngol Head Neck Surg. 2009;135(12):1219-24.

Endoscopic Management of Cerebrospinal Fluid Rhinorrhea

Milind V Kirtane, Hetal Marfatia Patel, Kashmira Chavan, Dhruv Satwalekar

INTRODUCTION

The surgical management of cerebrospinal fluid (CSF) rhinorrhea has traditionally been in the domain of neurosurgeons. With better understanding and with advancements in technology, a large number of cases are now being managed by the transnasal route with the endoscope. This chapter deals with the surgical management of anterior skull-base defects. However, frontal sinus defects, in the roof and posterior wall, that require an external approach have been excluded.

Cerebrospinal fluid rhinorrhea is the leakage of CSF through a communication of the subarachnoid space with the sinonasal cavity following a defect in the skull-base.

HISTORICAL ASPECTS

- *CSF rhinorrhea:* First described by Willis in 1682 and later demonstrated at autopsy by Miller in 1826.[1]
- *Transcranial repair of CSF leak:* First reported by Dandy in 1926.[2]
- *Extracranial approach to repair an anterior cranial fossa CSF leak via a naso-orbital incision:* First described by Dohlman in 1948.[2]
- *Transnasal approach:* Hirsch (1952) reported the repair of sphenoid leaks with septal flaps.[3] Later demonstrated by Vrabec and Hallberg (1964).[4]
- *Endoscopic repair of CSF leaks:* First performed by Wigand (1981).[5]

Since then, the transnasal endoscopic approach for repair of CSF rhinorrhea has gained popularity, given the high success rate and decreased morbidity associated with this approach.

PATHOPHYSIOLOGY

Physiology of Cerebrospinal Fluid Production

The total volume of CSF in a normal adult ranges between 90 mL and 150 mL. CSF is formed at a rate of 0.35–0.37 mL/minute (20 mL/hour or 350–500 mL/day).

Sites of Cerebrospinal Fluid Production

- *50–80%:* Choroid plexus in ventricles
- *30%:* Ependymal surface
- *20%:* Capillary ultrafiltration.

CSF thus produced, flows from the lateral ventricles to the third ventricle via the foramen of Monro, and further through the aqueduct of Sylvius into the fourth ventricle. It then flows out into the subarachnoid space via the foramina of Magendie and Luschka. CSF resorption takes place at the arachnoid villi and granulations projecting into the dural sinuses. The arachnoid villi act like a valve, preventing backflow of CSF into the subarachnoid space. Higher hydrostatic pressure drives the CSF unidirectionally into the dural sinuses.

The process of CSF production and absorption is shown in Flow chart 21.1.

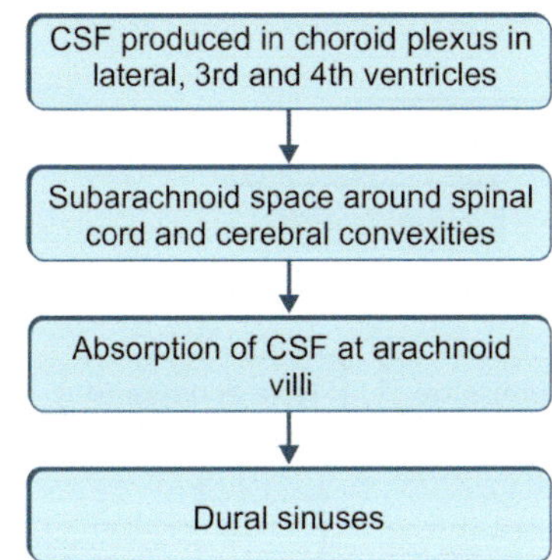

Flow chart 21.1: Process of cerebrospinal fluid production and absorption

Continuous production and absorption of CSF leads to a turnover of about 3–5 times a day. CSF pressure in the supine position is normally 5–15 cm H_2O. Neurologic symptoms may be seen when CSF pressure exceeds 15–20 cm H_2O.[6]

Classification of Cerebrospinal Fluid Leaks

Cerebrospinal fluid leaks can be classified on the basis of etiology, anatomic site, or underlying intracranial pressure. The etiology of CSF leaks is diverse.

Congenital

- Congenital skull-base defects with CSF leak
- Cerebrospinal fluid leak associated with congenital meningocele or meningoencephalocele
- Congenital hydrocephalus.

Acquired

Traumatic (most common reported cause of CSF leak: 70–80%):[7-9]

Iatrogenic trauma:
- Intranasal surgery (e.g, Intranasal ethmoidectomy)
- Endoscopic sinus surgery
- Skull-base surgery:
    - Transnasal endoscopic approach
    - Craniotomy.

Accidental trauma:
- Head injuries (open/closed)
- Post-traumatic hydrocephalus.

Inflammatory:
- Sinonasal polyps
- Invasive fungal sinusitis

- Mucoceles
- Skull-base osteomyelitis.

Neoplastic:
- Neoplasms involving the skull-base
    - Sinonasal malignancy
    - Nasopharyngeal carcinoma
    - Intracranial tumors.

Miscellaneous: Hydrocephalus.

Spontaneous: CSF leaks which occur in the absence of any distinct etiological factor are included in this category.

Ommaya et al.[10] were of the opinion that there are no cases which can truly be labeled as "spontaneous" and preferred to categorize them as nontraumatic leaks. They have classified nontraumatic CSF leaks into high pressure and normal pressure CSF leaks (Flow chart 21.2).

Sites of Cerebrospinal Fluid Leaks

The attachment of the middle turbinate divides the cribriform plate into medial and lateral lamellae which form the walls of the olfactory fossa. The dura in the region of the olfactory fossa is thin and is firmly attached to the underlying bone. The passage of the anterior ethmoidal artery and the olfactory filaments further weakens this area. This anatomy predisposes the region to the occurrence of CSF leaks, as any trauma in this area can easily result in dural tears. Most studies report the cribriform plate to be the most common site of defect in CSF rhinorrhea, followed by the roof of the ethmoid, sphenoid sinus, and the frontal sinus.[7,11,12]

Cerebrospinal fluid leaks secondary to accidental trauma: Traumatic CSF leaks usually occur at the fovea ethmoidalis or at the junction of the fovea ethmoidalis and the olfactory fossa.

Less common sites are the sphenoid sinus and frontal sinus.

Cerebrospinal fluid leaks secondary to iatrogenic trauma: The lateral lamella of the cribriform plate and the roof of the posterior ethmoids are common sites of injury following endoscopic sinus surgery.

Defects in the sphenoid sinus are more commonly seen following pituitary surgery.

Spontaneous leaks: Common sites for spontaneous CSF leaks are the cribriform plate (medial or lateral lamella) or the lateral wall of the sphenoid sinus, especially in a pneumatized lateral recess (Fig. 21.1).

Flow chart 21.2: Classification of cerebrospinal fluid rhinorrhea (Ommaya et al.[10])

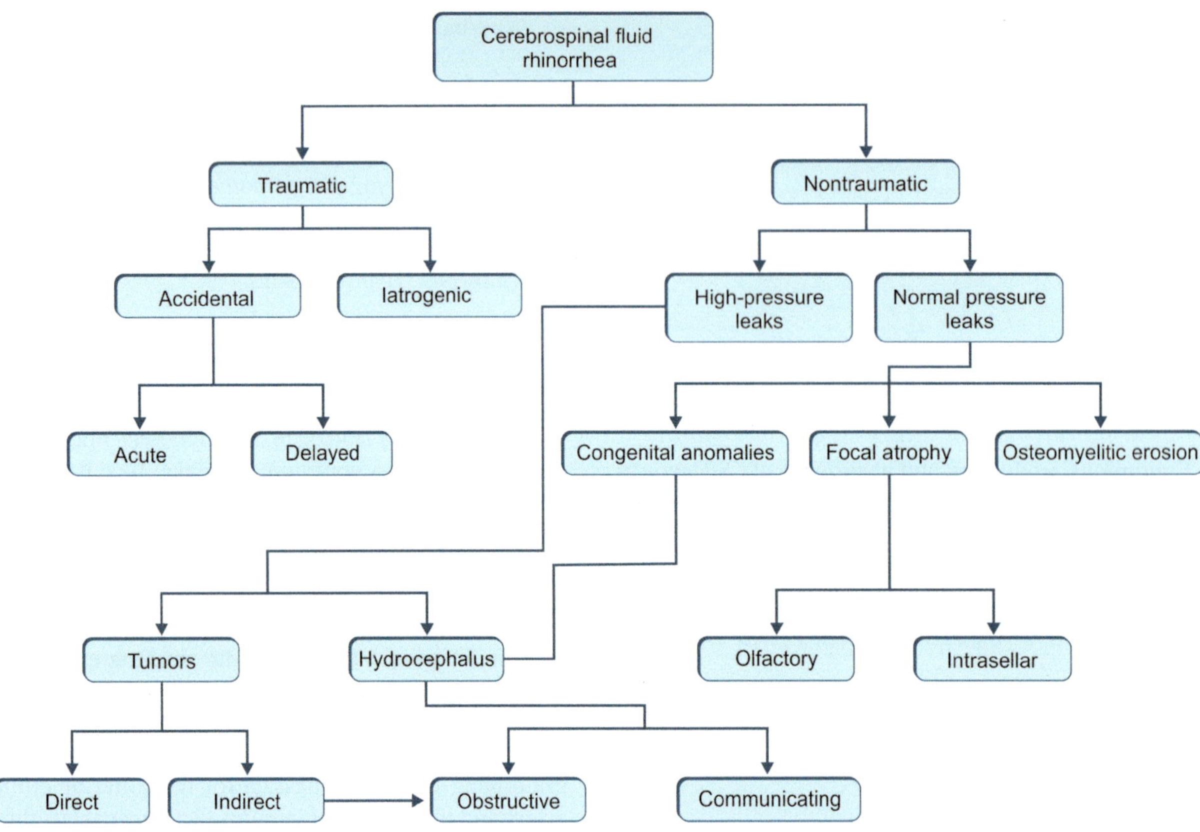

Congenital leaks: Congenital skull-base defects are commonly seen at the cribriform plate, in the region of the foramen cecum or the roof of the ethmoids.[13]

CLINICAL PRESENTATION

Patients with CSF rhinorrhea typically present with a history of watery nasal discharge, usually unilateral, which may be aggravated on bending forward or straining. In cases of sphenoid sinus leaks, the CSF may collect within the sphenoid sinus and drip through the nose when the patient bends forward (Teapot sign). Associated symptoms such as headache and visual disturbances, suggesting raised intracranial pressure, may be present. A past history of trauma may be present. Patients may also present with recurrent episodes of meningitis due to a pre-existing skull-base defect. A meningoencephalocele presenting as a nasal mass is also not uncommon. Patients with congenital defects may present with watery rhinorrhea, nasal obstruction due to an encephalocele or with meningitis.[13] Pneumocephalus[14] (Fig. 21.2) may occur following a large skull-base defect

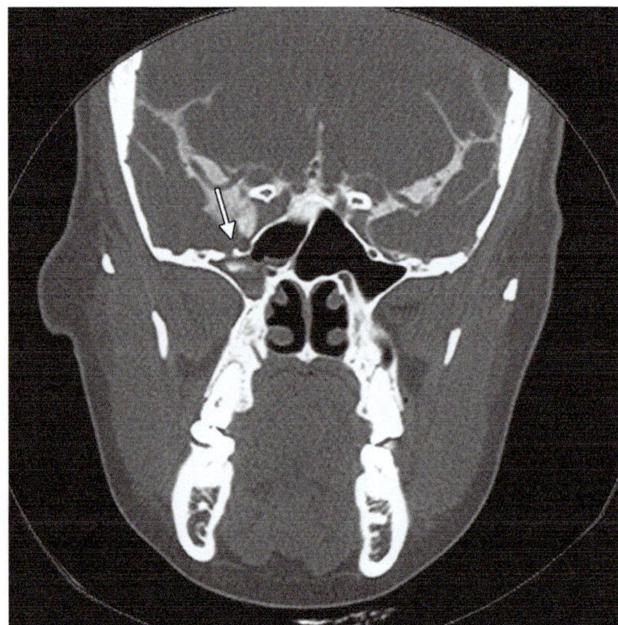

Fig. 21.1: Computed tomography cisternogram showing a defect in the lateral recess of the right sphenoid sinus (white arrow)

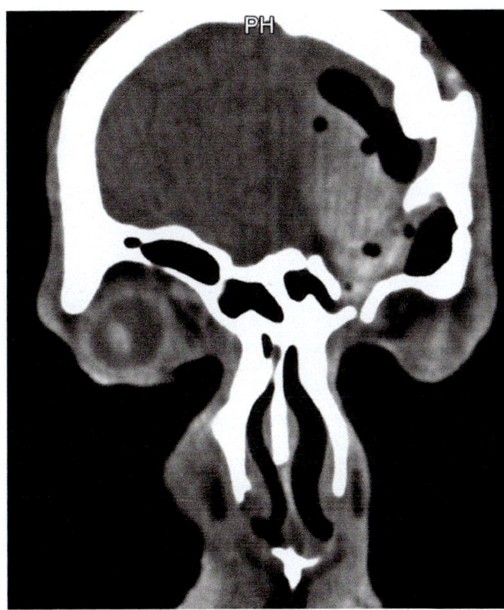

Fig. 21.2: Multiple skull fractures with pneumocephalus

TABLE 21.1: Clinical presentation in a case of cerebrospinal fluid rhinorrhea
• Active leakage of clear watery fluid from the nose
• Intermittent leak
• A past history of CSF leak
• Meningitis—one or more episodes
• Deafness secondary to meningitis
• Headache
• Persistent "cold"
• Mass in the nose

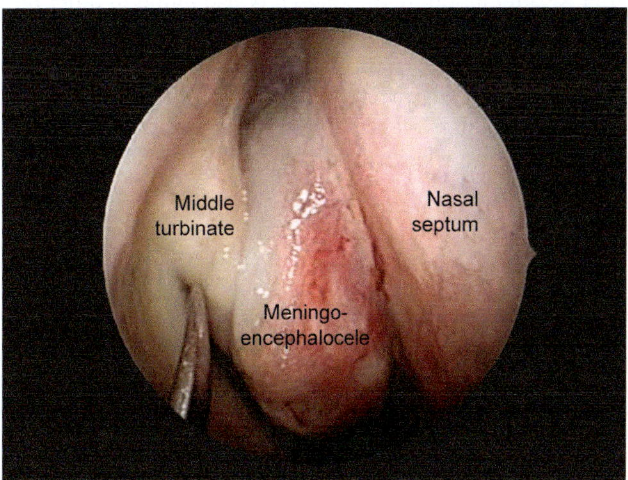

Fig. 21.3: Endoscopic view of a meningoencephalocele in the right nostril

due to transmission of pressure on coughing, sneezing, etc. Rarely, patients may present with hearing loss secondary to meningitis, and on investigating further into the cause of meningitis, the presence of a skull-base defect may be detected. Pressure-type headaches, pulsatile tinnitus, and balance abnormalities have been reported in patients with spontaneous CSF leaks.[6,15]

The "reservoir sign" may be positive (presence of intermittent rhinorrhea as the fluid accumulates in the paranasal sinuses and drains externally with changes in head position). The "halo sign", i.e. a ring of clear fluid surrounding a central blood stain may be elicited when CSF leaking from the nose mixed with blood is absorbed on a filter paper. Signs suggestive of meningitis, such as neck rigidity, may be elicited in cases presenting with an active episode of meningitis. Often physical examination may not reveal any positive findings, especially in patients with an intermittent leak. Table 21.1 shows the various clinical features that may be seen in patients of CSF rhinorrhea.

MANAGEMENT

Preoperative Assessment

Preoperative assessment of CSF leaks is directed toward confirming the diagnosis, localization of the site of the defect, assessing its size, and selecting the appropriate surgical approach. It involves interpreting CSF tests, diagnostic nasal endoscopy findings and imaging studies in conjunction.

Nasal Endoscopy

A nasal endoscopy done on an outpatient basis with adequate decongestion may reveal the skull-base defect or an associated pseudoencephalocele or meningocele (Fig. 21.3).

Biochemical Tests

Biochemical tests are useful to differentiate CSF from nasal secretions. However, localization of the leak is not possible on the basis of these tests.

Beta-2 transferrin test: Beta-2 transferrin testing is a highly specific and sensitive noninvasive method in identifying nasal fluid as CSF. Beta-2 transferrin is present only in perilymph, vitreous humor, and CSF. Beta-1 transferrin which is normally found in CSF is converted into beta-2 transferrin by cerebral neuraminidase. A very small quantity of nasal fluid is needed for beta-2 transferrin testing using newer laboratory techniques.[16] However, false negative results may be seen in the presence of high mucus content in the secretions, while false positive results are possible in patients with chronic alcohol abuse, chronic hepatic disorders, certain rare glycoprotein metabolism disorders, rectal carcinomas or with certain genetic variants of transferrin.[17,18]

Beta-trace protein: Beta-trace protein (βTP) is a brain-specific protein with a prostaglandin synthase activity found in the CSF. It is produced mainly in the leptomeninges and the choroid plexus[19] and is the second most abundant protein in CSF after albumin. Although it is also found in other body fluids, including serum, the concentration is much less as compared to CSF.[20] Quantitative nephelometric βTP assays can be performed in a few minutes which give it an advantage over the qualitative assay for beta-2 transferrin.[21] The beta-trace test has a specificity of nearly 100% and a sensitivity of 91.17%.[22]

Imaging

Radiological investigations provide key information regarding the location and size of the defect as well as the presence of any associated pseudomeningocele, meningoencephalocele, tumors or associated congenital anomalies. It is of utmost importance to precisely locate the site of CSF fistula whenever surgical intervention is considered. Numerous techniques, including computed tomography, magnetic resonance imaging, positive contrast (iophendylate) studies, radionuclide cisternography, preoperative or intraoperative injection of fluorescein dye, provide immense help to the operating surgeon to accurately localize the site and to determine the size of the defect.

High-resolution computed tomography: High-resolution CT (1–2 mm sections) in coronal and axial planes is often the only test required for localizing the defect site.[23] However, false positive results may be seen in cases with a history of previous skull-base surgery, wherein a bony defect may be seen in the absence of a true leak. Another difficulty encountered is the inability to distinguish between mucosal thickening, meningocele and CSF leaking from a distant defect which accumulates in a sinus, when opacification of a sinus is visualized in a plain CT scan.[12,24] Compression of the pituitary gland by a CSF filled herniating dura may lead to the appearance of an empty sella on CT, which can be confirmed on MRI (Fig. 21.4).

Magnetic resonance imaging and magnetic resonance cisternography: Magnetic resonance cisternography, a noninvasive technique can detect CSF leaks in multiple

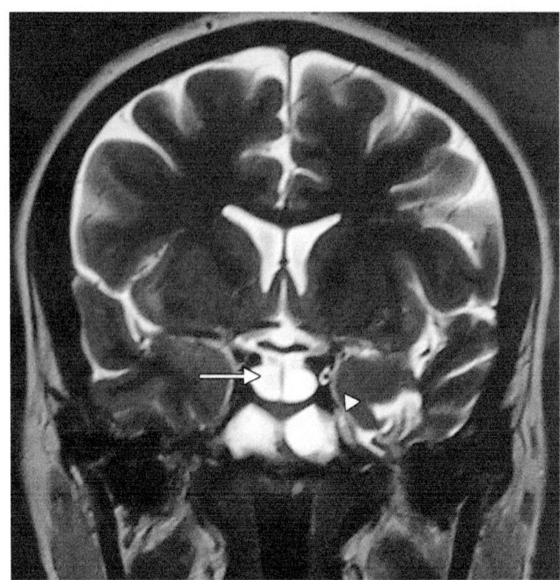

Fig. 21.4: Coronal T2-weighted MRI image showing an empty sella (white arrow) in a case of cerebrospinal fluid leak in the lateral recess of left sphenoid sinus (white arrowhead)

planes by the inherent bright signal of CSF on T2-weighted images. It helps in determining the uninterrupted CSF signal from the subarachnoid space into a meningocele or meningoencephalocele. MRI and MR cisternography are useful modalities to distinguish inflammatory tissue from meningoencephaloceles without radiation exposure.[12] A limited ability to delineate bony details on magnetic resonance imaging is however, a disadvantage, especially when surgical management is required.

Computed tomography cisternography: In cases of doubtful diagnosis, a CT cisternogram with intrathecal injection of a radio-opaque dye may be performed. In cases with active leaks, CT cisternography has been reported to have a success rate of detecting up to 87% cases.[23,25,26] Confirming the diagnosis of CSF rhinorrhea with a CT cisternogram may be difficult in cases where a patient does not have an active leak at the time of presentation, as leakage of the dye through the defect may not be visualized.[12,24,25,27] In such cases, cotton pledgets may be placed in the nasal cavity. These are later scanned, and if traces of dye are found on the pledgets, the diagnosis of CSF rhinorrhea is confirmed although the site of leak is not detected. CT cisternography is however, an invasive procedure associated with a slight risk for complications such as headache and infection, and is relatively contraindicated in patients with active meningitis or raised intracranial pressure. Low-osmolarity nonionic contrast agents such as iohexol and iopamidol have now replaced older compounds like metrizamide which were associated with higher incidence of side effects.[26]

Radionuclide cisternograms: Radionuclide cisternography involves placement of intranasal pledgets followed by intrathecal injection of Technetium-99. The imaging can be completed in hours to days after injection of the agent, depending on the half-life of the agent used, which increases its utility in cases of low-volume or intermittent leaks. Limitations of radionuclide cisternography include a high false positive rate, variable sensitivity, invasiveness, less spatial resolution and localizing ability, and a lesser specificity and ability to delineate fine anatomic details as compared to CT cisternography.[27,28]

Flow chart 21.3 shows an algorithm for performing radiological investigations to diagnose CSF rhinorrhea.

Intrathecal Fluorescein

Fluorescein can be injected intrathecally, preoperatively to establish the diagnosis of a CSF leak, or intraoperatively to accurately localize a skull-base defect. The procedure involves a lumbar puncture with intrathecal injection of 0.1 mL of 5% fluorescein diluted in 10 mL of the patient's CSF.[29] The demonstration of green-yellow fluid defines the site of CSF leakage. A blue light filter can improve the detection of fluorescein leaking from the defect. Multiple complications have been reported after intrathecal fluorescein administration, including seizures, dizziness, nausea, vomiting. These however, appear to be dose-dependent and are transient at lower concentrations.[29]

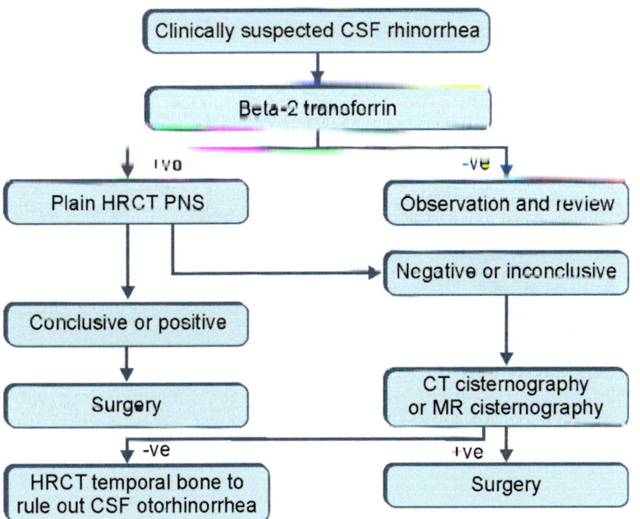

Flow chart 21.3: Algorithm for performing radiological investigations to diagnose CSF leaks

CONSERVATIVE MANAGEMENT

Conservative management is usually indicated in cases of post-traumatic CSF leaks. Conservative measures include bed rest with head elevation, avoidance of straining such as nose blowing, sneezing, coughing. Use of diuretics and stool softeners is also advocated.[11] Prophylactic antibiotics may also be given. Some authors however do not recommend use of prophylactic antibiotics due to the risk of developing antibiotic resistance.[6,30] A lumbar drain may be required for high-pressure leaks.[31] Traumatic CSF leaks often heal with conservative measures over a course of 7–10 days.

SURGICAL MANAGEMENT

Indications for Surgery

- Failure of conservative treatment
- Cerebrospinal fluid leaks which develop days or weeks after trauma
- Very large post-surgical defects
- High pressure leaks, which do not heal even on normalizing the intracranial pressure
- Persistent pneumocephalus despite cessation of leak.
- Spontaneous CSF leaks are unlikely to heal, and hence merit surgical repair.

Over the last 30 years, evolution of endoscopic surgical techniques has led to higher success rates and lower morbidity as compared to the traditional craniotomy approach. Hence endoscopic repair of CSF rhinorrhea is now the treatment of choice in most cases.

Endoscopic Repair of Cerebrospinal Fluid Rhinorrhea

Planning the appropriate approach to the defect site should be preceded by a detailed reading of the CT scan by the operating surgeon, and defining the site and size of the defect. This is best done with coronal sections on the CT scan. Axial sections may provide additional information, especially while planning an approach to the frontal recess.

Principles of Endoscopic Repair

The patient is placed in a supine position under general anesthesia. The area around the nose and the graft site (abdomen or thigh) is prepared and draped using aseptic precautions. The nasal cavity is decongested adequately using pledgets soaked in saline with adrenaline. Normal saline with 1:1,00,000 adrenaline is used for local infiltration.

Approaches to the Defect Site

Cribriform plate, roof of ethmoids: The cribriform plate consists of a medial and a lateral lamella separated by the attachment of the middle turbinate. The middle turbinate is thus a useful landmark to determine an approach to medial and lateral lamella defects.

In order to create adequate space to approach the medial lamella of the cribriform plate, the middle turbinate is gently lateralized and the area medial to the middle turbinate is decongested using adrenaline soaked pledgets (Figs 21.5A and B).

The lateral lamella (Figs 21.6A and B) and the roof of the ethmoids can be approached by passing the endoscope lateral to the middle turbinate. A complete ethmoidectomy is usually required to access the defect site. Trimming of the middle turbinate may be required occasionally if access is limited.

Sphenoid Sinus

The sphenoid sinus can be approached via a transethmoidal approach by performing a complete anterior and posterior ethmoidectomy. It can also be reached via a parasagittal approach in which the sphenoid ostium is identified medial to the superior turbinate, and a wide exposure is obtained by removing the anterior wall of the sphenoid sinus.

Approaching defects in the lateral recess of the sphenoid (Figs 21.7A and B) may however be difficult. An endoscopic transpterygoid approach to the lateral sphenoid recess has been described.[32] This approach involves performing a posterior ethmoidectomy. The sphenoid ostium is then identified and widened. The maxillary ostium is also widened, followed by removal of the posterior wall of the maxillary sinus. This gives access to the pterygopalatine fossa. The anterior wall of the sphenoid is then removed to expose the lateral recess of the sphenoid.

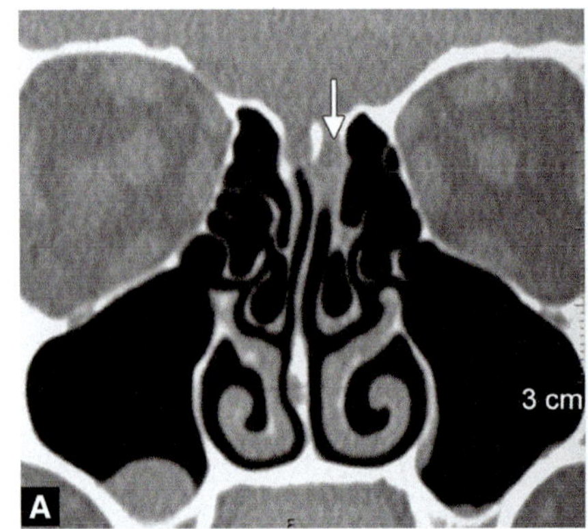
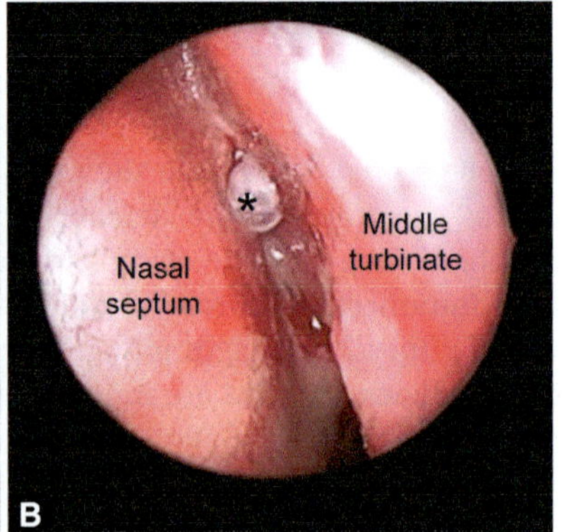

Figs 21.5A and B: (A) Computed tomography scan of a left medial lamella defect (white arrow); (B) Endoscopic view of the defect seen (*meningocele clearly visualized)

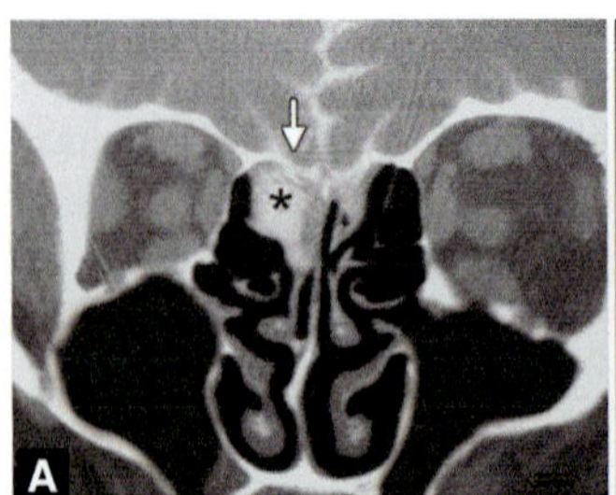
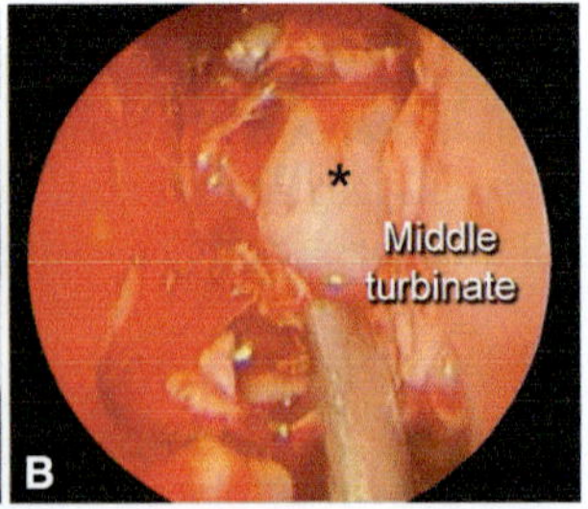

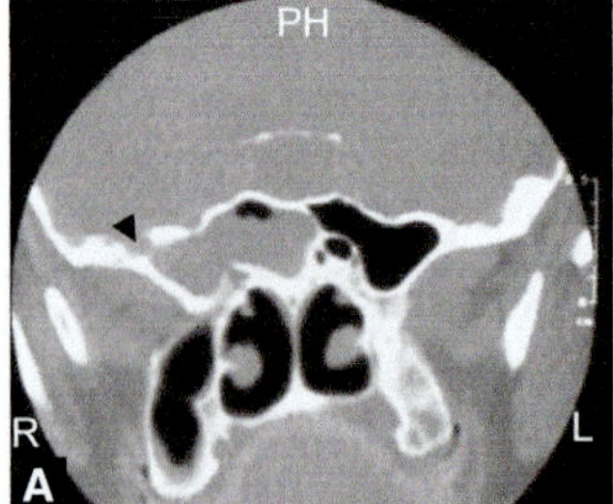
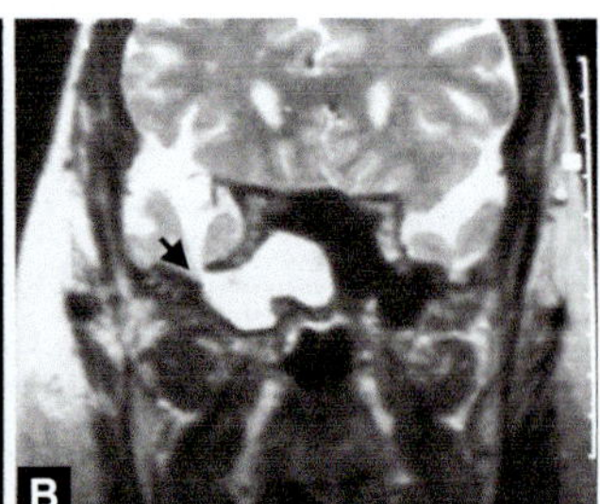

Figs 21.6A and B: (A) Computed tomography cisternogram demonstrating a right lateral lamella defect (white arrow) with a pseudomeningocele (asterix); (B) Endoscopic view after dissection showing the pseudomeningocele (asterix)

Figs 21.7A and B: (A) Computed tomography scan and (B) MRI images of defect in lateral recess of right sphenoid sinus with a meningoencephalocele prolapsing through the defect (black arrowhead)

The posterior end of the middle turbinate may be trimmed for better access.

Frontal Recess and Frontal Sinus

Although repair of defects in the roof and posterior wall of the frontal sinus require an external approach, frontal recess and certain frontal sinus defects can be repaired via the transnasal endoscopic approach. The basic principles for repair of these defects are similar to those of the other sites. However, the complex anatomy and awkward approach to this region makes endoscopic repair of these defects difficult.

Figures 21.8A to D demonstrates the repair of a frontal recess defect.

Since this chapter mainly deals with the endoscopic repair of CSF rhinorrhea, defects in the roof and posterior wall of the frontal sinus (which often require an external approach) have not been discussed.

While performing any of the techniques care should be taken to ensure that there is no obstruction to the outflow from the adjacent sinus openings to prevent iatrogenic sinusitis, especially in cases of frontal recess defects.

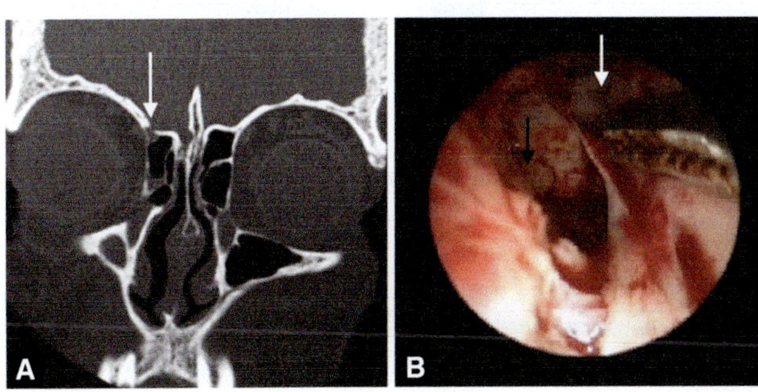

Figs 21.8A and B: (A) Computed tomography scan demonstrating a right frontal recess defect (white arrow); (B) Endoscopic view of the frontal recess defect (black arrow). The white arrow points towards the frontal ostium

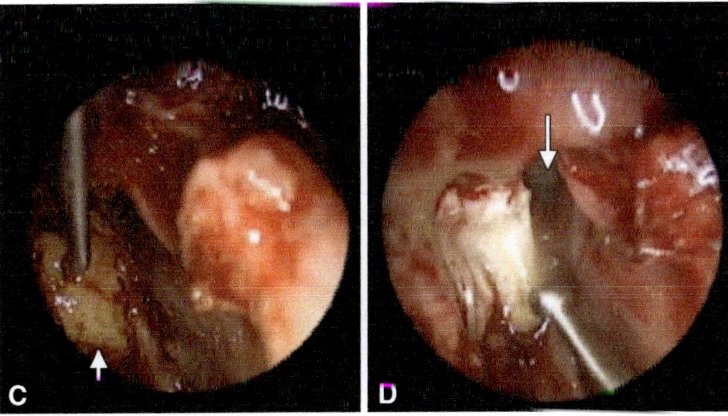

Figs 21.8C and D: (C) Defect sealed with fat (white arrow); (D) A layer of fascia held over the fat with fibrin glue. Note the patent frontal ostium (white arrow)

After adequate exposure has been obtained, the skull-base defect is localized and delineated. The mucosa surrounding the defect is removed to expose bone. This helps in better adherence of the graft material used for sealing the defect. If not removed, sinus mucosa continues to secrete mucus and may separate the graft from the recipient bed.[6] The underlying bone is then abraded slightly to provide a raw surface and stimulate osteoneogenesis.[6] A meningoencephalocele or arachnoid granulations prolapsing through the defect are cauterized with a bipolar cautery and excised. If the sac is not cauterized, intracranial hemorrhage may occur during attempts to reduce or excise the sac. In case of very large defects, the encephalocele may be reduced intracranially instead of excising, to prevent creating a larger dural defect, which may be difficult to close. In cases where multiple defects are present within the sphenoid sinus, the entire sphenoid sinus may be obliterated with fat. The Hadad-Bassagasteguy flap[33] may then be used to provide additional support, and can be held in place with fibrin glue. Gelatin sponge is then placed over the reconstruction for additional support.

Use of monopolar cautery should be avoided, especially adjacent to the optic nerve, carotid artery, skull-base or lamina papyracea.

Graft material: A variety of graft materials have been used for skull-base reconstruction. These include the use of local flaps such as middle turbinate osteomucoperiosteal flap,[34] or septal mucoperichondrial flap.[35] The Hadad-Bassagasteguy flap, a neurovascular pedicled flap of the nasal septal mucoperiosteum and mucoperichondrium based on the nasoseptal artery (branch of the posterior septal artery) is one such flap.[33] Free grafts from local nasal sites (e.g. septal mucoperiosteum, turbinate mucosa or septal cartilage), or from distant areas such as conchal cartilage, temporalis fascia, fascia lata, rectus sheath, abdominal or thigh fat, muscle, radial free forearm flaps[36] or calvarial bone may be used.[37] Dermal allograft,[38] lyophilized cadaver dura, bovine pericardium and exogenous materials, such as hydroxyapatite cement[39] or vicryl mesh[40] have also been used for reconstruction of skull-base defects. Various studies have proved that free grafts adhere to bone by 1 week[41] and vascularized fibrous tissue integrates into the free fascial graft by 2–3 weeks even in the absence of an overlying vascularized flap.[42]

Success rates of 92–96% have been documented irrespective of the graft materials used.[16,43-45]

Types of Reconstruction

Reconstruction of skull-base defects may be performed by using the overlay technique, underlay technique or a combination of both. The appropriate reconstruction technique chosen depends on the etiology, the location and size of the bony defect, and the underlying intracranial pressure.[46]

Underlay Technique

In the underlay technique the graft is placed between the dura and bone after elevating the dura from the margins of the skull-base defect (Fig. 21.9).

Overlay Technique

In the overlay technique, the graft material is placed over the skull-base bone (Fig. 21.9). An overlay graft over the skull-base bone may be sufficient in cases of small defects (< 5 mm).

Combined Underlay-Overlay Technique

Moderate sized (5–10 mm) defects and larger defects (> 10 mm) would usually require a combined underlay (graft placed between bony defect and dura) and overlay technique of graft placement.[47] A multilayered combined underlay and overlay soft tissue reconstruction may suffice for moderate sized defects (≥ 4 mm) with normal intracranial pressure. However, for large defects, a rigid underlay graft (cartilage or bone) with an overlay soft tissue graft may be required.[6]

The graft size should be slightly larger than the size of the defect[47] with the placement being such that there is no tenting or stretching.[45] Fibrin glue, a combination of fibrinogen, thrombin, and calcium cofactor, is commonly used to ensure that the graft is held in place and to provide an additional barrier to CSF leakage during wound healing. Microfibrillar collagen and gelatin sponge may be used to provide additional support. Nasal packs are used to provide temporary support.

The above mentioned repair techniques, however, need to be individualized depending upon the site and size of the skull-base defect.

Bath Plug Technique[48]

The skull-base defect is identified, defined and its size is determined. A fat plug larger than the defect is harvested from the abdomen, thigh or ear lobule. Fascia is also harvested at the same time. A 3-0 absorbable suture is passed along the length of the fat plug and knotted at one end of the plug. The fat plug is then introduced through the skull-base defect and gently pushed through the defect using a blunt instrument. Once the fat plug is completely introduced into the defect, a gentle pull is applied on the absorbable suture so that the fat plug is hitched at the defect providing a snug fit. A piece of fascia slightly larger in size than the size of the defect is slid along the absorbable suture to cover the fat plug and defect completely. Fibrin glue is used to reinforce the reconstruction, and the absorbable suture is cut. Gelatin sponge is then placed over the fascia for support.

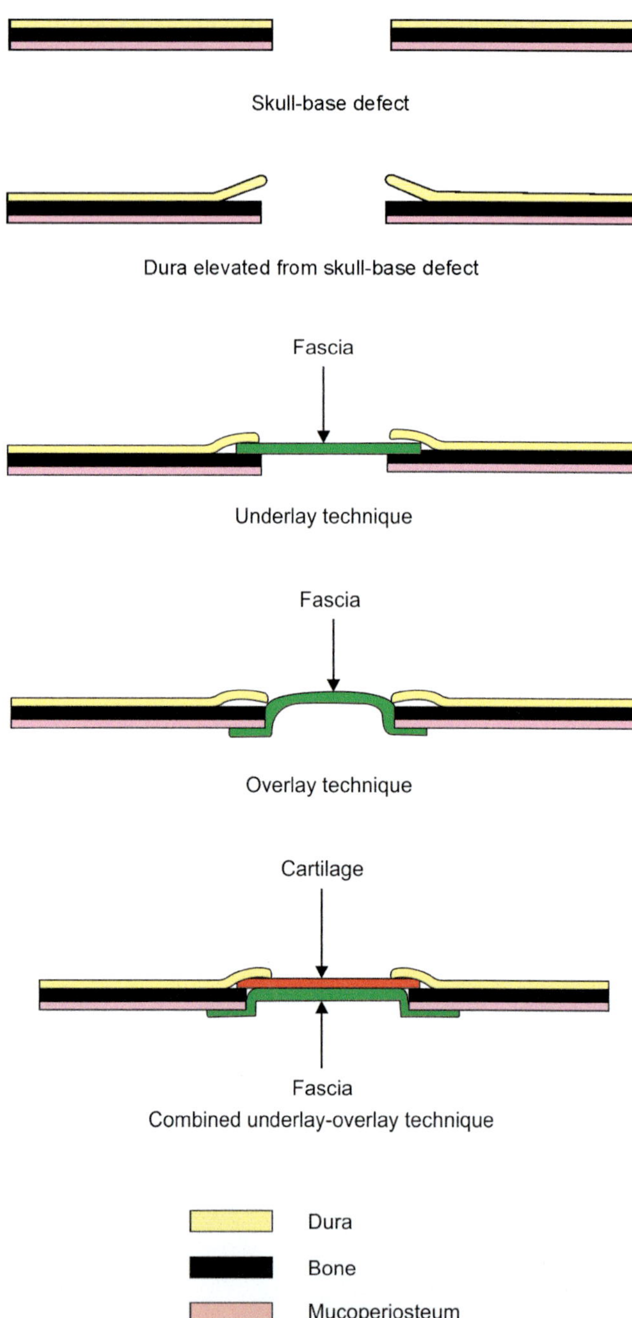

Fig. 21.9: Diagrammatic representation of techniques for repair of skull-base defects

Fascia, Cartilage, Fascia "Sandwich" Technique

In the presence of large defects, cartilage can be used to strengthen the reconstruction. A large piece of fascia is placed over the skull-base as an overlay. A premeasured piece of cartilage is placed over the fascia and pushed through the defect, carrying the fascia with it, so that a collar of fascia remains externally lying in contact with the bone (Fig. 21.10). Another piece of fascia is then placed over the cartilage as an overlay graft. A layer of fibrin glue is used to reinforce the adherence of the fascia to the cartilage and skull-base. This is further covered with gelatin sponge.

Bone pate: Multilayered closure of frontoethmoid and sphenoid sinus leaks using bone pate has been described.[49] The technique involves delineation of the skull-base defect followed by placement of a temporalis fascia graft in an underlay position. The bony defect is then filled with a second layer consisting of bone pate (obtained from the mastoid cortex) mixed with fibrin glue. This is further covered by an onlay free middle turbinate mucosal graft and gelatin sponge.

Drawbacks of Various Grafting Materials

Free cartilage or bone is associated with a risk of premature resorption. The inflexible nature of cartilage and bone makes it difficult to achieve a tight closure as the graft may not conform to the size and shape of the defect. This is especially true in cases of defects in the medial lamella of the cribriform plate where the space for placement of cartilage or bone is inadequate. Local pedicled flaps have a tendency to tent or pull away from the edge of the defect. This may result in inadequate approximation of the graft with the defect, thus affecting the final surgical outcome.[50] Chronic granulation tissue, inflammation, infection, and prolonged healing time have been seen with use of hydroxyapatite.[39] The high pressure CSF flow in cases with raised intracranial pressures may wash off the hydroxyapatite, and microfracturing of the cement may result due to transmitted brain pulsations, thus making it an unsuitable choice in such cases.

Nasal Packing

Either absorbable or non-absorbable material may be used for nasal packing to provide additional support to the graft. Nonabsorbable materials such as polyvinyl alcohol sponges are removed on the fifth postoperative day. However, no study has determined a difference in outcome with use of nasal packing.[9,51]

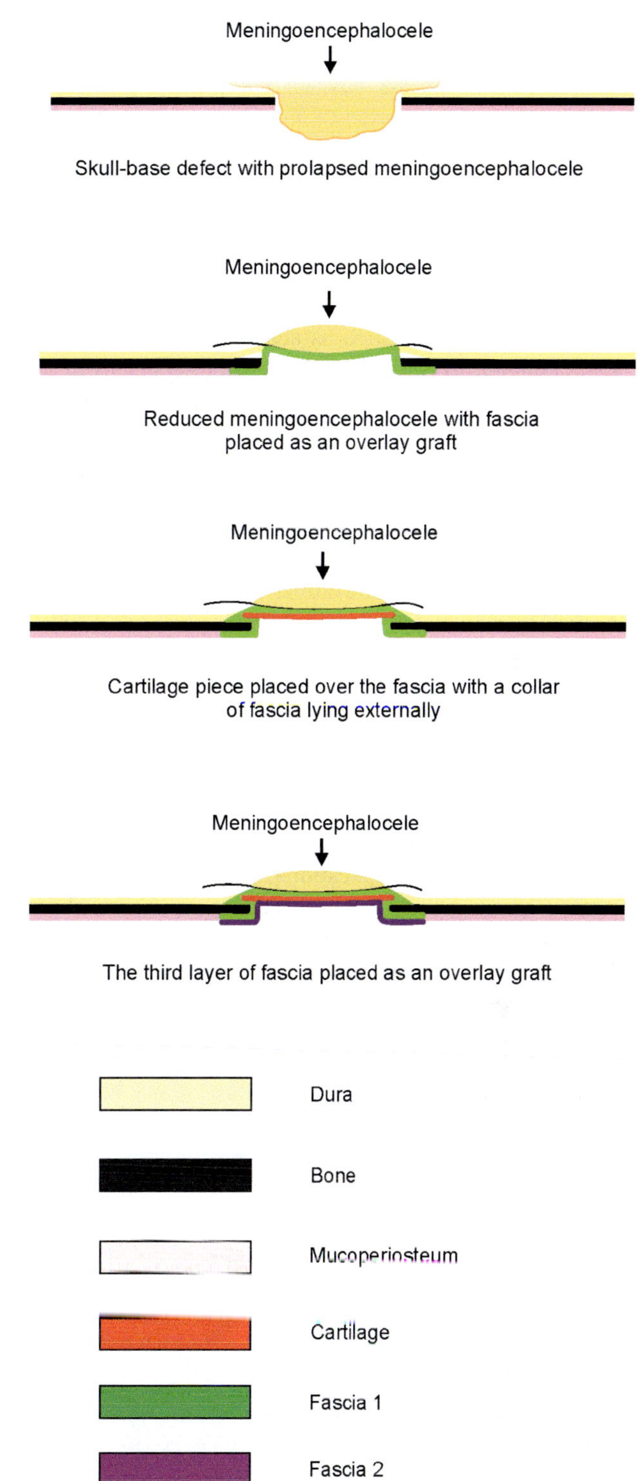

Fig. 21.10: Diagrammatic representation of the fascia-cartilage-fascia ("sandwich") technique for repair of skull-base defects

POSTOPERATIVE CARE

The patient should be advised complete bed rest with head elevation for a period of 5 days postoperatively. Non-absorbable nasal packs are usually removed on the fifth postoperative day. Nose blowing, strenuous activity, lifting of heavy weights and bending down is to be avoided for up to 6 weeks postoperatively.

Antibiotic prophylaxis may be given in the perioperative period and continued postoperatively till the nasal packs are removed.[11] A diuretic such as acetazolamide is prescribed postoperatively to decrease CSF pressure, especially in cases of raised intracranial pressures and spontaneous CSF leaks. Electrolyte monitoring and potassium supplementation are required with acetazolamide administration.

Use of a lumbar drain in cases of CSF leak is debatable. While some authors recommend routine use of a lumbar drain,[52] others report that lumbar drainage does not affect the outcome, and recommend a lumbar drain only in the presence of raised intracranial pressure or hydrocephalus.[50,51,53,54]

Follow-up CT scans are usually performed 3 months postoperatively to look for any obstruction in the sinus outflow tracts (Figs 21.11A and B).

POSTOPERATIVE COMPLICATIONS

Endoscopic CSF leak repair is associated with a low rate of complications.[51,52] Complications which may occur in the postoperative period include meningitis, brain abscess, subdural hematoma, olfaction disorders, and headache. Hegazy et al. in their meta-analysis have reported less than 1% incidence rate for each complication.[51]

Limitations of Endoscopic Techniques

- Defects located in the roof of the frontal sinus may require an osteoplastic flap with or without obliteration of the frontal sinus.
- Multiple/comminuted/large defects
- Coexistent tumors with intracranial extension which cannot be resected endoscopically.

Failure of Endoscopic Repair[32,55-57]

Success rates with endoscopic closure have been reported to be from 75.9% to 94% at the first attempt, increasing to 100% after a second attempt.[44,53,54,56-58]

Factors which may contribute to the potential failure of endoscopic repair of skull-base defects include:[52,55,56,58,59]

- Inability to successfully localize the defect
- Failure to identify coexisting defects
- Insufficient graft size
- Graft displacement
- Incomplete approximation of the graft to the skull-base defect
- Patient noncompliance with postoperative instructions
- Poor wound healing due to coexisting comorbid conditions
- Elevated body mass index
- Prior radiation therapy
- Infection.
- Development of new skull-base defects
- Very large skull-base defects.

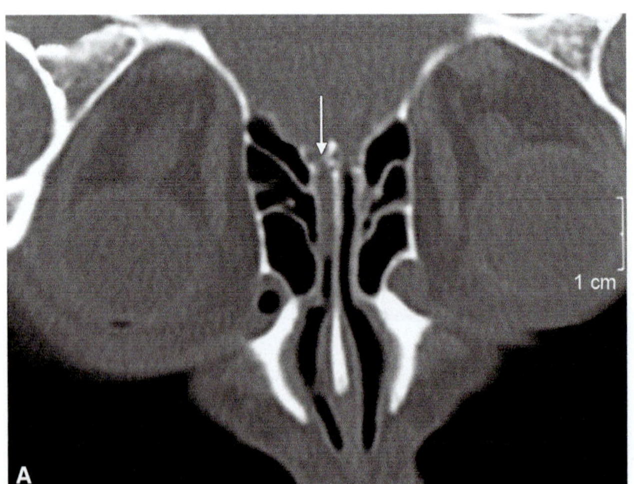 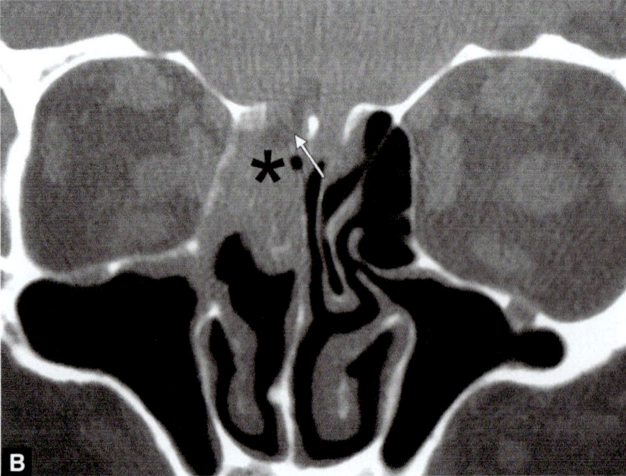

Figs 21.11A and B: (A) Computed tomography scan image of a right medial lamella defect repair (white arrow) showing a thick layer of fibrosis (3 months postoperatively); (B) Computed tomography scan image of a right lateral lamella defect repair (asterix) (3 months postoperatively). Note the hypodense shadow due to the fat plug used to seal the defect (white arrow)

A proper understanding of the etiology and mechanism of a CSF leak with accurate localization of the defect site, are factors which contribute to the planning of an appropriate surgical approach for CSF rhinorrhea repair. With the widespread practice of endoscopic surgery by otorhinolaryngologists, better technological know-how and lower morbidity as compared to external approaches, endoscopic repair is now a preferred option for the management of CSF rhinorrhea. Thus endoscopic repair is a reliable, safe and effective method in the management of CSF rhinorrhea.[48,56,59]

REFERENCES

1. Gross CW. The diagnosis and treatment of cerebrospinal fluid rhinorrhea. Trauma. 1975;45:11-4.
2. Dohlman G. Spontaneous cerebrospinal rhinorrhea case operated by rhinologic methods. Acta Otolaryngol Suppl. 1948;67:20-3.
3. Hirsch O. Successful closure of cerebrospinal fluid rhinorrhoea by endonasal surgery. AMA Arch Otolaryngol. 1952;56(1):1-13.
4. Vrabec DP, Hallberg OE. Cerebrospinal fluid rhinorrhoea. Arch Otolaryngol. 1964;80:218-29.
5. Wigand WE. Transnasal ethmoidectomy under endoscopic control. Rhinology. 1981;19(1):7-15.
6. Schlosser RJ, Bolger WE. Endoscopic management of cerebrospinal fluid rhinorrhea. Otolaryngol Clin North Am. 2006;39(3):523-38.
7. Lindstrom DR, Toohill RJ, Loehrl TA, et al. Management of cerebrospinal fluid rhinorrhea: Medical College of Wisconsin experience. Laryngoscope. 2004;114(6):969-74.
8. Lee TJ, Huang CC, Chuang CC, et al. Transnasal endoscopic repair of cerebrospinal fluid rhinorrhea and skull-base defect: ten-year experience. Laryngoscope. 2004;114(8):1475-81.
9. Kerr JT, Chu FW, Bayles SW, et al. Cerebrospinal fluid rhinorrhea: diagnosis and management. Otolaryngol Clin North Am. 2005;38(4):597-611.
10. Ommaya AK, Di Chiro G, Baldwin M, et al. Non-traumatic cerebrospinal fluid rhinorrhoea. J Neurol Neurosurg Psychiatry. 1968;31(3):214-25.
11. Lanza DC, O'Brien DA, Kennedy DW. Endoscopic repair of cerebrospinal fluid fistulae and encephaloceles. Laryngoscope. 1996;106(9 Pt 1):1119-25.
12. Shetty PG, Shroff MM, Sahani DV, et al. Evaluation of high-resolution CT and MR cisternography in the diagnosis of cerebrospinal fluid fistula. Am J Neuroradiol. 1998;19(4):633-9.
13. Woodworth BA, Schlosser RJ, Faust RA, et al. Evolutions in the management of congenital intranasal skull-base defects. Arch Otolaryngol Head Neck Surg. 2004;130(11):1283-8.
14. Wise SK, Harvey RJ, Patel SJ, et al. Endoscopic repair of skull base defects presenting with pneumocephalus. J Otolaryngol Head Neck Surg. 2009;38(4):509-16.
15. Rudnick E, Sismanis A. Pulsatile tinnitus and spontaneous cerebrospinal fluid rhinorrhea: indicators of benign intracranial hypertension syndrome. Otol Neurotol. 2005;20(2):166-8.
16. Papadea C, Schlosser RJ. Rapid method for beta-2 transferrin in cerebrospinal fluid leakage using an automated immunofixation electrophoresis system. Clin Chem. 2005;51(2):464-70.
17. Sloman AJ, Kelly RH. Transferrin allelic variants may cause false positives in the detection of cerebrospinal fluid fistulae. Clin Chem. 1993;39(7):1444-5.
18. Stibler H. Carbohydrate-deficient transferrin in serum: a new marker of potentially harmful alcohol consumption reviewed. Clin Chem. 1991;37(12):2029-37.
19. Urade Y, Katahama K, Ohishi J, et al. Dominant expression of mRNA for prostaglandin D synthetase in leptomeninges, choroid plexus and oligodendrocytes of the adult rat brain. Proc Natl Acad Sci USA. 1993;90(19):9070-4.
20. Hoffmann A, Conradt HS, Gross G, Nimtz M, et al. Purification and chemical characterization of beta-trace protein from human cerebrospinal fluid: its identification as prostaglandin D synthase. J Neurochem. 1993;61(2):451-6.
21. Arrer E, Meco C, Oberascher G, et al. Beta-Trace protein as a marker for cerebrospinal fluid rhinorrhea. Clin Chem. 2002;48(6 Pt 1):939-41.
22. Bachmann G, Nekic M, Michel O. Clinical experience with beta-trace protein as a marker for cerebrospinal fluid. Ann Otol Rhinol Laryngol. 2000;109(12 Pt 1):1099-102.
23. Lloyd MN, Kimber PM, Burrows EH. Post-traumatic cerebrospinal fluid rhinorrhea: modern high-definition computed tomography is all that is required for the effective demonstrated of the site of leakage. Clin Radiol. 1994;49(2):100-3.
24. Shetty PG, Shroff MM, Fatterpekar GM, et al. A retrospective analysis of spontaneous sphenoid sinus fistula: MR and CT findings. Am J Neuroradiol. 2000;21(2):337-42.
25. Chow JM, Goodman D, Mafee MF. Evaluation of CSF rhinorrhea by computerized tomography with metrizamide. Otolaryngol Head Neck Surg. 1989;100(2):99-105.
26. Manelfe C, Cellerier P, Sobel D, et al. Cerebrospinal fluid rhinorrhea: evaluation with metrizamide cisternography. Am J Roentgenol. 1982;138(3):471-6.
27. Stone JA, Castillo M, Neelon B, et al. Evaluation of CSF leaks: high-resolution CT compared with contrast-enhanced CT and radionuclide cisternography. AJNR Am J Neuroradiol. 1999;20(4):706-12.
28. Flynn BM, Butler SP, Quinn RJ, et al. Radionuclide cisternography in the diagnosis and management of cerebrospinal fluid leaks: the test of choice. Med J Aust. 1987;146(2):82-4.
29. Keerl R, Weber RK, Draf W, et al. Use of sodium fluorescein solution for detection of cerebrospinal fluid fistulas: an analysis of 420 administrations and reported complications in Europe and the United States. Laryngoscope. 2004;114(2):266-72.
30. Stankiewicz JA. Cerebrospinal fluid fistula and endoscopic sinus surgery. Laryngoscope. 1991;101(3):250-6.
31. Cooper PR. Skull fracture and traumatic cerebro-spinal fluid fistulas in head injury. In: Cooper PR (Ed). Head injury. Baltimore (MD): Williams and Wilkins; 1982.
32. Bolger WE, Osenbach R. Endoscopic transpterygoid approach to the lateral sphenoid recess. Ear Nose Throat J. 1999;78:36-46.
33. Hadad G, Bassagasteguy L, Carrau RL, et al. A novel reconstructive technique after endoscopic expanded endonasal approaches: vascular pedicle nasoseptal flap. Laryngoscope. 2006;116(10):1882-6.
34. Yessenow R, McCabe BF. The osteo-mucoperiosteal flap in repair of cerebrospinal fluid rhinorrhea: a 20-year experience. Otolaryngol Head Neck Surg. 1989;101(5):555-8.
35. Weisman RA. Septal chondromucosal flap with preservation of septal integrity. Laryngoscope. 1989;99(3):267-71.

36. Weber SM, Kim J, Delashaw JB, et al. Radial forearm free tissue transfer in the management of persistent cerebrospinal fluid leaks. Laryngoscope. 2005;115(6):968-72.

37. Bolger W, McLaughlin K. Cranial bone grafts in cerebrospinal fluid leak and encephalocele repair: a preliminary report. Am J Rhinol 2003;17(3):153-8.

38. Lorenz RR, Dean RL, Hurley DB, et al. Endoscopic reconstruction of anterior and middle cranial fossa defects using acellular dermal allograft. Laryngoscope. 2003;113(3):496-501.

39. Stankiewicz JA, Vaidy AM, Chow JM, et al. Complications of hydroxyapatite use for transnasal closure of cerebrospinal fluid leaks. Am J Rhinol. 2002;16(6):337-41.

40. Verheggen R, Schulte-Baumann WJ, Hahm G, et al. A new technique for dural closure–experience with a vicryl mesh. Acta Neurochir (Wien). 1997;139(11):1074-9.

41. Tachibana E, Saito K, Fukuta K, et al. Evaluation of the healing process after dural reconstruction achieved using a free fascial graft. J Neurosurg. 2002;96(2):280-6.

42. Fliss DM, Gil Z, Spektor S, et al. Skull-base reconstruction after anterior subcranial tumor resection. Neurosurg Focus. 2002;12(5):e10.

43. Lund VJ. Endoscopic management of cerebrospinal fluid leaks. Am J Rhinol. 2002;16(1):17-23.

44. Castelnuovo PG, Delú G, Locatelli D, et al. Endonasal endoscopic duraplasty: our experience. Skull-base. 2006;16(1):19-24.

45. Mattox DE, Kennedy DW. Endoscopic management of cerebrospinal fluid leaks and cephaloceles. Laryngoscope. 1990;100(8):857-62.

46. Schlosser RJ, Bolger WE. Nasal cerebrospinal fluid leaks: critical review and surgical considerations. Laryngoscope. 2004;114(2):255-65.

47. El Banhawy QA, Halaka AN, Altuwaijri MA, et al. Long-term outcome of endonasal endoscopic skull-base reconstruction with nasal turbinate graft. Skull-base. 2008;18(5):297-308.

48. Wormald PJ, McDonogh M. The bath-plug closure of anterior skull-base cerebrospinal fluid leaks. Am J Rhinol. 2003;17(5):299-305.

49. Chatrath P, Saleh HA. Endoscopic repair of cerebrospinal fluid rhinorrhea using bone pate. Laryngoscope. 2006;116(6):1050-53.

50. Dodson EE, Gross CW, Swerdloff JL, et al. Transnasal endoscopic repair of cerebrospinal fluid rhinorrhea and skull-base defect: a review of twenty-nine cases. Otolaryngol Head Neck Surg. 1994;111(5):600-5.

51. Hegazy HG, Carrau RL, Snyderman CH, et al. Transnasal endoscopic repair of cerebrospinal fluid rhinorrhoea: a meta-analysis. Laryngoscope. 2000;110(7):1166-72.

52. Senior BA, Jafri K, Benninger M. Safety and efficacy of endoscopic repair of CSF leaks: a survey of the members of the American Rhinologic Society. Am J Rhinol. 2001;15(1):21-5.

53. Komisar A, Weitz S, Ruben RJ. Cerebrospinal fluid dynamics and rhinorrhea: the role of shunting in repair. Otolaryngol Head Neck Surg. 1983;91(4):399-403.

54. Casiano RR, Jassir D. Endoscopic cerebrospinal fluid rhinorrhea repair: is a lumbar drain necessary? Otolaryngol Head Neck Surg. 1999;37:33-6.

55. Wise SK, Harvey RJ, Neal JG, et al. Factors contributing to failure in endoscopic skull-base defect repair. Am J Rhinol Allergy. 2009;23(2):185-91.

56. Castillo L, Jaklis A, Paquis P, et al. Nasal endoscopic repair of cerebrospinal fluid rhinorrhea. Rhinology. 1999;37(1):33-6.

57. Schick B, Ibing R, Brors D, et al. Long-term study of endonasal duraplasty and review of the literature. Ann Otol Rhinol Laryngol. 2001;110(2):142-7.

58. Cassano M, Felippu A. Endoscopic treatment of cerebrospinal fluid leaks with the use of lower turbinate grafts: a retrospective review of 125 cases. Rhinology. 2009;47(4):362-8.

59. Mao VH, Keane WM, Atkins JP, et al. Endoscopic repair of cerebrospinal fluid rhinorrhea. Otolaryngol Head Neck Surg. 2000;122(1):56-60.

CHAPTER 22

Complications of Endoscopic Sinus Surgery

Satish Jain, Gaurav Shankar Medikeri

INTRODUCTION

Mosher in 1929 wrote regarding the ethmoid sinuses, "Any surgery in this region should be simple, but has proven one of the easiest ways to kill a patient".

Endoscopic sinus surgery (ESS) is considered by many to be the most exciting development of the decade in otolaryngology. The aim is to restore the natural mucociliary clearance mechanism, drainage, and aeration of the sinuses by a minimally invasive technique, maintaining as much of the normal anatomy as possible.

Stanckiewicz[1] himself had reported a complication rate of 5% in his first 90 cases which subsequently dropped to a mere 0.7% in the next 90 cases signifying the slow learning curve of the procedure. With more and more surgeons picking up the endoscope today, there is a fertile ground for complications to occur, which is why this chapter is very important.

This chapter will give an overview on what complications can occur, how to manage them and also how to prevent them. The purpose of this chapter is only to make the endoscopic surgeon aware of the possible complications and their subsequent management and not to daunt or create trepidation for the surgeon.

CLASSIFICATION OF COMPLICATIONS OF ENDOSCOPIC SINUS SURGERY

There is more than one way to classify complications of ESS.

I. Based on the site of complication they can be classified into (Table 22.1):

- Intranasal complications
- Intraorbital complications
- Intracranial complications

II. Based on the time frame when the complication occurs they can be classified into (Table 22.2):

- Intraoperative complications
- Postoperative complications
  - Immediate
  - Delayed

RISK FACTORS FOR COMPLICATIONS IN ENDOSCOPIC SINUS SURGERY

- Age greater than 65 years
- Disease involving sphenoid or frontal sinuses
- Revision surgery
- Dehiscent lamina papyracea, skull-base, optic nerve or carotid artery
- Asymmetric fovea, olfactory fossa or lateral lamella
- Altered course of anterior ethmoid artery or artery running in the mesentery (Table 22.3).
- Use of powered instrumentation
- Pan sinus opacification (complete whiteout)
- Lack of air shadow before reaching skull-base on computed tomography (CT) scan.

ORBITAL COMPLICATIONS

Orbital complications though rare can be extremely calamitous if they do occur during ESS. Some of the

TABLE 22.1: Classification of complications based on site

Intranasal complications	Orbital complications	Intracranial complications
Bleeding	Periorbital ecchymosis	Cerebrospinal fluid fistula/rhinorrhea
Adhesions	Orbital emphysema	Pneumocephalus
Crusting	Nasolacrimal duct injury	Injury to great vessels/Hemorrhage
Osteitis	Intraorbital hematoma	Meningitis
	Extraocular muscle injury or entrapment	Brain abscess
	Direct optic nerve damage	Encephalocele
		Frontal lobe damage
		Anosmia

TABLE 22.2: Classification based on time frame of complication

Intraoperative	Postoperative
• Fat herniation	• Bleeding
• CSF leak	• Adhesions
• Intraorbital hemorrhage	• Epiphora
• Optic nerve injury	• Periorbital emphysema
• Medial rectus damage	• Anosmia
• Injury to the ICA	• Frontal recess stenosis
	• Crusting
	• Neuropathic pain
	• Infection
	• Osteitis
	• Meningitis

Abbreviations: CSF, Cerebrospinal fluid; ICA, Internal carotid artery

TABLE 22.3: Description and frequencies of variations of anterior skull-base[2] (n = 75)

	Number	Percentage
Ethmoid asymmetry	64	85.4
Asymmetry in contour	8	72 .7
Asymmetry in height	2	18.2
Combined	1	9.1
Anterior ethmoid artery		
Course through ethmoid cells	31	41.3
Runs along skull-base	44	58.7
Lateral lamella		
Normal	69	92
Lateralized or protruded	6	8
Olfactory fossa		
Type I	15	20
Type II	59	78.7
Type III	1	1.3

commonly seen orbital complications include intraorbital hematoma, extraocular muscle injury or entrapment, ocular dysmotility, orbital emphysema, nasolacrimal duct injury, and direct optic nerve damage. About 16–50% of the major complications involve the orbit although orbital injuries occur in less than 1% of all ESSs.

Nasolacrimal Duct Injury

Damage to an anatomic structure neighboring a sinus is a continuous plausibility throughout ESS. Maxillary antrostomy can cause prompt injury to the nasolacrimal duct (NLD) or lamina papyracea. This is particularly common with a hypoplastic maxillary sinus, which is seen in silent maxillary sinus syndrome. In such cases, the uncinate tightly sticks to the lamina papyracea, intensifying the danger of injury to the orbit in the event of use of a sickle knife. In such cases, unless the uncinate is displaced far from the lamina papyracea, the lamina papyracea might be effortlessly cracked and a surgical instrument might be embedded into the orbit.

There are two scenarios where the NLD may be injured. During uncinectomy and during widening of the maxillary antrostomy anteriorly. If the NLD be injured, it is best to allow the NLD to sit unbothered and not control it. Bolger et al.[3] reported that the 15% occult injury to the NLD provoked no epiphora postoperatively in spite of the fact that no intraoperative management was performed. Epiphora from nasolacrimal duct injury is evaluated to happen in 0.3–1.7% cases.

One of the techniques to avoid injury to the NLD is to stay posterior to the maxillary sinus ostium. After identifying the maxillary sinus ostium after an uncinectomy, the antrostomy should be made posteriorly, as there is no need to go anteriorly where the NLD is housed. Our approach now is to use a reverse-cutting (forceps) anteroinferiorly as the distance between the uncinate and the instrument is farthest with this angulation. The surgeon must stop using the reverse-cutting when he encounters hard bone. When trying to remove the uncinate by detaching the anterior attachment of the uncinate, one has a higher probability of entering into the orbit around the area of the uncinate attachment. Even if the lamina papyracea is violated, observation for proptosis, bleeding, edema, and ecchymosis may be the only management needed.

Management of nasolacrimal duct injury depends on the timing of diagnosis of the complication. If diagnosed intraoperatively, then the surgeon has options such as watchful waiting or planned frequent irrigation or syringing of the NLD to prevent fibrosis and subsequent stricture formation of the NLD or to perform a standard dacryocystorhinostomy (DCR) procedure at the same time. If the surgeon is unaware of the complication intraoperatively and the patient presents with epiphora in the postoperative period, then an endoscopic DCR is the definitive management.

Periorbital Ecchymosis

It is not always that a periorbital ecchymosis signifies an anterior or posterior ethmoid artery bleed. It may also occur due to a fractured or dehiscent lamina papyracea which can cause periorbital bruising due to the subperiosteal extravasation of blood.

Management

In the event of a periorbital ecchymosis in the absence of any vascular mishap, the patient can be managed conservatively as more often than not this condition settles on its own in a few days. The patient should be instructed not to blow his/her nose for a period of 1–2 weeks. The patient can develop orbital emphysema on failure to comply. The patient must be preferably put on a broad spectrum antibiotic for a period of 1 week.

Intraorbital Hemorrhage

Two types of hemorrhage have been described in literature, the first being a slow hemorrhage which is typically venous or capillary and the second being of rapid onset which is arterial. Spontaneous hematoma is usually venous, iatrogenic is arterial and traumatic may be either. The main difference between the two is the higher intraorbital pressures occurring in the arterial bleeds whereas there is no difference in the diagnostic features or the management of the two conditions.

The most commonly described reason for orbital hematoma throughout ESS is complete transection of the anterior ethmoid artery (Fig. 22.1) and ensuing withdrawal

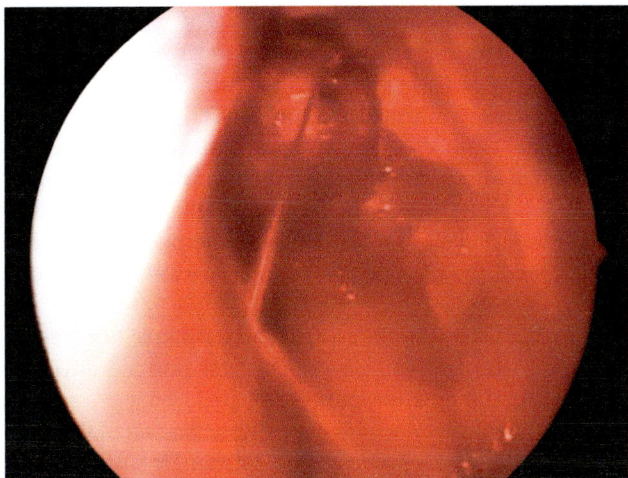

Fig. 22.1: Anterior ethmoid artery bleed

of the artery into the orbit. Expanded intraorbital pressure or vasospasm of the central retinal artery then causes diminished vision due to retinal or optic nerve ischemia. Animal models[4] of central retinal ischemia infer that irreversible visual loss may happen within 100 minutes. Then again, clinical reports of lasting visual loss have occurred within 1 hour. Early identification and treatment is the key since perpetual sequelae, for example vision loss, is reversible or preventable.

The orbit is encompassed by hard bony walls on all sides with the exception anteriorly, where fascial planes hold the globe in position. It has a volume of roughly 20 cm². The globe is underpinned by the extraocular muscles, which are suspended by some ligaments to the orbit. Expanded intraorbital force accordingly causes proptosis, yet the measure of globe projection is restricted by these tendons and ligaments. As forces approach mean arterial pressure, diminished blood vessel perfusion of the retina and optic nerve occur, and venous outflow may likewise be hindered. To discharge the globe anteriorly for brief pressure relief, division of the medial or lateral canthal associations is needed.

Within the orbit the anterior and posterior ethmoid branches are given off from the ophthalmic artery, which pierce the lamina papyracea to enter the roof of the paranasal sinuses and run in a bony canal along the roof of the ethmoids to perforate the lateral lamella of the cribriform plate and enter the olfactory fossa intracranially.

The approximate landmarks for the anterior branch are 24 mm from the anterior orbital margin, posterior ethmoid being another 12 mm from the anterior ethmoid and the optic nerve being 6 mm from the posterior ethmoid.

In roughly 91% cases, the anterior ethmoid lies along the skull-base or a millimeter or two below the skull-base in which case it is safe but in the remaining cases, the artery may be lying loose in a mesentery in which case it becomes vulnerable to damage during ESS. The chances of the mesenterial anterior ethmoid artery are greatly increased in the presence of a pneumatized supraorbital cell.

This can be confirmed on a coronal CT scan wherein we see the classic "Kennedy's nipple" sign at the level of confluence of the medial rectus and superior oblique muscles. On a coronal scan, the anterior ethmoid artery roughly corresponds to the ground lamella section whereas the posterior ethmoid corresponds to the section of the anterior wall of the sphenoid sinus.

Signs and indications that infer orbital damage or bleeding are excessive pain (higher than regular postoperative pain after ESS), diplopia, proptosis, and periorbital ecchymosis. Findings such as reduced/loss of vision, fixation of the globe, and tonometric pressures above 40 mm Hg are suggestive of orbital compression syndrome and require prompt and efficient management as this condition can potentially give a permanent visual loss.

Fundal examination findings in the event of an intraorbital hemorrhage include retinal vascular shutdown and optic nerve pallor but is unindicative of permanent optic nerve damage. The best way to test the optic nerve activity is by the swinging flashlight test (afferent pupillary defect). This indicates that the intraorbital pressure is greater than the systolic pressure. If left unchecked, the retina becomes pale with the appearance of a cherry red spot on the macula.

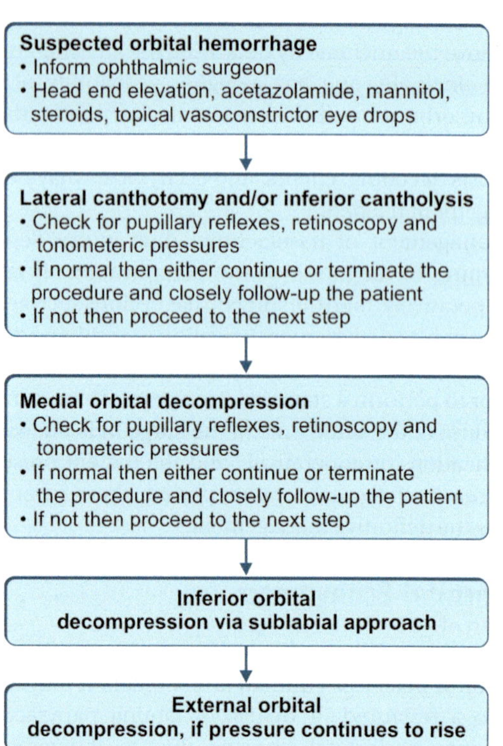

Flow chart 22.1: Algorithm for the management of orbital hemorrhage

Management

In the event of an orbital hematoma (Flow chart 22.1), an ophthalmic surgeon must be immediately informed and the initial management involves head end elevation, removal of any nasal packing and instillation of topical vasoconstrictor eye drops (Timolol drops 0.5%, 1–2 drops topically twice daily) and systemic steroids in order to reduce the intraocular pressure. Mannitol (20%, 1–2 g/kg over 30 minutes; has rapid onset of action) and acetazolamide (500 mg IV; has slow onset of action) also can help to significantly reduce the intraocular pressure.

It is best to avoid nasal packing or to keep it to as minimal as possible as it stagnates the blood within the orbit and prevents its escape thus increasing the intraorbital pressure.

If this modality of management fails, then the surgeon must himself go ahead with a lateral canthotomy and/ or inferior cantholysis in order to decompress the globe anteriorly to further accommodate the rising pressure within the orbit. This procedure can reduce the pressure by around 14–30 mm Hg and is the simplest and the most rewarding of the procedures as far as pressure relief is concerned.[5]

Lateral canthotomy and cantholysis begins by infiltrating the lateral canthus with 2% lignocaine with 1 in 1 lakh adrenaline at the junction of the upper and lower eyelid. A sharp scissors is then used to cut the lateral canthus up to the junction of the orbital rim. The lateral canthal tendon is then identified after retracting the lower lid anteroinferiorly and is cut thus releasing the orbit anteriorly; hence reducing the pressure. The wound is then addressed secondarily once the hematoma has been dealt with and the cosmetic outcome of a secondary suturing is excellent.

Further rise in pressure mandates an endoscopic medial orbital decompression which allows the blood to drain into the ethmoids if the artery continues to bleed. In the rare situation of further rise in intraorbital pressure, inferior orbital decompression into the maxillary sinus via the sublabial approach can be done. External orbital decompression should be carried out only as last resort approach when all other modalities of management have failed. Under no circumstances should one attempt to catch or cauterize the bleeding vessel within the orbit, as this may worsen the scenario by further traumatizing the intraorbital structures.

Extraocular Muscle Injury

Extraocular muscle injury although rare, almost always occurs due to inadvertent handling of powered instrumentation. The patient usually complains of diplopia as a presenting feature in this scenario. There are two muscles which are most commonly involved in decreasing order of incidence, medial rectus and inferior rectus.

The medial rectus originates from the annulus of Zinn and travels anteriorly to be inserted onto the sclera. This is the reason why the medial rectus is well protected within the orbit with the periorbital pad of fat (Fig. 22.2) lying medial to it in the anterior ethmoidal air cells. In the posterior ethmoid group of air cells, it is just lateral to the lamina papyracea, thus making it more vulnerable to injury.

Medial rectus injury has been classified into 4 categories by Huang et al.[6] Once a diagnosis of extraocular muscle injury has been made, further evaluation involves imaging with gadolinium enhanced magnetic resonance imaging (MRI). Not only does an MRI give high resolution images of the muscle fiber bundles with their innervating motor neurons, but it also is able to delineate different stages of the injury as well. Initial stages show the presence of muscle edema or intramuscular hemorrhage whereas later scans show muscle atrophy or complete volume loss depending on the presence of partial or complete transection of the muscle respectively. Management of an extraocular muscle injury falls within the domain of an ophthalmologist.

Management

The management of rectus muscle injury is based on two principles. First, to restore the adduction function of the muscle, and second, to minimize the amount of fibrosis and contractile forces experienced by the antagonizing musculature; both these principles aiming for one common goal—to re-establish a binocular single visual field.

The exploration of the wound must be carried out within a period of 3–4 weeks in order to reduce the chances of fibrosis and scar contracture. The only indication for immediate exploration is entrapment of the muscle.

Microdebrider associated injury is usually accompanied with volume loss of the muscle, and unfortunately despite the best attempts, the prognosis remains guarded. Some of the options for the treatment of medial rectus injury include oblique muscle transpositions, weakening the antagonist lateral rectus muscle by using botulinum toxin[7], and muscle-to-muscle anastomosis, with or without an interposition graft or hang-back adjustable sutures.

Periorbital Emphysema

Damage to the lamina papyracea can lead to periorbital emphysema if the patient blows his/her nose, coughs, and sneezes or vomits postoperatively. This leads to accumulation of air within and outside the orbit (Fig. 22.3).

Management

A patient with a diagnosed crack or damage to the lamina papyracea must be closely watched for a crunchy feel of the periorbital area postoperatively. This is similar to that of bursting a bubble wrap. The patient must be instructed not to blow his/her nose but to suck and spit instead. The patient must sneeze with an open mouth. In the event of emphysema, the patient must be put on a broad spectrum antibiotic. Spontaneous resolution is the rule rather than the exception with watchful waiting.

Optic Nerve Injury

Optic nerve injury is a rare complication of ESS but nonetheless "THE" most devastating of the complications. The optic nerve is most prone to damage in the presence of an Onodi cell which lies in close proximity to the optic nerve

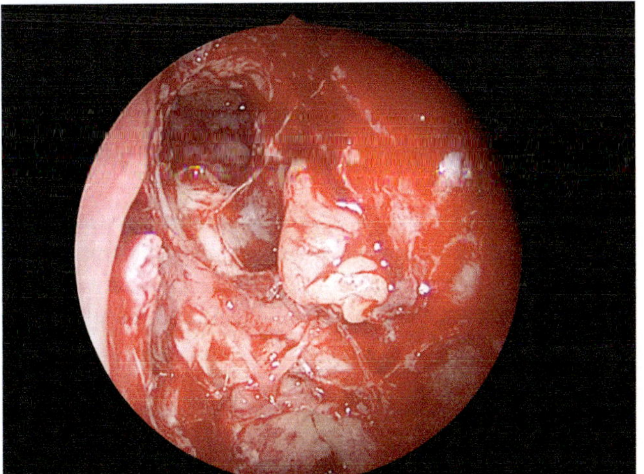

Fig. 22.2: Orbital fat prolapse near the frontal recess

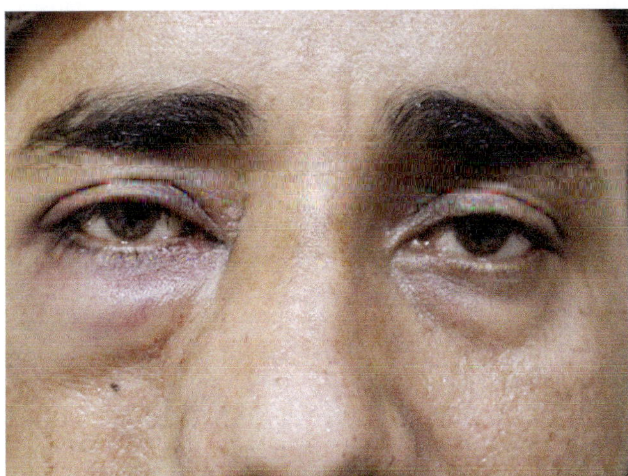

Fig. 22.3: Periorbital emphysema occurring after the lamina papyracea was breached and the patient had bouts of sneezing postoperatively. This usually settles within a week

and the nerve could also be dehiscent within the cell, which further increases its risk of being damaged. Onodi cells may be present in 10% of the population. The thickness of the bone over the maximum area of bulging of the optic canal is 0.28 mm, and in 12% of the patients there is a dehiscence.[8]

Optic nerve injury is of two types—direct, wherein there is direct trauma to the optic nerve or indirect, wherein there are transmitted forces on the optic nerve such as compression due to a intraorbital hematoma.

Optic nerve injury within 1 cm of the globe causes direct damage to the optic nerve before the entry of the central artery of retina and hence, the disturbances are immediately visible on the fundus. Injury to the optic nerve beyond the entry of the central artery, like in the posterior ethmoid cell which is the more common scenario in ESS, causes no immediate changes within the fundus and may take 3–4 weeks for the changes to appear.

The mechanism of optic nerve damage secondary to intraorbital hematoma has already been discussed.

Assessment of Optic Nerve Injury

There are two scenarios wherein optic nerve injury can occur—first when the patient is under general anesthesia and second, when under local anesthesia. The assessment in these two scenarios are different.

Intraoperatively, under general anesthesia, optic nerve injury can be confirmed with the rapid swinging flash light test, wherein the surgeon flashes a light rapidly from one pupil to another and should not find any difference between the two pupil sizes in a normal eye. This is due to the equal amount of light being transmitted in both the optic nerves.

However, in the case of an optic nerve injury, the surgeon can identify the weaker pupil, as both pupils appear dilated when light is flashed into the defective eye. This is because the affected optic nerve is not carrying the same amount of light as the opposite eye and hence would observe a paradoxical pupillary dilatation on swinging the light into the weaker eye. Hence this test identifies the relative differential light transmission between the two optic nerves through the direct and consensual light reflexes.

When under local anesthesia, assessment involves comparing the visual acuity of the patient with that of the documented preoperative visual acuity in the patient.

Color vision, especially for red color has been shown to be the earliest predictor of optic nerve injury. Patient typically reports the color as faded.

Visual field examination can be carried out and may help in localizing the site of optic nerve damage. Patient may also complain of diplopia if the annulus of Zinn has been disrupted anteriorly.

Imaging involves getting a MRI and a CT scan in most cases. MRI delineates the nerve and surrounding edema better than CT scan, whereas in cases of a bony spicule impinging on the nerve a CT is of more value.

Management

Management can be either medical or surgical depending on the pathogenesis of the injury.

Medical management includes administering high doses of methylprednisolone with a loading dose of 1 gm intravenous and a maintenance dose of 250 mg intravenous sixth hourly. The largest series on traumatic optic neuropathy management has been published by the International optic nerve trauma study[9] which has reported an improvement in 54% patients with steroid administration for a follow-up period of 3 months.

In case of a bony spicule impinging on the nerve then the spicule has to be removed endoscopically at the earliest possible time. In the case of an intraorbital hematoma compressing on the optic nerve, orbital decompression may have to be done if all other methods have failed to decompress the orbit as discussed previously.

Indications for optic nerve decompression
- Failure to improve vision after 48–72 hours of methylprednisolone
- Progressive visual loss despite steroid therapy
- Total blindness with CT evidence of optic nerve compression.

Prognostic factors
- Time elapsed since trauma until the management
- Degree of visual loss and CT evidence of canalicular or pericanalicular fracture.

PREVENTION OF ORBITAL COMPLICATIONS

Preoperative Steps to Prevent Complications

- A history of previous surgery or biopsy, presence of a sinonasal tumor, maxillofacial trauma should immediately alert the surgeon and he/she must be expectant of altered sinonasal anatomy or a pre-existing dehiscent lamina papyracea.
- Visual acuity and eye movements must preferably be charted in every case undergoing ESS to avoid inadvertent lawsuits.
- Preoperatively, the surgeon must pay specific attention to the CT scans, especially to rule out the presence of

a hypoplastic maxilla or a dehiscent lamina papyracea (Fig. 22.4). The anterior ethmoid artery must be outlined using the landmarks mentioned above. The presence of a suprabullar cell must alert the surgeon to the possibility of an anterior ethmoid artery in a mesentry (Figs 22.5 and 22.6). Whilst coronal scans are the most helpful in terms of appreciation of the surgical anatomy pertaining to the ESS procedure, the axial scans reveal the orbital anatomy in both antero-posterior and medial to lateral planes.

Intraoperative Steps to Prevent Complications

- The surgeon must have a bloodless field in order to identify the anatomical landmarks with utmost confidence. This involves the role of the surgeon as well as the anesthetist. Proper technique of infiltration to constrict the sphenopalatine artery (SPA) at the sphenopalatine foramen and the anterior ethmoid artery near the axilla of the middle turbinate are important in creating a dry surgical field. Hypotensive anesthesia also plays a vital role in achieving the same.
- The surgeon must learn to identify the lamina papyracea early on and make the lamina work as a constant landmark throughout the surgery thus keeping it as the lateral boundary of dissection.

- The head of the debrider should never put pressure on the lamina but should stay a couple of millimeters away from the lamina. Avoid use of the microdebrider in areas of dehiscence as the powerful combination of the suction and the sharp blade of the debrider can cause catastrophic consequences, should periorbital fat or muscle get entangled in it.
- In the presence of extensive disease in the region of the anterior ethmoidal artery on a CT scan, it is preferable to clear the disease with an intact bulla technique so as to safeguard the artery while exploring the frontal sinus and later opening the bulla and delineating the artery slowly in the presence of less disease.

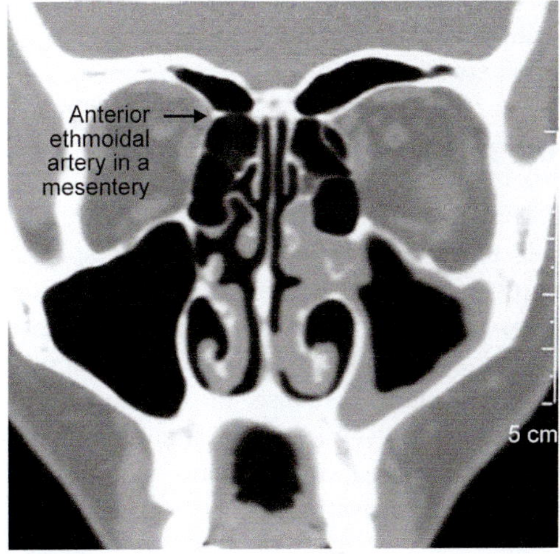

Fig. 22.5: Observe the anterior ethmoid artery hanging freely in a mesentery. This scenario is very common in the presence of a suprabullar cell

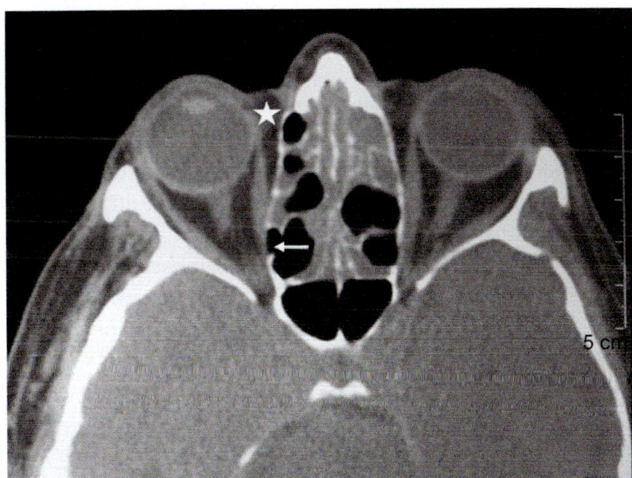

Fig. 22.4: Observe the dehiscent lamina papyracea (white arrow) with the close proximity of the medial rectus with the lamina papyracea in the posterior ethmoidal cells. Also note the presence of periorbital fat (white star) between the lamina papyracea and the medial rectus in the anterior ethmoidal cells. Hence, fat herniation (Stanckiewicz sign) will only be seen on damage to the lamina in the anterior ethmoidal air cells and not when it is damaged in the posterior ethmoid air cells. Preoperative identification of a dehiscent lamina papyracea especially in the posterior ethmoid cells is very important to avoid inadvertent damage to the medial rectus

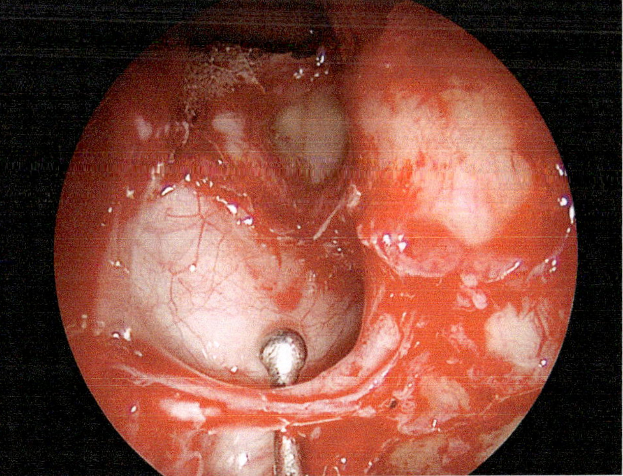

Fig. 22.6: Intraoperative finding of anterior ethmoidal artery in the mesentery which was identified preoperatively on the CT scan

- The debrider must be used with caution in the presence of an anterior ethmoid artery in a mesentery on the CT scan (Fig. 22.6).
- Precaution must be taken while working along the lamina papyracea in the posterior ethmoidal cells due to the close proximity of the lamina to the medial rectus muscle without any intervening fat (Fig. 22.4).

INTRACRANIAL COMPLICATIONS IN ENDOSCOPIC SINUS SURGERY

In today's scenario, increasing surgical experience and better equipment has made intracranial complications rare. However, despite the impressive safety record of ESS, complications though occasional, do occur and shall be discussed here (Table 22.4).

Cerebrospinal Fluid Rhinorrhea

Cerebrospinal fluid (CSF) rhinorrhea can occur following ethmoidectomy, frontal sinus surgery or sphenoidotomy with an incidence of 0.5%. There is a 10% risk of developing meningitis after CSF rhinorrhea. The most consequential factors leading to CSF leak are failure to appreciate the anatomic landmarks because of the surgeon's lack of experience or because ill-defined anatomic landmarks are obscured by bleeding, the presence of space-occupying lesions, and anatomic variations.

Risk Factors for Cerebrospinal Fluid Rhinorrhea

- Poor skills and training
- Distorted anatomical landmarks
- Repeated surgeries
- General anesthesia
- Excessive bleeding

Intraoperatively a CSF leak can be identified on the table when the surgeon sees a clear fluid arising from the skull-base which washes away blood. Postoperatively, biochemical

TABLE 22.4: Intracranial complications
• Cerebrospinal fluid fistula/rhinorrhea
• Pneumocephalus
• Injury to great vessels/hemorrhage
• Meningitis
• Brain abscess
• Encephalocele
• Frontal lobe damage
• Anosmia

confirmation can be helpful. CSF glucose is higher than other nasal secretions; CSF protein levels are lower than that of nasal secretions and CSF has higher chloride levels compared to nasal secretions. Although these are well known facts, none of these tests can definitively rule out CSF rhinorrhea. Presently, only the beta transferrin levels are the most sensitive and specific test available to rule of CSF rhinorrhea safely. The desialylated isoform of transferrin without neuraminic acid is only present in CSF which can be identified by immunofixation electrophoresis (IFE). A complete review of the diagnostic methods of CSF rhinorrhea is discussed in Table 22.5. The 0.1mL of 10% fluorescein is mixed with 10 mL of the patient's CSF and then slowly injected intrathecally over 45–60 minutes. Although no special light is required, a blue filter enables the surgeon to readily identify the leak.

In the event of suspicion of a CSF leak intraoperatively, certain maneuvers can be performed to help identify the leak. These include valsalva maneuver, lowering the head end of the table, compression of bilateral internal jugular veins, intrathecal injection of dye, ringer lactate solution or air. The advantage of the intrathecal dye injection also helps in ascertaining a water tight seal at the end of the closure.

When a CSF leak is detected intraoperatively (Fig. 22.7), there are three options for repair, intracranial, extracranial, or transnasal endoscopic surgical approach. Of these approaches, in this endoscopic era, the role for the intracranial or extracranial approaches has been limited to selective cases. The advantages offered by the endoscopic approach are not only in terms of a reduced morbidity but also preservation of the olfactory function which is lost in the transcranial approach. Today, the endoscopic approach is the least invasive of all the approaches and is successful in 95% of the cases. The endoscope is a magnificent tool in locating the leak especially with the use of an intrathecal dye such as iohexol. Possible side effects of the dye include minor meningeal irritation, numbness and weakness of the lower extremities, opisthotonos, and seizures but are infrequent and reversible. Magnetic resonance cisternography has the advantage of not requiring a contrast administration.

Management of Cerebrospinal Fluid Leaks

Intraoperative CSF leaks should be sealed immediately to reduce the chances of meningitis postoperatively rather than waiting for them to close spontaneously, which would involve longer hospitalization for bed rest and possibly a spinal tap or lumbar drain.

Conservative management involves:
- Bed rest
- Serial lumbar punctures
- Subarachnoid lumbar drains

TABLE 22.5: Diagnostic methods of cerebrospinal fluid (CSF) leakage

Diagnostic methods		Usefulness	Potential limitations
Imaging methods	CT cisternography	• Localization of fracture line or intracranial air.	• High cost and limited access to machine • Radioactive tracers in CT scanning or scintigraphy are potentially dangerous
	MRI	• Defining the prolapsed meninges and CSF in the adjacent sinuses.	• Fails to demonstrate persistent violation of the leptomeninges with CSF leakage and may miss some fractures • Demonstrating leakages with high sensitivity and less than 1 mm spatial resolution.
Intrathecal and topical fluorescein technique		• Localization of the fistula.	• Specific endoscope is needed and potential complications are possible.
Biochemical tests	Glucose oxidase test	• Easy to perform, fast, cheap and widely available method in detection of the CSF in the nasal discharge.	• Low diagnostic sensitivity and specificity • False negative results in cases of bacterial contamination or false positive results in diabetic patients.
	beta-2 trf test	• Reliable, non-invasive in the diagnosis and management of patients with suspected CSF leakage • Specific CSF marker that has replaced surgical techniques as the test standard • The assay required 10 µL of sample.	• Results of beta-2 trf test are obtained with delayed availability of test (120–150 min) due to use of electrophoretic technique • Difficult to perform, more expensive and labor-intensive than betaTP. • Patients with alcoholic disease and chronic states have an increased serum beta-2 trf.
	betaTP test	• Quantitative assay can be performed in 20 min on a nephelometer • Non-invasive, highly sensitive, quick and low-cost method in detection of CSF rhinorrhea in nasal secretions • At least 200 µL of sample is required for a single measurement.	• Problem with assessment of the accurate cut-off values as a major determinant of diagnostic significance • Still for research use only • Patients with renal insufficiency and bacterial meningitis have an increased serum and decreased betaTP values in CSF.

Abbreviations: CT, Computed tomography; MRI, Magnetic resonance imaging; beta-2 trf, Beta-2 transferrin; betaTP, Beta-trace protein

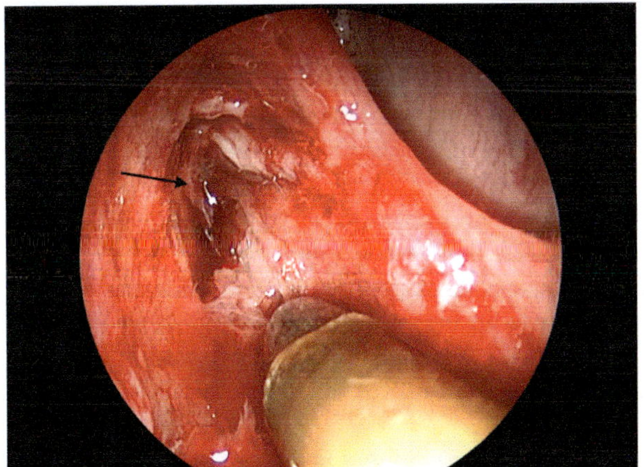

Fig. 22.7: Observe the clear fluid (black arrow) appearing from the lateral lamella of the cribriform plate near the frontal recess. This is one of the most common areas of an iatrogenic CSF leak

The use of prophylactic antibiotics is debatable.

If conservative management of postoperative fistulae fails, and the leak is visible, endoscopic repair may be attempted. Treatment failures can undergo repeated endoscopic repair. If unsuccessful, or if the leak is not visible, an external or intracranial approach may be necessary.

The stunning results of the endonasal endoscopic approach make it the most preferred approach for repair of CSF leaks with the exception being defects of the posterior table of the frontal sinus and defects larger than 5 cm in size.

Materials used to seal a CSF leak:

- Temporalis fascia
- Septal or turbinate mucosa
- Muscle
- Fat
- Fascia lata.

Almost any type of living tissue membrane may be used to patch a fistula, including temporalis fascia, septal or turbinate mucosa, muscle, fat and fascia lata. The muscle and fascia are harvested through a standard incision in the scalp hair posterior and superior to the pinna. The fascia is pressed and dried to improve manipulation. The fistula repair is then approached endoscopically, while bleeding is rigorously controlled. The graft is placed over the fistula and tucked into the skull-base, ethmoid, or cribriform plate which is known as the 'bath plug' graft. Muscle is placed on the top of the fascia followed by gelatin foam packing for support. A layer of oxidized cellulose is placed between the graft and the nasal pack to prevent sticking and undue removal of the graft during pack removal. A nasal trumpet serves the dual purpose of providing an airway and supporting the gelatin foam. It should remain in place for 5 days. Patient is nursed in a 30° head up position and must avoid straining.

If a mucosal graft is used, the mucosa is carefully elevated from the surrounding bone for at least 5 mm in all directions because residual mucosa will prevent adhesion of the mucosal graft to the underlying bone. If there is a significant defect in the dura, the intracranial side is supported with abdominal fat or a musculofascial graft from the temporalis muscle. Often, a free graft of mucoperiosteum is obtained from the contralateral nasal septum, which will itself remucosalize in 3–4 weeks. A pedicle graft from the ipsilateral septum (Hadad flap) can be used if a large or vascularized graft is required. The graft is subsequently placed over the defect with the edges tucked under the perimeter of the surrounding mucosa. The use of microfibrillar collagen around the graft helps secure it. A lumbar spinal drain may be used to reduce the CSF pressure and the flow of leakage in large fistulae. Lumbar spinal drains may be used in sphenoid sinus leaks for 24–120 hours after surgery to reduce the CSF pressure, preserve the position of the graft, and facilitate the process of adhesion. In addition, after operative procedures, patients are advised bed rest with the head of the bed elevated. Stool softeners are used to avoid straining, and strenuous activity should be limited for 4–6 weeks.

Sphenoid CSF leaks may prove difficult to repair because of poor visualization. The leak may be controlled primarily with fibrin glue and gelatin foam packing. One thousand units of thrombin and 5 cm^3 of 10% calcium chloride are combined in one syringe and then mixed with one syringe of cryoprecipitate to make fibrin glue. This substance may be injected into the sphenoid sinus after removal of the complete mucosa of the sinus; once the glue is gelatinized, the sphenoidotomy opening is plugged with gelatin foam. Alternately, a fistula within the sphenoid sinus may be repaired with a free graft technique or with an obliterative technique using free abdominal fat. Self-setting hydroxyapatite bone cement has also been used for direct repair of the defect and is effective for normal pressure CSF fistulae, a category in which most postsurgical fistulae belong. Long-term studies show an absence of fibrous encapsulation, minimal inflammation, and an absence of foreign body or giant cell formation. A long-term benefit of hydroxyapatite cement involves the progressive replacement of the implants with new bone by a combination of resorption and osteoconduction. Vascularized bone ingrowth at the periphery of the implant enhances the long-term stability of the reconstructed area. Because the hydroxyapatite cement must be applied in a dry field to promote setting, adequate hemostasis and control of the CSF egress from the fistulae is required before application. Frequently a middle turbinectomy may need to be performed if the middle turbinate obstructs visibility or interferes with graft manipulation.

Pneumocephalus

The presence of air within the cranial cavity is known as pneumocephalus or cranial aerocele. It can occur as a complication of functional endoscopic sinus surgery (FESS) when a connection has been created between the external environment and the epidural, subdural or subarachnoid space. The most common site of damage causing a pneumocephalus is the cribriform plate at the site where the anterior ethmoid artery pierces the skull-base. Tension pneumocephalus occurs when the intracranial air exceeds 65 cm^3.

The main mechanisms involved in the occurrence of pneumocephalus are:

- *Ball valve mechanism:* In this mechanism, the high pressure nasopharyngeal air is pushed into the cranial cavity secondary to nose blowing, coughing or sneezing. Similarly, when the anesthetist uses bag and mask to ventilate the patient postoperatively, he/she can create a tension pneumocephalus and hence must avoid the use of bag and mask postoperatively.
- *Inverted bottle mechanism:* Drainage of the CSF through the subarachnoid space creates a negative pressure within the space and hence sucks the air in the nasal cavity to normalize the pressure difference.
- The use of intraoperative nitrous oxide has also shown to cause an increase in the intracranial pressure in the presence of a closed cranial cavity with intracranial air. However, this resolves with the cessation of nitrous use.

Common manifestations of pneumocephalus include:
- Headache
- Altered mental status
- Obtundation
- Dizziness
- Behavioral change
- Confusion

- *Bruit hydro-aerique:* This is a characteristic feature of pneumocephalus wherein the patient hears a succussion splash with the movement of the head.
- CSF rhinorrhea
- Meningismus
- Seizures
- Hemiparesis

The imaging modality of choice is a CT scan (Fig. 22.8)—which can detect air pockets as small as 0.5 cm³. X-rays also have been used previously due to their easy availability and cost effectiveness; however, a CT scan can give a quantitative analysis regarding the amount of air present intracranially.

Management

Currently there are three main options for decompression:
- *Ventriculostomy:* This is the most common modality of management of a pneumocephalus.
- *100% oxygen inhalation:* This acts by replacing the nitrogen within the intracranial space which is the main component of a pneumocephalus. Removal of nitrogen then reduces the intracranial pressure thus decompressing the intracranial space.
- Needle aspiration of the space is an option which can be done through a burr hole. Occasionally, a needle aspiration might be carried out on an emergency basis prior to imaging in the setting of a tension pneumocephalus.

The patient must be nursed in the supine position so as to prevent air entry into the cranial cavity. Occasionally, the intracranial air may be resorbed after the skull-base defect has been sealed by a blood clot or a granulation and the pneumocephalus may spontaneously resolve with conservative management.

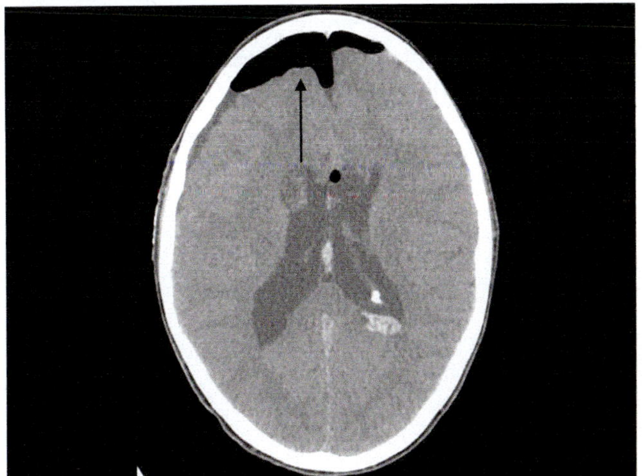

Fig. 22.8: Post CSF leak, patient had 2 bouts of vomiting and developed confusion, drowsiness. A CT scan was taken which showed the presence of air in the cranial cavity (black arrow) and hence a diagnosis of pneumocephalus was made

Once decompression has been achieved, an airtight multi-layered reconstruction of the skull-base must be carried out and adequate support must be provided to the flap for a period of at least 10 days.

Injury to Great Vessels/Hemorrhage

The fovea ethmoidalis is especially thin and unguarded at the connection point of the vertical bony shelf of the middle turbinate. Likewise, in the medial ethmoid sinus, the roof is dainty, and the dura may be adherent. Negligible trauma here may reason bleeding of the intradural meningeal or subarachnoid branches of the anterior cerebral artery. Intracranial bleed initiated by harm to the internal carotid artery and anterior cerebral artery can be shocking, on the grounds that there is no satisfactory exposure to expedite the quick control of bleeding. Various landmarks for the carotid artery are mentioned in Table 22.6.

Trauma to the cribriform plate may be detrimental to the anterior communicating artery and its feeding vessels, in light of the fact that they are in close adjacency. Spasm of these vessels can have savage outcomes, creating central nervous system (CNS) dysfunction and even demise.

Intracranial bleeding recognized intraoperatively brought on by injury to the internal carotid artery or the anterior cerebral artery requires surgical packing and neurosurgical intervention, with likely instantaneous anterior craniotomy. A neuroradiologist might help to reduce blood loss and prolong the patient's life by passing an inflatable catheter for intravascular tamponade. Critical injury to the CNS is debilitating. The individuals who survive, experience a disturbance of olfactory filaments with olfactory loss and might have prolonged neurologic deficits.

Carotid injury has devastating consequences as bleeding occurs in a relatively inaccessible area. The endoscopic surgeon has only one hand to use as the other hand is occupied with the endoscope. Any attempt to reduce the bleeding by means of hypotensive anesthesia can be met with cerebral hypoperfusion and can in turn leave the patient with a neurological deficit. Lastly, there is an increased risk of embolization or pseudoaneurysm occurrence.

The carotid bleed that occurs within the sphenoid sinus (Fig. 22.9) is from the anterior genu of the cavernous carotid.

TABLE 22.6: Anatomic landmarks for various segments of the internal carotid artery

Segment	Anatomic landmark
Paraclinoid	Medial clinoid
Anterior genu	Medial pterygoid
Horizontal segment	Vidian nerve
Ascending carotid	Eustachian tube

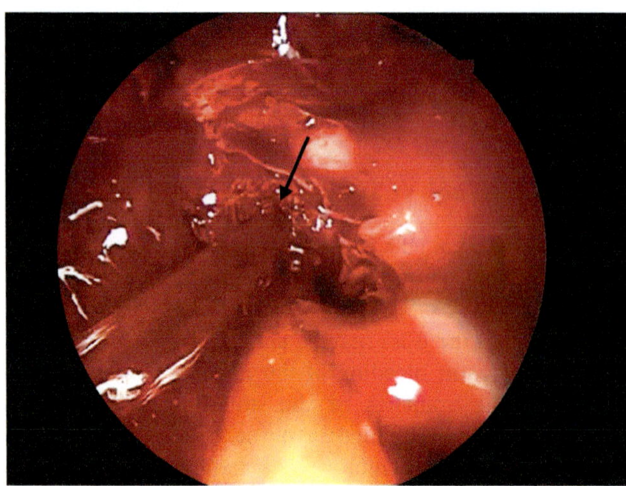

Fig. 22.9: Observe the pressure with which the carotid artery (arrow) bleeds making it very difficult to visualize the operative field or to control the hemorrhage

Vertical septae within the sphenoid sinus should not be pulled, but they can be cut with sharp instruments such as the Blakesly Tru-cutting forceps as the septae can be attached to the carotid artery. The carotid artery can be dehiscent in 20% of cases in the sphenoid sinus and hence blind instrumentation within the sphenoid sinus can be met with devastating consequences.

In the event of an internal carotid bleed, the surgeon must use two suctions and visualize the rent in the carotid artery (Fig. 22.9) by placing the suction directly over the rent. Then the nasal cavity can be packed with ribbon gauze or polyvinyl alcohol sponge. Oxidized cellulose balls are then directly placed over the bleeding vessel to buy time to shift the patient to neuroradiology. Once the bleeding is under control, the patient must be shifted to the neuroradiology suite immediately, wherein the neurosurgeon and the neuroradiologist decide on the further management options. Some of the options include (Table 22.7) embolization by means of coils or balloons. However, these options depend on the presence of good cross circulation through the circle of Willis. A cover stent may be placed which encircles the circumference of the vessel from the inside and covers the bleeding point in the vessel. It also has the added advantage of preventing a pseudoaneurysm.

Implications of Carotid Injury

- Torrential blood loss leading to hemodynamic compromise
- Cerebral anoxia
- Stroke

TABLE 22.7: Surgical options for control of the internal carotid artery (ICA) bleeding point

- Bipolar cauterization of the carotid laceration
- Circumferential ligation of the vessel
- Digital compression of the ICA in the neck
- Compressive packing
- Suture repair of the lacerated ends
- Reconstruction of the artery after clipping with aneurysmal clips

- Thrombosis or embolism of carotid artery
- Carotico-cavernous fistula
- Death.

A contrast CT scan in the immediate postoperative period screens the patient for untoward complications such as intracranial hematoma or an hemorrhage. The patient obviously has to be admitted in the intensive care unit and continuously monitored. Any epistaxis in such a case must be endoscopically investigated in the postoperative period. Long-term follow-up must be carried out with serial angiograms in order to remain vigilant for a pseudoaneurysm.

Meningitis

This is a common complication once the mucosa-bone-dura barrier is broken. Two outcomes occur after the barrier is broken, meningitis which occurs in the acute setting and cerebral abscess which occurs in the chronic setting.

Routes of Spread of Infection

- Direct extension through a dural tear
- Along perivascular and vascular channels through a thrombophlebitic phenomenon
- Through the septal lymphatics leading to the perineural spaces of the olfactory fibers.

Common Presenting Features

- Headache
- Fever
- Nuchal rigidity
- Vomiting
- Cranial nerve palsy
- Behavioral changes
- Seizures
- Abnormal mental status
- Confusion
- Lethargy
- Deficits in responsiveness
- Focal neurologic deficits.

Commonly Involved Organisms

- *Streptococcus pneumoniae*
- Gram-negative bacilli other than *Haemophilus influenzae*
- *Neisseria meningitides*
- Streptococci
- *Staphylococcus aureus*
- *Listeria monocytogenes*
- *Cryptococcus* is seen in AIDS patients.

Diagnosis

Diagnosis is mainly by lumbar puncture which will demonstrate the organism involved, raised counts with a predominance of neutrophils, marked increase in protein to greater than 250 mg/dL, normal to marked decrease in glucose levels (less than 40 mg/dL) and an elevated opening pressure of greater than 180 mm of H_2O.

Prior to a lumbar tap, a contrast enhanced CT scan is advised which will be normal in case of meningitis but will show ring enhancement in the presence of an abscess. Patients with meningitis will present with dural enhancement on contrast enhanced MRI.

Management

The treatment of meningitis mainly involves the administration of antibiotics which can penetrate the blood brain barrier. Initially a broad spectrum antibiotic is chosen as empiric therapy and later when the culture report arrives, the antibiotic of choice is chosen based on the sensitivity report.

Common Sequelae

- Seizure disorder
- Hearing loss
- Cranial nerve deficit
- Death.

Brain Abscess

Intracranial abscess is a rare but potentially fatal complication of ESS. They are of many types, extradural, subdural, intraparenchymal and Pott's puffy tumor. Routes of spread of infection are similar to those of meningitis. The most common areas involved in the brain are the frontal and frontoparietal lobes.

Symptomatology varies with the site of the abscess and the time duration since its occurrence. A patient might display diffuse migraine, furthermore an unpretentious change in nature. Then again, a more fulminant picture might include intense migraine, queasiness, emesis, fractiousness, and laziness. Visual field deformities are likewise regular.

Focal neurological deficits may occur in an abscess resulting in hemiparesis or hemiplegia. On the other hand temporal lobe lesions may not be so evident in symptomatology. Almost all patients will have raised intracranial tension (ICT), which can be identified clinically by papilledema. Hence, a fundoscopy becomes mandatory as a lumbar puncture is contraindicated in the presence of raised ICT for the fear of brain herniation.

Imaging modality of choice is an iodine enhanced contrast CT scan. Serial CT scans can be used to follow the lesions after treatment has been initiated.

Commonly isolated organisms are *Streptococcus milleri, Staphylococcus aureus, Bacteroides spp., Peptostreptococcus spp., Propionibacterium spp., Streptococcus sanguis, Peptococcus spp., Fusobacterium spp.,* and *Haemophilus spp.*

A broad spectrum antibiotic which can cross the blood brain barrier is the preferred empirical therapy until culture results become available.

Aspiration of the abscess cavity or drainage through a clean route through a burr hole craniotomy may be attempted with a neurosurgical colleague. A Penrose drain may be left *in situ* and intrathecal antibiotics may be administered with a ventricular cannula. Steroids and anticonvulsants are administered along with the antibiotics.

Frontal Lobe Damage

Failure to recognize a skull-base injury can lead to damage to the brain tissue, especially with the use of powered instruments. There are two common areas where skull-base injury is very common, the first being the area between the anterior and posterior ethmoid roof and the second being in the region of the frontal recess wherein the bone behind the frontal ostium may be injured. Patients typically present with a personality change or irritability, particularly associated with a CSF leak, or may also present with features of meningitis.

These patients must be taken up immediately for repair of the CSF leak as mentioned above and must be followed on a regular basis with serial psychiatric evaluation. Usually these patients do well with psychiatric treatment for a period of about 3–6 months.

Anosmia

This is often one of the most neglected of complications which is a consequence of lack of respect for the olfactory mucosa extending from the olfactory cleft up to the medial surface of the middle turbinate or a little lower. Preservation of olfactory mucosa begins in the preoperative period itself wherein the surgeon must start the patient on steroids to know if there is any chance of reversing the anosmia which the patient already has as a consequence of the sinonasal disease. If the anosmia reverses with steroids, then the surgeon can presume that the anosmia is reversible with surgery and the same can be conveyed to the patient. If the anosmia or hyposmia does not reverse with a course of oral steroids, then the prognosis for the reversal after surgery is bleak and the same must be explained to the patient. The author prefers to use a deflazacort trial to check for the reversibility of existing anosmia, especially in the presence of polyps medial to the middle turbinate.

In the presence of polyposis medial to the turbinate during surgery, the surgeon must accomplish a thorough ethmoidectomy to create sufficient space so as to lateralize the middle turbinate, which will then allow the use of a powered instrument in the cleft between the septum and the turbinate. This clearance allows the nasal steroid spray to reach the olfactory cleft which otherwise would be inaccessible.

INTRANASAL COMPLICATIONS OF ENDOSCOPIC SINUS SURGERY

Intranasal complications of ESS, though minor are a very common incidence. Majority of these complications occur due to the lack of clear anatomical knowledge or due to the lack of respect for mucosa resulting in erratic tissue healing. These complications are sometimes inevitable in every endoscopic surgeon's career and hence one must be aware of the complications and must improve their skills to avoid them. In the inadvertent scenario of their occurrence, he must learn how to manage them with the least morbidity to the patient. It is this attention to fine detail that helps a surgeon go a long way in going from one end of the spectrum of the learning curve described by Stankiewicz to the other end.

Bleeding

Bleeding can be either intraoperative or postoperative. Intraoperative bleeding mainly occurs from three main sources:

1. *The sphenopalatine artery:* This artery can bleed at certain specific locations during surgery. There are three specific locations where the SPA can bleed. The first is wherein the middle turbinate branch of the lateral segment of the SPA enters the middle turbinate at the posterior end of the middle turbinate. This bleeding can occur when the surgeon excises more than half of the middle turbinate. Second region is at the site of maxillary antrostomy where in the surgeon extends the antrostomy posteriorly and encounters the main trunk of the artery coming through the sphenopalatine foramen. This is the reason why the surgeon must perform the sphenopalatine block to

vasoconstrict the SPA preoperatively. The third location is when the surgeon encounters the septal branch of the SPA when he widens the sphenoidotomy inferiorly. Hence, it is preferable to widen the sphenoid ostium medially first towards the septum.

2. *The anterior ethmoid artery:* Bleeding from this artery is often feared by many an endoscopic surgeons. The trouble with the anterior ethmoid artery bleed is not the blood loss which occurs but it is the fear of retraction of the vessel into the orbit and continuous bleed within the closed orbital space. This can cause a compressive optic neuropathy and subsequent visual loss which if left unchecked can become permanent. The details of the management have been covered under orbital complications of FESS.

3. *The posterior ethmoid artery:* Bleeding can occur from this vessel if the skull-base in the region of the posterior ethmoid is thinned out due to the intrinsic pathology such as tumors or long-standing polyposis or fungal rhinosinusitis. The posterior ethmoid artery is protected by the thicker posterior skull-base when compared to the anterior ethmoid artery which is covered by relatively thinner bone in the anterior part of the skull-base.

In the authors' experience however, such bleeds are minor and can be controlled easily with tactful skill if the surgeon is well versed with the anatomy of the artery and the skull-base. A vasoconstrictor sponge or bipolar cautery can be used to control the intranasal bleeder once it has been localized endoscopically. However, occasionally, when the bleeder is not entirely visible, a bismuth iodoform paraffin paste pack can be placed in the nasal cavity.

Adhesions and Synechia Formation

These are mainly the consequence of lack of respect for the mucosa and the following fibrosis leading to adhesions between opposing surfaces. Prevention of synechia begins intraoperatively itself where in the surgeon must create adequate space to work within the middle meatus so as to minimize mucosal trauma. This can be achieved with adequate decongestion with topical sponge packs and infiltration. Two raw opposing mucosal surfaces must always be separated with a polyvinyl alcohol sponge to prevent adhesions. In the event of a floppy middle turbinate, it can be separated from the lateral wall by placing a polyvinyl alcohol sponge in the middle meatus in the postoperative period for a week. Other techniques such a suture fixation of the middle turbinate, bolgerization between the middle turbinate and the septum or application of fibrin glue between the septum and the middle turbinate, enhance the chances of the middle turbinate healing in the medial position and thus keeps the middle meatus widely patent.

Some authors have used mitomycin C to prevent adhesions and have found no significant difference in the synechia formation despite its use.

A major role in the prevention of synechia is to ensure proper nasal douching. A lot of confusion exists regarding the frequency with which the patient must douche the nose and as to when he must start douching. A good time to start douching the nose would be a day after pack removal as crusting begins in this period. Sufficient wound debridement carried out at regular intervals also helps relieve the sensation of nasal obstruction and helps prevent synechiae formation. Weekly debridement for four weeks is recommended for optimal clearance of crusts. However, overenthusiastic douching too can lead to problems such as troublesome bleeding and pain.

Nasal douching with the head low position has been advocated to be the best position for irrigating the frontal and maxillary is sinuses. A larger volume of irrigating fluid measuring about 200 mL is used to successfully irrigate the frontal sinus. Tonicity of the irrigating material used does not have a major role in increasing mucociliary clearance.

Crusting

A certain amount of crusting is a normal phenomenon after any intranasal surgery. However, when the patient experiences discomfort and nasal block, or develops infection secondary to crusting, then it is deemed pathological. The main reason behind excessive crusting is damage to the mucosa which renders the mucociliary mechanism ineffective. Thus, the mucociliary blanket remains static and dries out due to excessive airflow and leads to crust formation. This crusting in turn leads to discomfort and feeling of nasal obstruction and may also progress to secondary infection following stasis of secretions.

Osteitis

This is another complication which occurs due to exposure of the bone. The patient complains of dull nagging pain which is not relieved by any medication and ultimately subsides on its own. Giving the mucosa its due respect is key to prevention of this complication.

PEARLS AND PERILS FOR SAFE ENDOSCOPIC SINUS SURGERY

Complications in the career of an ESS surgeon, whether major or minor, are inevitable especially when the surgeon has a lot of cases to his credit. The only way to reduce the rate of complications is to learn not only from one's mistakes but also from other's mistakes. These are some tips for the novice endoscopic surgeon to cut down on the complications in the training period.

Preoperative Management for Optimal Surgical Field

The technique for reducing complications begins from the preoperative period as soon as the diagnosis is made. In case of polyposis medial to the middle turbinate, the surgeon must give the patient a course of steroids so as to reduce the size of the polyps, reduce vascularity and reduce capillary bleeding which improves visibility. In the presence of active infection it would be prudent to start a course of antibiotics and perform regular douching. Additional comorbidities must be investigated for, which play a role in moderating hemostasis such as hypertension, liver disease and vitamin K deficiency. Bleeding diathesis must be ruled out and a detailed history of any drug intake pertinent to bleeding such as aspirin or warfarin must be obtained.

Study the CT Scan Diligently

Studying the CT scan is of utmost importance so as to identify situations with potential complications so that the surgeon is prepared to deal with the situations intraoperatively. The CT scan is like a three-dimensional road map for the endoscopic surgeon to perform a 'virtual' endoscopic surgery in his mind before venturing into the actual surgery.

There are some pertinent points that a surgeon should note on the CT scan, such as the level of the cribriform plate and the Keros classification. The Keros classification gives a rough idea of the potential risk for skull-base injury. The presence of a lamina papyracea dehiscence has grave implications if missed preoperatively and hence must be made note of. Presence of an Onodi cell and optic nerve dehiscence should be identified. The neurovascular relations of the sphenoid sinus and the level of the skull-base must be identified. The lowest level is that of the sphenoid roof as the skull-base has a slope from anterior to posterior and from lateral to medial. The frontal outflow tract must be recognized if medial or lateral depending on the attachment of the uncinate. This will avoid undue instrumentation in the frontal recess and prevent fibrosis and also prevent damage to the skull-base. The surgeon must have the patient's CT scan on a view box in front of him during surgery so as to facilitate any cross reference intraoperatively.

Prepare the Intraoperative Field

Intraoperatively, the surgical field has to be enhanced for better hemostasis and visualization which will in turn reward the surgeon with reduced mucosal trauma and fewer complications. The patient must be put in the head up position so as to reduce the venous ooze during surgery. Adequate infiltration and application of local decongestant will provide the surgeon with more space to operate and allows better instrumentation. Hypotensive anesthesia helps control arterial bleeding. A mean blood pressure of 60 mm Hg and a pulse rate of 60 per minute are ideal during surgery.

Identify Landmarks

The main feature which differentiates an extraordinary sinus surgeon from a mediocre one is the ability to create landmarks when it seems like there are not any. There are certain landmarks in ESS which are relatively constant and are present even in revision cases.

The middle turbinate is the most important landmark in the entire surgery and must always be in the surgeon's vision. The axilla of the middle turbinate is an important landmark to the frontal recess and the middle meatus.

The lamina papyracea is the lateral most limit in endoscopic sinus surgery and all the cells medial to the lamina must be cleared throughout its length to ensure complete removal of all the cells.

The inferior turbinate is another important landmark, the maxillary sinus ostium being just above the genu of the inferior turbinate.

The frontal recess lies between three main landmarks, the frontal beak, the lamina papyracea and the middle turbinate. One must go in between these three landmarks and will automatically reach the frontal sinus instead of recklessly probing around and creating a mucosal massacre. The anterior ethmoidal artery has a relatively constant landmark. It lies exactly one cell behind the frontal recess (Fig. 22.10). The point where it enters the cranial cavity is the weakest point of the anterior skull-base. It is well known that if the anterior ethmoid artery bleeds, then the chances of a coexisting CSF leak are high as the trauma required to damage the skull-base at this point is much less than that needed to damage the anterior ethmoid artery.

The septum and the superior turbinate along with the posterior choana form important landmarks for the identification of the sphenoid. It is very easy for a beginner to get confused between an Onodi and the sphenoid sinus. One must expect an Onodi after studying the CT scan.

Be Meticulous in your Surgery

The surgeon must handle tissue with care and gently remove all bony spicules so as to avoid granulations which occur if

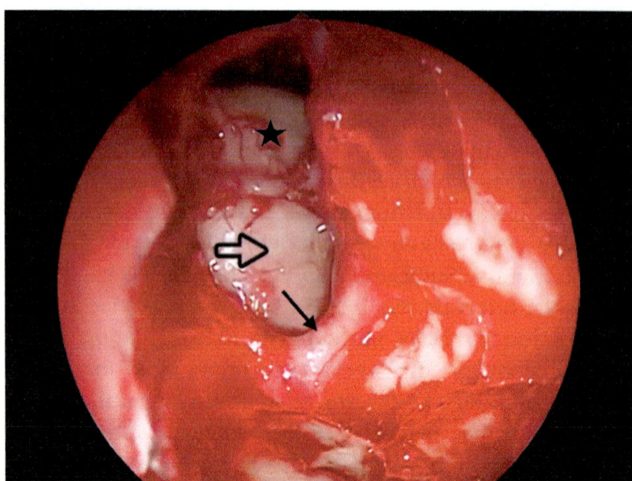

Fig. 22.10: Normal location of the anterior ethmoid artery (Black arrow) on endoscopy. It lies one cell (hollow arrow) behind the frontal ostium (star).

bone bits are left behind. Mucosa must never be pulled lest it may peel away. Always use a sharp cutting instrument to cut the mucosa. Ensure hemostasis at the end of your surgery by asking the anesthetist to reverse the hypotensive anesthesia. There must be no bleeding in the presence of normotensive anesthesia if the surgeon wants to prevent bleeding in the postoperative period.

Learn from your Mistakes

Any surgeon doing a large volume of cases will invariably encounter complications in their career and one must not be deterred by them but must learn from their previous mistakes so as to not repeat them again. This means that once a complication has been encountered, the surgeon automatically becomes cautious about it in the future and prevents that complication from occurring again. However, under most ideal conditions, complications do happen and one must be able to manage them promptly and efficiently.

REFERENCES

1. Stankiewicz JA, Lal D, Connor M, Welch K. Complications in endoscopic sinus surgery for chronic rhinosinusitis: a 25-year experience. Laryngoscope. 2011;121:2684-701.
2. Ali A, Kurien M, Shyamkumar NK, Selvaraj. Anterior skull base: High risk areas in endoscopic sinus surgery in chronic rhinosinusitis: A computed tomographic analysis. Indian J Otolaryngeal Head Neck Surg. 2005;57(1):5-8.
3. Bolger WE, Parsons DC, Mair EA, et al. Lacrimal drainage system injury in functional endoscopic sinus surgery. Incidence, analysis, and prevention. Arch Otolaryngol Head Neck Surg. 1992;118:1179-84.

4. Ramakrishnan VR, Palmer JN. Prevention and management of orbital hematoma. Otolaryngologic Clinics of North America 2010;43(4):789-800. doi:10.1016/j.otc.2010.04.006.

5. Yung CW, Moorth RS, Lindley D, et al. Efficacy of lateral canthotomy and cantholysis in orbital hemorrhage. Ophthal Plast Reconstr Surg. 1994;10:137-41.

6. Hwang SY, Flanders M, Desrosiers M. Endoscopic ocular muscle surgery. Operative Techniques in Otolaryngology-Head and Neck Surgery 2008;19(3):205-8. doi:10.1016/j.otot.2008.09.012.

7. Hong JE, Goldberg AN, Cockerham KP. Botulinum toxin A therapy for medial rectus injury during endoscopic sinus surgery. Am J Rhinol. 2008;22(1):95-7.

8. Kainz J, Stammbekger H. Danger areas of the posterior rhinobasis. An endoscopic and histoanatomical study. Laryngo-Rhino-Otology. 1991;70:479-86.

9. Levin LA, Beck RW, Joseph MP, Seiff S, Kraker R. The treatment of traumatic optic neuropathy: the International Optic Nerve Trauma Study. Ophthalmology. 1999;106:1268-77.

CHAPTER 23

Image-guided Sinus Surgery

TN Janakiram

INTRODUCTION

Intranasal surgery has under gone tremendous change and evolution throughout the last century. Although modern endoscopes and monitors provide a magnified and panoramic view of the operative field, several limitations continue to exist the largest of which is the inability to see through bone or tissue to predict what anatomy lies just beyond the penetration of the visible light (Fig. 23.1).

Navigation displays patient specific anatomy even where the endoscope is unable to provide the whole picture. Navigation system has become an integral part of the armamentarium for performing endoscopic sinus surgery and beyond. It acts as a road map in tracking various structures during surgery, thus reducing surgical time and apprehension of the surgeon in dealing with the critical areas. It is specially useful in revision fess and in surgery of frontal recess and skull base.

HISTORY

The earliest neuronavigational device was described in 1908[1] and utilized rigid frame for fixing the head, and a system of levers and pulleys to predict the location of intracranial structures based on external landmarks of skull. The application of plain radiography to stereotaxy was described by Spiegel and Wycis in 1940s.[2]

The era of modern image guidance began in 1970s with the incorporation of computed tomography. The CT base system described by Bergstrom and Greitz[3] in 1976 utilized a fixed metal ring worn by the patient during both the scan and the procedure.

TECHNOLOGY AND PRACTICAL USE

Although the specific solutions offered by the different commercially available systems vary, the basic tenets of

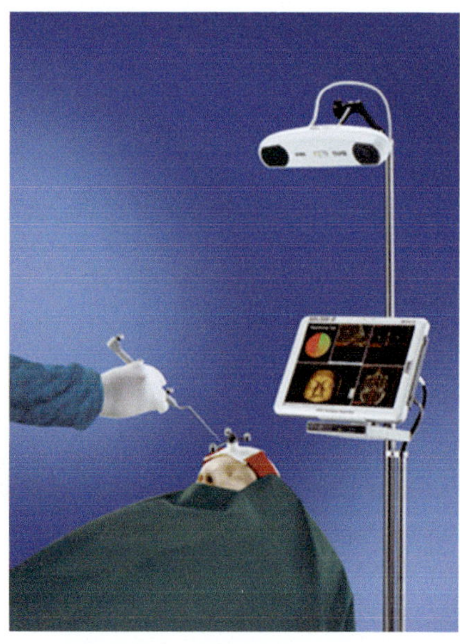

Fig. 23.1: Endoscope and monitor

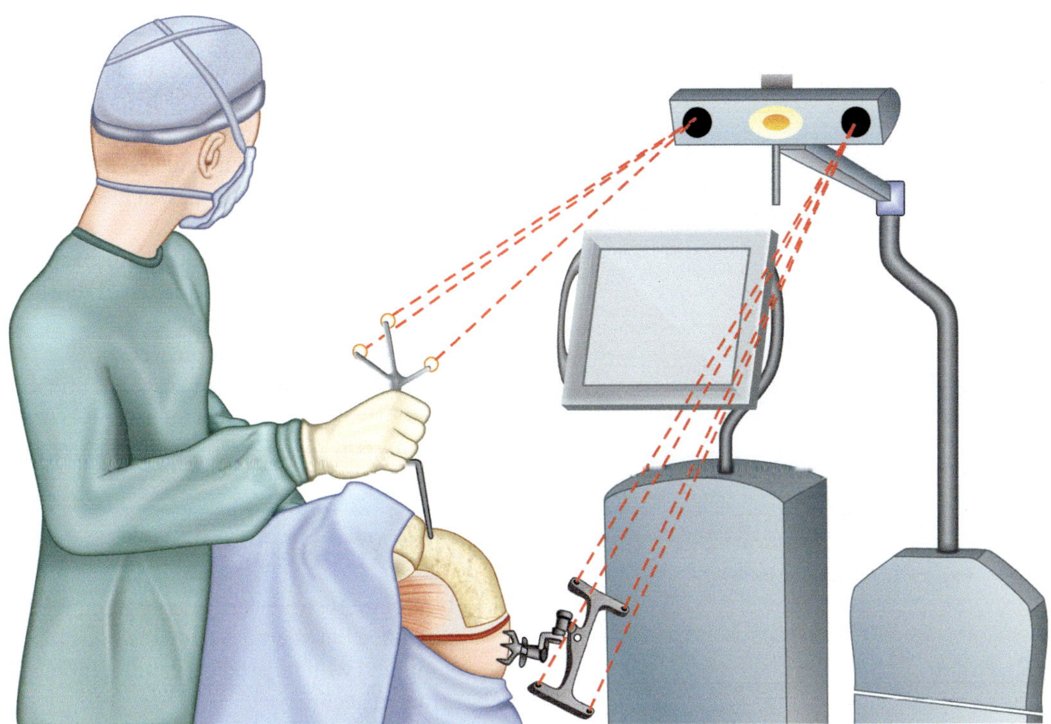

Fig. 23.2: Practical use of endoscope

image guidance, are similar. The hardware component houses the computer workstation, a monitor for image display, and an interactive component that communicates between the surgical team and the computer. The tracking device interfaces between the patient and the computer and enables navigation to be performed during the surgery. Modern systems are based on either line-of-sight or electromagnetic technology. Line-of-sight technology utilizes light-emitting diodes and infrared communication between the computer workstation and the tracking device, whereas electromagnetic technology achieves this with radiofrequency emission (Fig. 23.2).

The patient undergoes appropriate imaging study; specific protocols for these scans are utilized typically with 1 mm thick slices around the area of the surgical field. The images are transferred to the computer workstation and reviewed by the surgical team preoperatively to confirm that the indicated study was performed with the correct formatting and the anatomical area of interest is well displayed.

Once the patient is brought into the operating room and anesthetized, registration and calibration are performed. Registration is defined as the three-dimensional correlation of radiographic images with the surgical anatomy.

STEPS TO GET STARTED WITH THE NAVIGATION SYSTEM

1. Load the CD into the CD ROM drive
2. Mark four reference points on the patient (lateral orbital walls nasion and the columella).
3. The camera is aligned with patient tracker which gives a green signal in the patient model.
4. Registration is done using the navigation probe and placed over the four marked points which initiates a green clock on the panel.
5. Navigation probe is now used to confirm a point with an error less than 0.5 units. The navigation panel unit is now ready for use (Fig. 23.3).

CLINICAL INDICATIONS FOR NAVIGATION SURGERY

The endoscopic approach to the sella is facilitated by image guidance including confirmation of the anterior face of the sphenoid sinus, sellar floor, sphenoidal portion of internal carotid artery and optic nerves. Specific situations where image guidance has greater utility include:

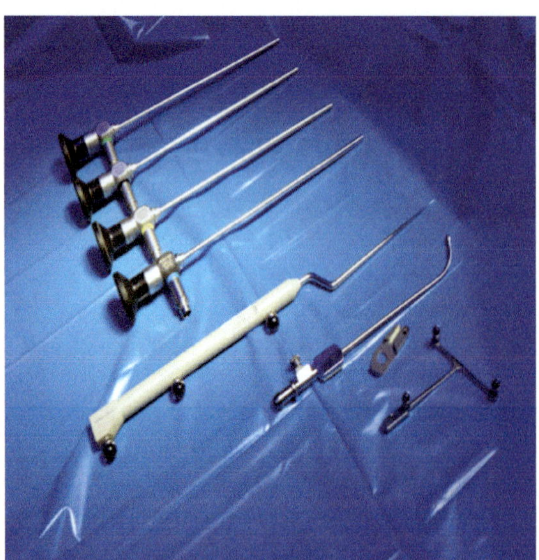

Fig. 23.3: Navigation probe

Revision Surgery

The anatomical disorientation that can occur in revision surgery may result from adhesion formation, removal of normal surgical landmarks, and the presence of reconstruction material.

Anatomical Variants

Anatomical variants associated with increased surgical complexity during the surgery include:
- Poor pneumatization of the sphenoid sinus (conchal variant)
- Presence of multiple intersinus septa
- Dehiscence of internal carotid artery or optic nerve
- Medial location of the cavernous portion of the internal carotid artery
- Presence of aberrant posterior ethmoidal air cells within the sphenoid sinus (Onodi cells)
- Surgery in pediatric patients
- Combined sinonasal disease including inflammatory chronic sinusitis.

Extended Procedures

In lesions with extrasellar extension, the required bony opening can be defined by image guidance.

SURGICAL ADVANTAGES

- Visual display and enlargement of critical anatomical structures
- Planning capability for minimally invasive accesses, resulting in improved surgical outcome through reduced trauma
- Minimization of risk through definition of landmarks and their reliable visualization
- Reduced surgery time through more rapid procedure
- Reduced costs as a consequence of shorter surgery times
- Safety check during surgery
- Documentation of all surgical steps
- Training and education of surgeons and/or staff
- The navigation is complimentary to the CT allowing the surgeon to orient himself in three different planes intraoperatively.

LIMITATIONS

- *Accuracy:* Accuracy in image guidance referred to the difference between the true positions of a point in space compared with its predicted radiographic postion. Errors in accuracy:
  - Target registration error refers to the difference between the anatomical point and its radiographic position
  - *Fiducial localization error:* It is the difference between the position of a fiducial point and its predicted radiographic location following registration, which in turn is calculated by image-guidance software in terms of root mean square value.
- *Anatomical disorientation:* The potential for anatomical misleading information is inherent to all image-guidance system; especially those based on preoperative image studies. Several factors including limitations in accuracy, structural shifting and registration error may result in disparity between intraoperative findings and the information conveyed by the image-guidance system.
- *Cost:* The cost associated with image guidance is both fixed capital expense and those incurred with use.

REFERENCES

1. Horsley V, Clarke RH. The structure and the function of cerebellum examined by new method. Brain. 1908;31:45-124.
2. Spiegel EA, Wycis HT, Marks M, et al. Stereotaxic apparatus for operations on the human brain. Science. 1947;106(2754):349-50.
3. Bergstrom M, Greitz T. Stereotoxic computed tomography. AM J Roentgenol. 1976;127:167-70.

CHAPTER 24

Nasal Packing Materials

Siddharth Chaudri

INTRODUCTION

Nasal packing has always been an essential part of any nasal or sinus surgery. Most surgeons feel the need to pack the nose after the surgery for various reasons such as hemostasis and maintaining the new position of the structures that are altered due to surgery, thus preventing adhesions.

Conventional or nonabsorbable nasal packing has been used for decades in the postoperative period with the duration of packing varying from 24 to 48 hours. This period has always been extremely uncomfortable for the patient as it causes suffocation, dry throat due to mouth breathing, watery eyes, headache; apart from the discomfort and risk of bleeding during pack removal.

It is these disadvantages, which have led to the usage of absorbable packing materials which do not close the nostrils completely, maintain hemostasis more effectively, and relieve the patient of the discomfort of removal of packs. These materials are being used more frequently in various centers, but they also have disadvantages related to wound healing, such as granulation tissue formation, crusting, delayed wound healing and adhesions.

In this chapter, we shall discuss the various types of packing materials including conventional nonabsorbable nasal packs, common absorbable nasal packs, and the more sophisticated advanced absorbable materials which do not have the disadvantages of crusting and synechia formation.

Difference between Dissolvable and Removable Nasal Packing

Sinus surgeons can use either traditional removable or more modern dissolvable nasal packing after surgery. Both kinds of packing absorb blood and support structures in the nose while the sinuses heal. Removable nasal packing, however, must be taken out of the nose 24 to 48 hours after surgery. This removal can be very painful because the healing tissue is disturbed as the nasal packing is removed. Dissolvable nasal packing goes away after a few weeks, eliminating the need for pack removal.

NONABSORBABLE NASAL PACKING MATERIALS

Vaseline or Paraffin Ribbon Gauze Packing

This has been traditionally used for decades in nasal and sinus surgery, the main advantages being that it is cheap and easily available.

However, this has traumatic effects on the nasal mucosa and surgical wounds. Moreover, removal of the nasal packs is uncomfortable for patients and there is also a higher risk of nasal bleeding during and after pack removal.

BIPP Ribbon Gauze Packing

Bismuth iodoform paraffin paste (BIPP) offers an additional advantage of being inert, hence the chances of infection are less. However it also shares the same disadvantages of vaseline ribbon gauze packing.

In both the above methods the mucosal trauma and pack removal discomfort can be reduced by inserting the loops of the roller packs into a finger glove.

Merocel Packing

Merocel nasal packs (self-expanding oxycellulose) are constructed of a unique sponge material using an exclusive formula. The small cell structure of Merocel provides a smooth surface, which maximizes comfort while minimizing tissue in growth. The high tensile strength of the sponge material prevents shedding or tearing. The packs are supplied compressed for ease of insertion and will expand as fluid is introduced, giving time for accurate positioning. It is also available with an integral airway to facilitate nasal airflow during use.

Features

- Biocompatible lint and fiber-free sponge material
- Superior liquid absorption and wicking
- Supplied compressed for ease of insertion
- Extremely soft and pliable cell structure

Hence, it is less uncomfortable and the incidence of bleeding is less during pack removal.

ABSORBABLE NASAL PACKING MATERIALS

There is no real risk to using most of the commercially available "dissolvable" pacing materials after nasal and sinus surgery. These include Gelfoam, Merogel and newer materials like NasoPore, Chitosan packs and NexPak. They are all usually absorbed in about two weeks.

The use of surgicel is debatable, as this takes a bit longer to be absorbed; crusting causes concern about its possibility of promoting synechia formation.

Gelfoam

This packing material has benefits in terms of both cost, and efficacy on hemostasis. However, Gelfoam causes thick clots and fibrinous bridges which do not get absorbed quickly encouraging synechia and stenosis after wound healing.

Surgicel and Fibrillar

This is the most effective hemostatic agent but has disadvantages of long-term crusting and synechia formation. However, the use of Surgicel (oxidized regenerated cellulose) as a nasal pack can be effective especially in patients with hematological malignancies with coagulopathies.

Surgicel is applied as a single or double layer and applied to the bleeding area in the nasal cavity. Fibrillar has the consistency of cotton and can be used more precisely to apply pressure on the bleeding areas.

When wet, they adhere to the nasal mucosa, reducing epistaxis but maintaining airflow. Surgicel and fibrillar are usually absorbed or get extruded out after some time. This method avoids the discomfort associated with conventional nasal packs and the traumatic raw areas upon removal. Surgicel and fibrillar also have bactericidal action against a wide range of gram-positive, gram-negative and even anerobic organisms.

FloSeal

The optimal form of nasal packing after endoscopic sinus surgery still has not been established. Although wide variations exist among sinus surgeons, the goals are adequate hemostasis, rapid healing, and patient comfort. Preliminary studies indicated that FloSeal, a novel absorbable hemostatic paste used as a nasal pack, was associated with minimal postoperative discomfort and effective hemostasis.

Absorbable hemostatic agents are associated with a high degree of patient comfort and provide hemostasis comparable with traditional techniques. However, FloSeal has the disadvantage of being very expensive.

Fibrin Glue

Endoscopic sinus surgery (ESS), especially when combined with turbinectomy and/or with submucous resection of the septum, may involve postoperative bleeding that might end with nasal packing. Fibrin glue also causes effective hemostasis. Drainage and ventilation of the paranasal sinuses are not impaired. There are no allergic reactions to the glue. Aerosol application of fibrin glue can be readily performed in ESS, requires no special treatment (antibiotics), and appears to have an adequate hemostatic effect. Hence, the use of this second-generation glue in ESS appears to stop nasal bleeding well and to be relatively safe and convenient.

Merogel

The woven fleece form of this nasal packing can be used in its dry state to absorb up to 10 times its weight in liquids and help control minimal bleeding. When hydrated, the biopolymer gradually transforms into a muco-adhesive gel after approximately 24–48 hours. It separates mucosal surfaces and gradually dissolves after approximately 2 weeks, eliminating painful nasal packing removal. Surgeons have observed better healing in clinical studies.

Not only does this nasal packing eliminate the pain of painful packing removal, but they also include a therapeutic material called hyaluronic acid that helps sinus wounds heal faster. This material helps keep the wound moist, reduces adhesions (scarring), and decreases healing time.

NEWER ABSORBABLE NASAL PACKS

NasoPore

NasoPore nasal dressing is made of a fully synthetic biodegradable fragmentable foam. It is indicated for use after nasal surgery. It absorbs fluids, provides pressure to and supports the surrounding tissue.

This biologically inert foam is a highly interconnected porous structure with a rapid and high absorbent capacity (up to 25 times its weight). It separates mucosal surfaces during the critical, early days of post-sinus surgery when mucosal swelling is heightened. By keeping mucosal tissue separated, it prevents formation of postsurgical adhesions in nasal cavities.

It provides gentle compression after surgery. By absorbing nasal fluids and blood, it slowly starts to fragment whilst still offering sufficient wound support during the critical healing period. During this period, it does not swell and so will not hinder natural drainage. After fragmentation it drains from the nasal cavity via natural pathways without any pain (Figs 24.1A to C).

Daily spraying with saline solution is recommended in the first week after surgery, to fasten the fragmentation and to reduce the risk of infection.
- Easily manipulated to allow optimum placement within the nasal cavity.
- It can also be used to medialize the middle turbinate, and septum, preventing lateralization.
- The unique structure has a proven high absorption capacity, being able to absorb up to 25 times its original weight.
- As there is no need for postoperative removal, it is atraumatic and comfortable for patients.
- Independent trials show that NasoPore may also function as a potential drug delivery carrier.

Fluid and temperature cause fragmentation of NasoPore, which starts after 12 hours. Hence, it is designed to give compression during two days and completely wears off in 7–14 days.

NasoPore is built of biocompatible materials so there is no problem when reabsorbed. Also it can be adjusted easily to clinical needs and be easily divided by cutting for bilateral use.

PosiSep and PosiSepX (Chitosan Nasal Packing)

PosiSep and PosiSepX are dissolvable intranasal splints made of chitosan, an aminopolysaccharide derivative of chitin which is made from the exoskeletons of crustaceans (Figs 24.2A and B).
- PosiSep transforms from a sponge to a gel when moistened.
- PosiSepX expands to occupy space within the nasal cavity when moistened.

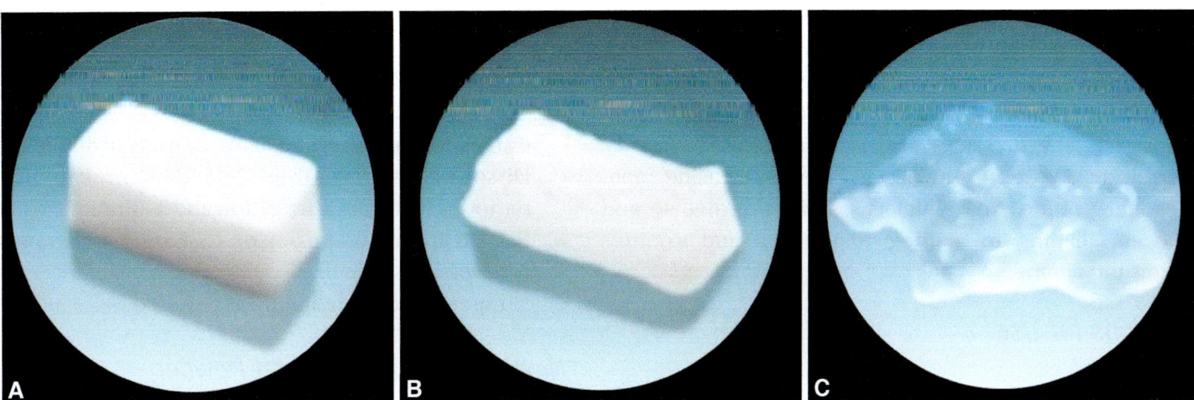

Figs 24.1A to C: (A) NasoPore; (B) When in contact with fluid; (C) Postfragmentation (*Courtesy:* NasoPore®; The fully degradable Nasal Dressing for improved wound healing ; NexusNovus 2013, Polyganics)

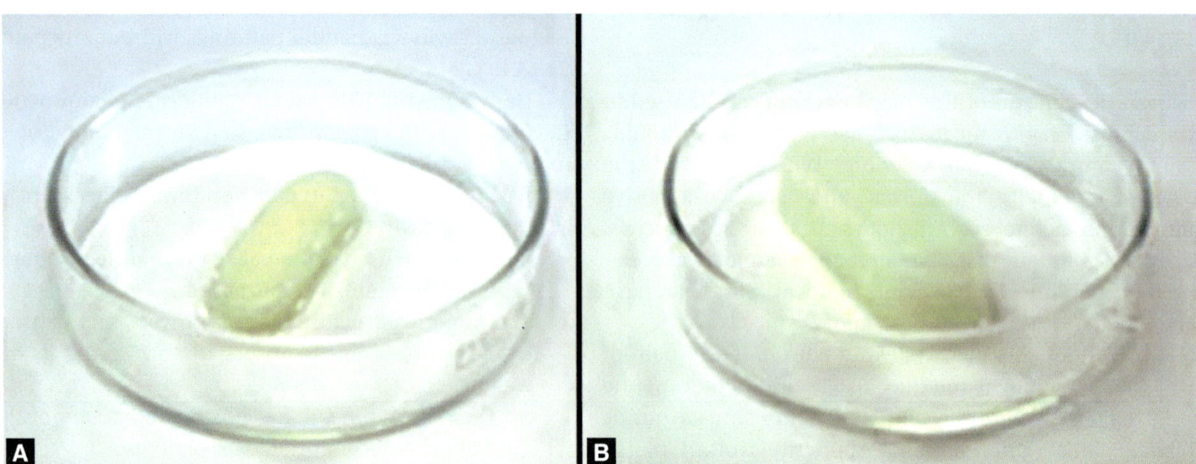

Figs 24.2A and B: Absorbable nasal packs: (A) PosiSep; (B) PosiSepX (*Courtesy:* PosiSep® Hemostatic Dressing/Intranasal Splints; Hemostasis Global, Bleeding Control Technologies)

- PosiSep and PosiSep X are indicated for use as intranasal splints intended to minimize bleeding and edema and to prevent adhesions between the septum and the nasal cavity. They are placed in the nasal cavity after surgery or trauma.
- Dissolves naturally or can be easily removed with gentle irrigation and aspiration
- Biocompatible—made of chitosan-based polymers
- Minimizes bleeding and edema after surgery
- Foam easily conforms to nasal anatomy
- Easy to apply—no mixing or additional preparation time necessary
- No special storage conditions required.

Description

The PosiSep line is constructed of a patient-comfortable sponge which is manufactured from naturally occurring chitosan polymer particles and polysaccharide binders. Chitosan has well-known hemostasis properties and, when combined with carboxymethylcellulose and hydroxyl-ethylcellulose binders, forms a foam-type dressing that has an affinity to absorb and hold water. PosiSep and PosiSepX hemostat dressings have the identical material composition. The dressings are used for topical wounds. They quickly dehydrate blood cells, thereby causing rapid hemoconcentration of platelets, serum proteins and fibrinogen, leading to clotting that limits and controls bleeding and edema.

Indications for Use

PosiSep and PosiSepX hemostat dressings are topical dressings for the temporary treatment of bleeding wounds such as surgical wounds (postoperative, donor sites, dermatological), cuts and lacerations and for the treatment of mild bleeding from topical ENT surgical wounds and nose bleeds.

NexStat, NexFoam and NexPak

NexStat topical hemostat powder and NexFoam topical hemostat sponge are easy-to-use plant-based products proven efficacious to speed clotting. Both products are indicated for the treatment of mild bleeding from topical ENT surgical wounds and nose bleeds.

NexPak is also made from the same plant based polysaccharide as NexStat and NexFoam, but NexPak is indicated as an intranasal splint intended to prevent adhesions in the nasal cavity after surgery or trauma while minimizing bleeding and edema.

Method of action: Bleeding cessation is accomplished by rapid dehydration and subsequent hemoconcentration of blood in contact with NexFoam Sponge. The concentration of clotting factors enhances the endogenous clotting mechanisms.

- Biocompatible—made from 100% plant-based polysaccharides
- Can be trimmed or shaped for a variety of applications
- Dissolves naturally over 7–14 days or can be easily removed with gentle irrigation and aspiration
- Easy to apply—no mixing or additional preparation time is necessary
- No special storage conditions required.

NexStat Topical Hemostat Powder

It is easy to apply and naturally dissolves from the sinus cavity generally within about a week. Easy to use applicator allows

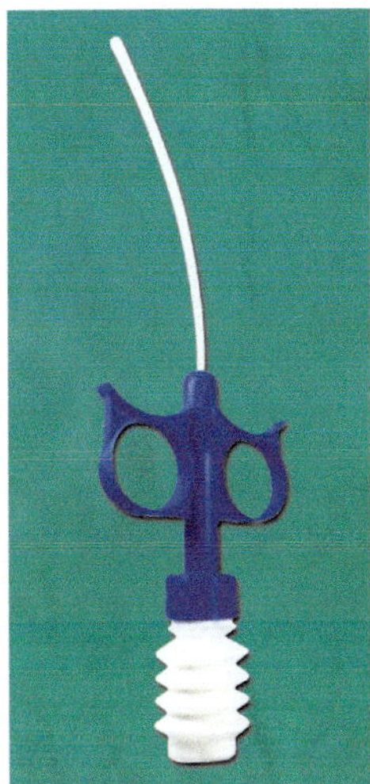

Fig. 24.3: NexStat topical hemostat powder applicator (*Courtesy:* NexStat® Topical Hemostat Powder; Hemostasis Global, Bleeding Control Technologies

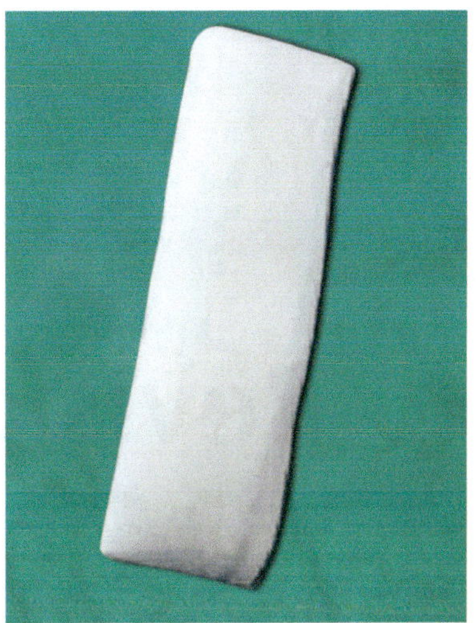

Fig. 24.4: NexFoam topical hemostat sponge (*Courtesy:* NexFoam® Topical Hemostat Sponge; Hemostasis Global, Bleeding Control Technologies)

precise application for hard-to-reach surgical wounds (Fig. 24.3)

- Versatile—multiple flex tips provided for each application
- No mixing or additional preparation time necessary
- No special storage conditions required.

NexFoam Topical Hemostat Sponge

It is versatile and can be conformed to virtually any shape or size (Fig. 24.4).

NexPak Topical Hemostat Sponge (Fig. 24.5)

- Compressible foam easily conforms to nasal anatomy.
- Easy to apply—no mixing or additional preparation time necessary.
- No special storage conditions required.

Fig. 24.5: NexPak topical hemostat sponge (*Courtesy:* NexPak® Intranasal Splint; Hemostasis Global, Bleeding Control Technologies)

ACKNOWLEDGMENTS

- Merocel® Nasal packs, Medtronic
- Surgicel® and Fibrillar® Absorbable Hemostat, ETHICON 360
- MeroGel® Bioresorbable Nasal pack, Medtronic
- NasoPore®; The fully degradable Nasal Dressing for improved wound healing; NexusNovus 2013, Polyganics
- PosiSep® Hemostatic Dressing/Intranasal Splints; Hemostasis Global, Bleeding Control Technologies
- NexStat® Topical Hemostat Powder; Hemostasis Global, Bleeding Control Technologies
- NexFoam® Topical Hemostat Sponge; Hemostasis Global, Bleeding Control Technologies
- NexPak® Intranasal Splint; Hemostasis Global, Bleeding Control Technologies.

CHAPTER 25

Revision Endoscopic Sinus Surgery

Milind V Kirtane, Swapna Patil, Sharmela Sondhi

INTRODUCTION

With an increasing focus on spending, in terms of cost of care to patients and society, revision endoscopic sinus surgery (RESS) has a very significant economic impact on the global healthcare scenario. Functional endoscopic sinus surgery has its share of patients requiring revision procedures, and in some cases, more than a single revision procedure. The burden is on healthcare providers to justify the need for these interventions, as every RESS procedure carries a risk of complications like intracranial and orbital trauma as well as a potential long-term risk of disruption of mucociliary clearance and change in olfaction.

This chapter deals with identifying the causes of failure of surgery or persistence of disease and the best approach for revision surgery.

When assessing the patient with a recurrence of sinus disease, the goal must be to identify the underlying cause, if possible. These causes can be classified as:[1]

- *Environmental factors:* Smoking or tobacco consumption in any form, exposure to pollutants, smoke, dust, allergens like pollens or molds, etc.
- *Host factors:* Systemic causes like Samter's triad (defined as asthma, aspirin sensitivity and nasal polyposis), cystic fibrosis, ciliary dysfunction, chronic granulomatous disease and neoplasia, and also patient non-compliance postoperatively.
- *Iatrogenic factors:* Inadequate or poor surgical technique, inadvertent mucosal stripping, osteitis or inadequate postoperative management including medical therapy.

The environmental and host factors may lead to chronic inflammation of the mucosa and alter the mucociliary clearance pathways. This necessitates adequate control of these factors, if not total elimination, before contemplating a revision surgery. Though environmental and host factors cannot be overlooked, this chapter will focus more on surgical factors.

INDICATIONS FOR REVISION SINUS SURGERY[2]

Most frequently encountered indications for a revision surgery are:

- *Incomplete previous surgery*
  - Retained ethmoid cells
  - Deviated nasal septum causing obstruction to drainage of sinuses
  - Retained uncinate process
- *Complications of previous surgery*
  - Mucocele formation
  - CSF leak not detected during previous surgery
  - Synechiae leading to ostiomeatal blockage

- *Persistent disease*
  - Recurrent attacks of acute sinusitis
  - Chronic rhinosinusitis, with or without polyps
  - Allergic fungal sinusitis
  - Neoplastic disease.

Failure of primary surgery may be a result of incomplete dissection, poor surgical technique, inadequate postoperative medical therapy, or inadequate postoperative cavity management, when the host and environmental factors are excluded. It could also result from excessive mucosal stripping which leads to exposed bony surfaces causing osteitis or neo-osteogenesis. Bony inflammation acts as a nidus for local production of inflammatory mediators, resulting in persistent mucosal disease, thus interfering with mucosal healing.[3-5] Mucosal stripping also leads to excessive scarring, which may lead to lateralization of the middle turbinate with subsequent blockage of the ostiomeatal complex, synechiae formation, and circumferential stenosis of ostia.

- *Synechiae* or adhesions may develop following a primary nasal surgery if raw areas are created facing each other (Fig. 25.1). These often lead to mechanical obstruction to outflow and may alter mucociliary clearance pathways. Adhesions to the middle turbinate can lead to its lateralization. Middle turbinate lateralization can be prevented by placing middle meatal spacers, stents or by bolgerizing the turbinate.[6-8]

Bolgerization[7,8] induces iatrogenic adhesion formation between the middle turbinate and the nasal septum, thus preventing its lateralization and subsequent obstruction to the sinus outflow tract. It can be achieved by artificially creating corresponding raw areas on the medial surface of the middle turbinate and the nasal septum, either by using a sickle knife or electrocautery. It can also be achieved by

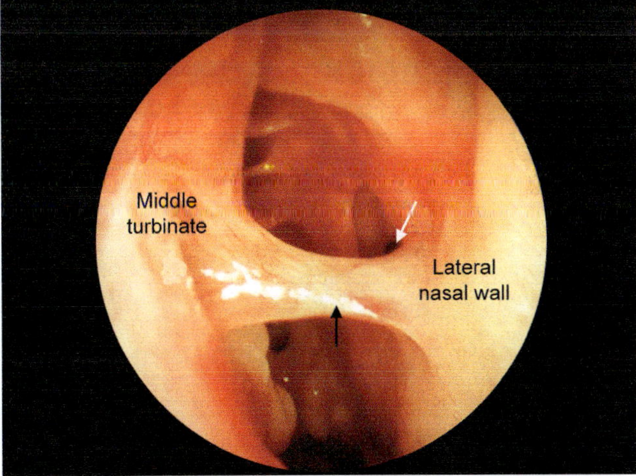

Fig. 25.1: Synechiae (black arrow) between middle turbinate and lateral nasal wall. The maxillary ostium can be visualized posteriorly (white arrow)

suturing the middle turbinate to the nasal septum by an absorbable suture.

Rather than dealing with synechiae, it is better if a surgeon avoids mucosal stripping and creating raw surfaces to avoid synechiae formation altogether. After excising synechiae, a nasal stent or a silastic sheet should be placed between the two raw surfaces to prevent redevelopment of synechiae. The stent can be removed after 4–6 weeks.

The difficulties faced in a revision surgery can be mainly due to:
- Scarring
- Loss of landmarks
- Anatomical dehiscence
- Bleeding.

Scarring, along with loss of landmarks, can be quite challenging even to an experienced endoscopist. The close proximity of numerous vital structures adds to the difficulty. The challenge lies in identifying the remnant landmarks and abiding by them to prevent further complications. Comprehensive and thorough medical and surgical therapy remains the keystone of the management of revision ESS cases as multiple factors are involved in disease persistence.

DIAGNOSIS AND PREOPERATIVE EVALUATION

Arriving at a decision about when to perform a revision surgery is important, so as to avoid unnecessary complications that may occur as a result of a revision surgery in a case that could have been managed by medical therapy alone. The associated environmental and host factors should also be taken care of prior to surgery. For example, in a patient complaining of headaches inspite of "adequate surgery", it would be wise to rule out all other possible causes before coming to a diagnosis of rhinogenic headache to be re-operated upon.

Diagnostic Nasal Endoscopy

A diagnostic nasal endoscopy plays a key role in aiding the surgeon to decide the need for revision surgery. It helps identify any structural abnormalities, incomplete surgery, retained secretions, blocked passages and synechiae.

Imaging Studies

Computed Tomography (CT) Scan

Understanding the complex anatomy of the paranasal sinuses and their drainage pathways becomes easy if the surgeon is familiar with reading CT scans. Imaging studies are of the utmost importance in revision cases where the endoscopic landmarks are obscure. CT scan sections in the coronal, axial and sagittal planes help in preoperative surgical planning. A thorough scrutiny of the preoperative CT scan should be performed to:

- Define the anatomical landmarks and integrity of boundaries like lamina papyracea, skull-base
- Assess draining of the frontal recess pathway
- Identify a partially resected uncinate process
- Identify resected turbinates or a lateralized middle turbinate
- Compare with previous CT scans.

Magnetic Resonance Imaging (MRI)

MRI is useful for the differential diagnosis of soft tissues in the involved paranasal sinuses, as it can distinguish a tumor from retained secretions. It is also helpful in the imaging of orbital and intracranial complications of sinusitis and detection of a meningocele or meningoencephalocele prolapsing through a breach in the skull-base.

CT-MRI Fusion

Image fusion creates images with both CT and MRI characteristics allowing better definition of the lesion and the surrounding bony and soft tissue anatomy, thus facilitating more comprehensive and minimally invasive endoscopic surgery with low morbidity.[9]

Three-dimensional Computed Tomography Angiography (3DCTA)

3DCTA is of assistance in the management of complex skull-base lesions. Combining CT images with angiography helps establish the location, patency, and relationship of major blood vessels to the lesion.

▌TECHNIQUES OF REVISION SURGERY

General Considerations

Preoperative preparation of patients with a course of local and systemic steroids, along with appropriate antibiotics, helps to minimize bleeding, by reducing the inflammation of the surgical bed.

Secretions may be sent for culture and antibiotic sensitivity testing, so that specific antibiotics can be started in the pre- and perioperative period.

Local infiltration with 2% xylocaine with 1:2,00,000 adrenaline can provide a good operative field. Normal saline with adrenaline (1:1,00,000 concentration) may be used in patients under general anesthesia. Pledgets soaked in cold saline can be used for a vasoconstrictive effect, if adrenaline is contraindicated.[10] A combination of sphenopalatine block with the greater palatine block leads to significant vasoconstriction in the posterior portion of the nasal cavity and reduces bleeding.[2] Well-controlled hypotensive anesthesia will further ensure a clear operative field.

Anatomical Landmarks for Revision Surgery[11]

Anterior Arch: It is the angle formed between the postero-superior aspect of the lacrimal bone and the anterior attachment of the middle turbinate (Fig. 25.2). It proves to be the most important and consistent landmark even when the middle turbinate has been resected. It defines the anterior border of the cribriform plate.

- *Maxillary sinus ostium:* If not visualized, the maxillary ostium can be exposed by removing remnants of the uncinate process. If it is covered by mucosa, visualizing a bubble of air on probing in the area, may indicate the location of the ostium. Identifying the maxillary ostium (Fig. 25.3) leads the surgeon towards the next two landmarks.
- *Lamina papyracea (Fig. 25.3):* This is the lateral-most limit of dissection. The ethmoid roof can be traced by following the lamina papyracea superiorly.
- *Ridge:* The junction of the medial orbital wall and the orbital floor forms the ridge. An imaginary line at the level of ridge can be extended posteriorly towards the anterior face of the sphenoid sinus area (Fig. 25.3). This line is a useful landmark to differentiate between the posterior ethmoid cells, which lie superolateral to it, and the sphenoid sinus, which lies inferomedially.

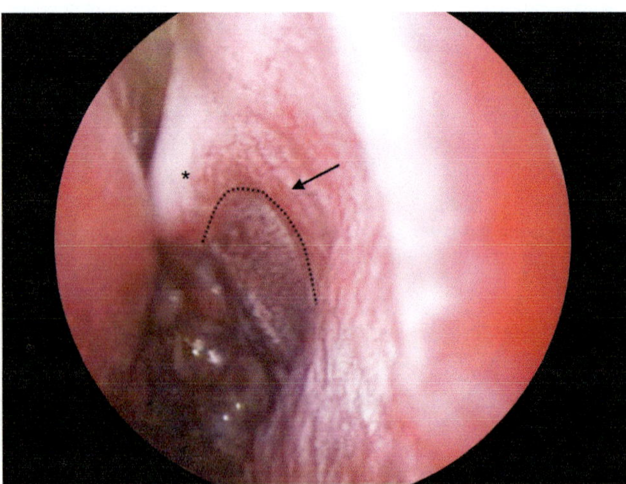

Fig. 25.2: Endoscopic image showing the anterior arch (black dotted line) in an operated left nasal cavity with the area of lacrimal bone (black arrow) and the middle turbinate remnant (*)

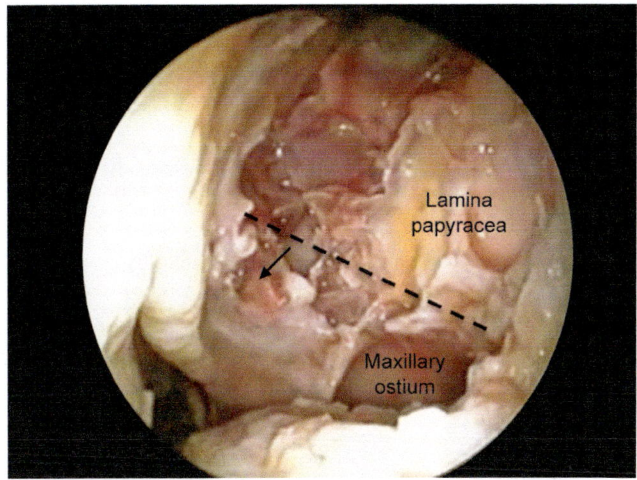

Fig. 25.3: Endoscopic image of the left nasal cavity showing the lamina papyracea and the maxillary ostium. The ridge is demonstrated by a black dashed line. The black arrow showing the expected position of the sphenoid ostium

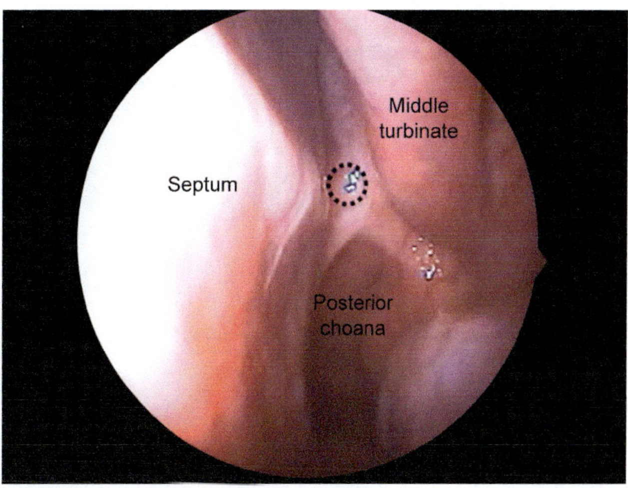

Fig. 25.4: Endoscopic image of the left nasal cavity showing the position of the sphenoid ostium (dotted circle) above the posterior choanal arch

- *Posterior choanal arch:* This is especially helpful in revision cases, to locate the sphenoid ostium, which may be obscured by disease. The sphenoid ostium lies about 1–1.5 cm above the posterior choanal arch, just away from midline (Fig. 25.4).
- *Roof of sphenoid:* It forms the skull-base and is continuous anteriorly as the ethmoidal roof, and hence is a useful guide for the superior limit of dissection.
- *Anterior ethmoidal artery:* When identified, it is a guide for the frontal recess and the frontal ostium (Fig. 25.5), which lie anterior to it.

Maxillary Sinus Revision Surgery

Novice endoscopists begin their journey in FESS with the so-called simpler maxillary sinus to operate on. As a result, revision surgery of maxillary sinus may be required, if the primary surgery has been inadequate.

- A partially resected uncinate process should be sought for, if persistent maxillary sinus disease is observed inspite of a widely patent maxillary ostium.
- If the middle meatal antrostomy is performed in the posterior or anterior fontanelle and is not in continuity with the natural ostium, some of the mucus coming out of the natural ostium can flow back via the surgical antrostomy into the sinus. Due to this "circulus" phenomenon, the incompletely cleared mucus is constantly recycled, and becomes a seat for bacterial growth, usually *Staphylococcus* or *Pseudomonas spp.*[11] This may also occur if an accessory ostium is present,

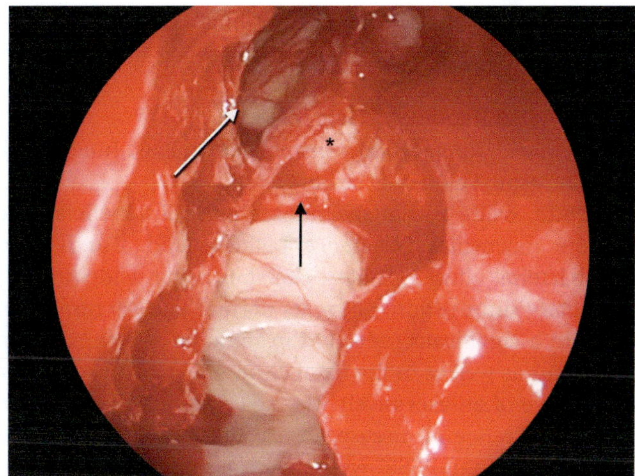

Fig. 25.5: Endoscopic image showing the relationship of the anterior ethmoidal artery (black arrow) separated from the frontal sinus opening (white arrow) by a single cell (*)

and is not connected to the widened natural ostium (Fig. 25.6).

- In certain cases of recurrent attacks of acute sinusitis where temporary relief is experienced with antibiotics, but the infection recurs later, a mechanical obstruction should be suspected.

The problems to be dealt with in revision surgery of the maxillary sinus are:

- Adequately performed inferior meatal antrostomy, but obstructed ostiomeatal complex.

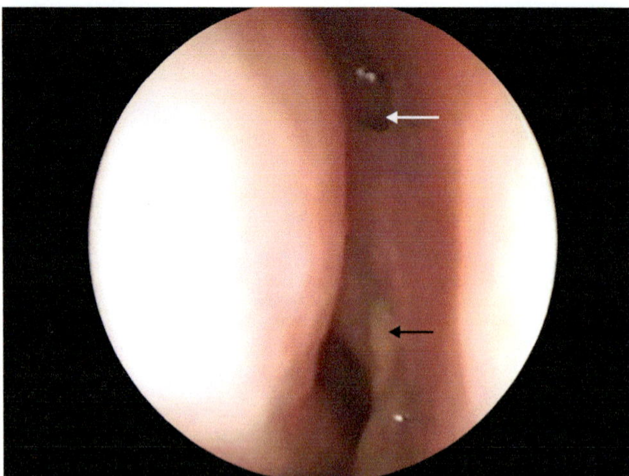

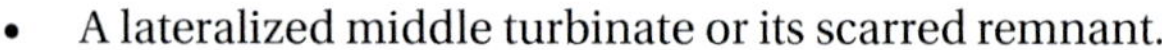

Fig. 25.6: Endoscopic image showing an accessory maxillary ostium (white arrow) and the natural maxillary ostium with a polyp (black arrow)

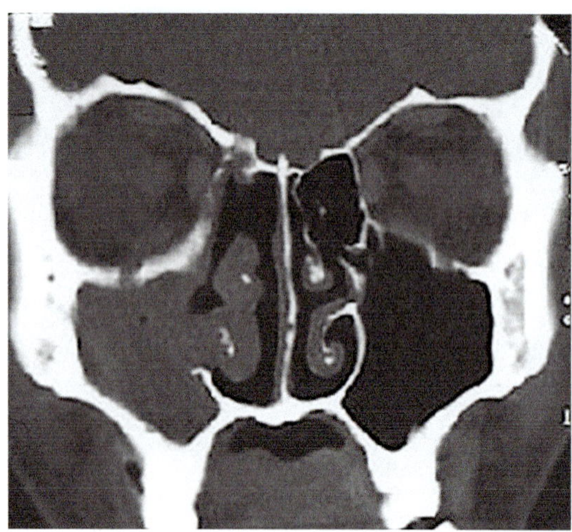

Fig. 25.7: Radiological image of an excessively widened right maxillary ostium with recurrence of disease

- A lateralized middle turbinate or its scarred remnant.
- Incomplete uncinectomy.
- Osteogenesis at the site of antrostomy.
- Persistent frontal sinus disease draining into maxillary sinus.
- Missed infraorbital (Haller) cell.
- Retained foreign body, inspissated mucus, fungal ball, bony spicules, dental cement, etc.

Nitric oxide within the sinuses plays a beneficial role in the mucociliary clearance pathway and also has an antibacterial effect.[12] It has been shown that widening the maxillary sinus ostium above its normal size (20 mm^2) can lead to a significant reduction in nitric oxide levels within the sinus as well as in the nasal cavity.[12] Figure 25.7 shows a CT image of an excessively widened right maxillary ostium with recurrence of disease. Hence the introduction of the concept of "mini FESS", where uncinate process is removed without disturbing the size of the maxillary ostium.[12] Other studies have concluded that although uncinectomy with ostium-preservation, or uncinectomy with ostium enlarging techniques show similar long-term recovery of the middle meatal and ostiomeatal complex area, uncinectomy along with an antrostomy may be slightly superior with regards to early mucosal recovery and ostium patency.[13]

In cases where fibrosis may be inevitable after surgery, local rotational flaps to cover the exposed bony edges of the maxillary sinus ostium have been used to prevent reclosure of sinus ostia, or at least to ensure minimal degree of patency of the ostia.[14]

The location of the maxillary sinus ostium makes it difficult to view the interior of the sinus by a 0 degree telescope. Use of angled scopes like 45 or 70 degree scopes helps to look at interiors, especially the floor of the sinus, making a surgeon's task easier. Viewing of the anterior wall may still be difficult, even with angled scopes, and may require a sublabial approach.

A thorough saline wash with a curved tip cannula should be given to remove any debris sitting in the floor or other inaccessible areas of the maxillary sinus.

Frontal Sinus Revision Surgery

Boundaries of the frontal recess are:
- *Lateral:* Lamina papyracea.
- *Medial:* Middle turbinate attachment.
- *Anterior:* Agger nasi.
- *Posterior:* Ethmoidal bulla.

Access to the frontal recess may be made difficult by the presence of many air cells such as agger nasi cell, the supraorbital ethmoid cell, frontoethmoidal cells, interfrontal sinus septal cell, suprabullar cell, frontal bullar cell.[1] The frontal recess is also closely related to the anterior ethmoidal artery, the anterior cranial fossa, olfactory area and the orbit, hence increasing the risk of complications while working in this region. The complex drainage pathway of frontal sinus, and difficulty in its clearance due to close proximity to various vital structures makes it prone to recurrence or persistence of disease.

The surgeon has to take special care to preserve the mucosa of the frontal recess area as this is more prone to stenosis, which is the commonest reason necessitating a revision surgery of the frontal sinus. Figures 25.8A and B shows iatrogenic frontal stenosis.

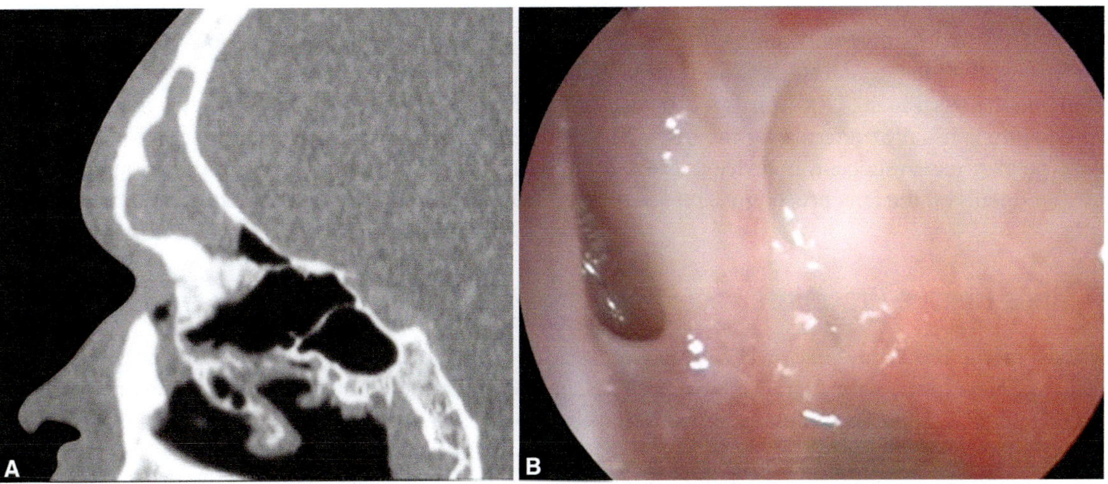

Figs 25.8A and B: CT scan (A) and endoscopic view (B) demonstrating postoperative frontal sinus stenosis

Causes of failure of frontal sinus surgery:[15,16]

- Stripping of mucosal lining causing neo-osteogenesis, and thus stenosis of the frontal recess
- Scarring, causing narrowing of the recess
- Lateralization of middle turbinate
- Inadequately resected uncinate process (superior portion)
- Inadequately dissected agger nasi cell, frontal recess cells
- Polyposis obstructing the pathway.

Use of angled scopes (45 or 70 degree) becomes necessary for complete clearance of the frontal recess and to visualize the frontal ostium.

The frontal recess lies posterior to the agger nasi cell. Clearance of Kuhn's frontoethmoidal cells may occasionally be required for adequate exposure. The area can be gently cleared in a back to forward motion using a blunt probe, removing the bony spicules and preserving as much of the mucosa as possible. It is best if a surgeon avoids leaving behind bare denuded area of bone, which stimulates osteogenesis.

Procedures such as Draf type II and III, with or without frontal sinus drill-out, frontal sinus rescue procedures, frontal sinus trephining may be performed at the time of revision surgery, if required.

Draf Procedures[17]

Draf I procedure (Fig. 25.9) is an endoscopic frontal recess approach and involves complete removal of the anterior ethmoid cells, uncinate process and any obstructing frontoethmoidal cells to facilitate drainage of the frontal sinus ostium into a patent frontal recess. It is a conservative approach for chronic frontal sinus disease involving the frontal recess. Care must be taken to preserve mucosa to prevent stenosis.

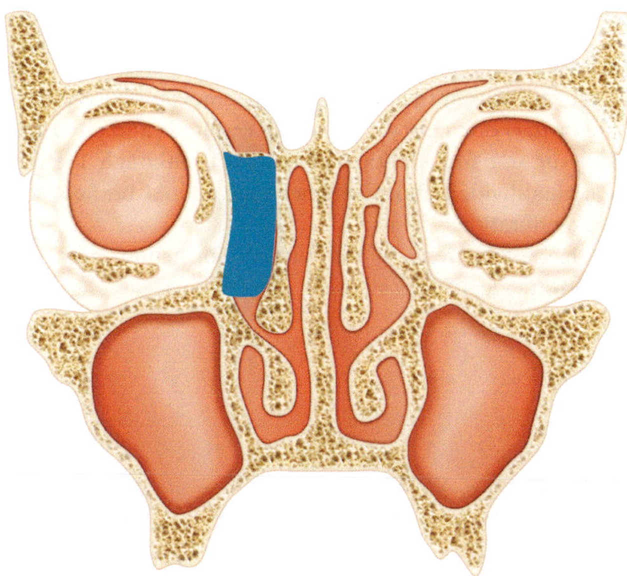

Fig. 25.9: Schematic diagram of endoscopic frontal recess approach (Draf I) procedure (Adapted from Draf[17])

Draf II procedure (Fig. 25.10), also known as endoscopic frontal sinusotomy, is done in cases where a conservative approach has failed or recurrence of disease occurs after a clearance. It involves resection of the floor of the frontal sinus from the lamina papyracea laterally to the middle turbinate medially (IIA), or to the nasal septum medially (IIB), with clearance of disease from the anterior face of the frontal recess.

Draf III procedure (Fig. 25.11) or the modified Lothrop's procedure is done by removing the floor of frontal sinuses bilaterally along with the inferior part of interfrontal septum, superior part of the nasal septum and anterior portions of the middle turbinates. Both the frontal sinus cavities are merged and opened into the nasal cavity.

This procedure is usually preferred for the more chronic and severe type of disease, especially in revision cases.[16,17]

For further details on the Draf procedures, please refer to the Chapter 7.

Frontal Sinus Rescue Procedure

A frontal sinus rescue procedure may be performed in cases where a previously performed middle turbinate resection has resulted in a lateralized middle turbinate remnant causing frontal sinus outflow tract obstruction.[18,19]

This involves advancing a mucoperiosteal flap into the frontal sinus neo-ostium to try and restore sinus functionality. Details of the procedure have been described in the chapter 'Endoscopic Surgery of the Frontal Sinus'.

As the frontal recess area is prone to post-operative narrowing and stenosis, stenting of the frontal sinus outflow tract can help in maintaining the patency in revision cases. Stents may be made of a variety of materials and are usually kept *in situ* for a period of 6 weeks, although literature remains divided about whether they should be kept for a longer duration.[20-22]

However, crusting and biofilm formation may be a disadvantage of using stents.[23]

Revision Surgery of the Ethmoid Sinuses

The numerous, but inconsistent number of cells in the ethmoid labyrinth makes it difficult for a surgeon to know if all the cells have been cleared during surgery. Recurrence of ethmoid disease is not uncommon, necessitating revision surgery.

Causes for Recurrence of Ethmoid Disease[2]

- Retained cells or septae during previous surgery
- Recurrent inflammation and scarring of residual mucosa
- Osteitis of the retained bony septae
- Lateralization of middle turbinate causing obstruction of ethmoid cells
- Retained superior part of uncinate process
- Unresected agger nasi cell

Important cells while clearing an ethmoidal complex disease are:
- Onodi cell
- Haller cell
- Anterior most ethmoidal cell (agger nasi)
- Superior most ethmoidal cell
- Frontoethmoidal cell.

The lateral boundary of the ethmoidal labyrinth, i.e. the lamina papyracea, and the roof, i.e. the skull-base, can be

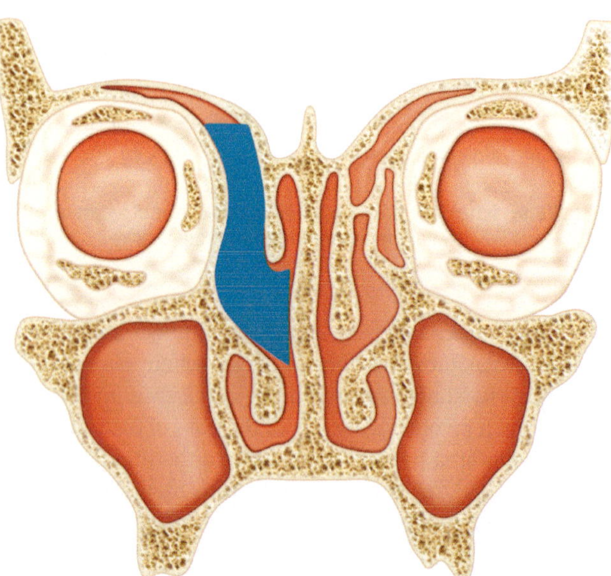

Fig. 25.10: Schematic diagram of endoscopic frontal sinusotomy (Draf IIA) procedure (Adapted from Draf[17])

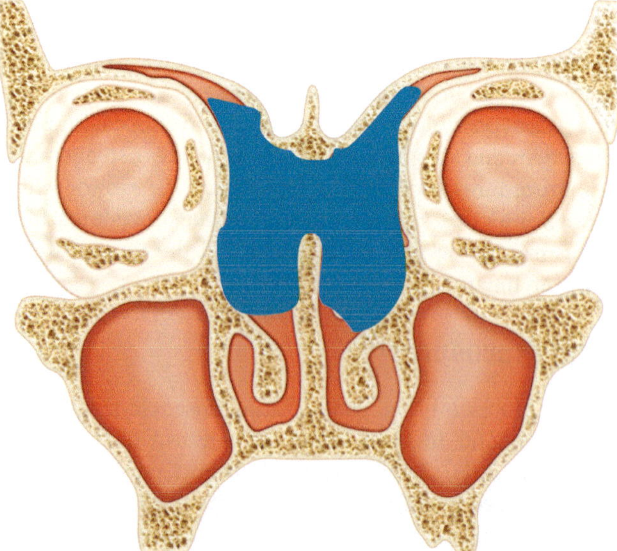

Fig. 25.11: Schematic diagram of the Draf III (endoscopic modified Lothrop) procedure

markedly thinned out due to previous surgery or chronic disease. The roof of the ethmoids slopes downwards from anterior to posterior and can be followed upwards and anteriorly after locating the sphenoid sinus roof. Care should be taken to avoid trauma to these walls during a revision surgery. The posterior limit of dissection is the anterior wall of the sphenoid sinus.

During a revision ethmoidectomy, remanants of the uncinate process or agger nasi should be removed. Retained bony septae and areas of diseased ethmoid mucosa should be cleared, preserving as much healthy mucosa as possible. The diseased mucosal edges can be trimmed finely with the help of a microdebrider or a tru-cut forceps. A drill with suction-irrigation, may at times be required to clear bony septae which may be thickened due to osteitis. Mucoceles, which may occur as a result of scarring following previous surgery should be drained and marsupialized. Skull-base defects created as a result of previous surgery may have to be sealed.

Revision Surgery of the Sphenoid Sinus

Persistent sphenoid disease and sphenoid ostium stenosis are less frequently seen in patients undergoing revision endoscopic sinus surgery.[24,25] However, revision surgery of the sphenoid sinus may pose a difficulty to the operating surgeon due to the absence of landmarks and the presence of important structures like the optic nerve and the internal carotid artery in the vicinity.

Causes for a Revision Sphenoid Sinus Surgery

- Failure to locate the sphenoid ostium during primary surgery: A surgeon may mistake a posterior ethmoid cell (onodi cell) for the sphenoid sinus and open it instead. This may be avoided if the CT scan images are studied in detail before the surgery.
- A circumferentially opened ostium can stenose due to osteitis or inadequate postoperative cavity management.
- At times, although the sphenoid sinus is opened, the natural ostium may have been left out from the new ostium created. This may lead to recirculation of mucous flow and a need for revision surgery.
- Scarring of the superior turbinate leading to obstruction of the sphenoid ostium.
- Persistent inflammation of posterior ethmoidal cells or retained posterior ethmoid partitions.
- Recurrent polyposis or fungal ball occluding the natural ostium: Inflammatory sphenoid lesions such as fungal balls may increase the risk of postoperative ostial stenosis, especially in cases when postoperative surveillance or debridement is difficult or impossible.

The sphenoid sinus can be approached via a transethmoidal approach by performing a complete anterior and posterior ethmoidectomy. It can also be reached via a parasagittal approach, in which the sphenoid ostium is identified medial to the superior turbinate after lateralizing the middle turbinate. However, locating the sphenoid ostium may be difficult during a revision surgery owing to the loss of landmarks. Other landmarks may be used as a guide in such cases.

Landmarks to locate the sphenoid ostium during revision surgery:
- *Superior turbinate (whenever present):* The ostium can be located medial to the superior turbinate.
- Following the ridge posteriorly (Fig. 25.3)
- *Posterior choanal arch:* The ostium usually lies 1–1.5 cm above the arch (Fig. 25.4).

The internal carotid artery and optic nerve lying in the posterolateral wall of the sphenoid sinus may be dehiscent, and may be damaged if the sphenoid sinus is opened inaccurately. A mushroom punch or downward directed Kerrison's punch can be used to widen the ostium. Powered and cutting instruments should be handled with care. Widening should always be done in an inferior and medial direction to avoid injury to vital structures and also to avoid circumferential widening. The ostium may be enlarged in the lateral direction, always after palpating the bone.

The posterior branch of the sphenopalatine artery lies about 1.5 cm below the sphenoid ostium, hence care should be taken while widening it inferiorly. In case of bleeding, it can be controlled by bipolar cauterization.

Raising a mini-nasoseptal flap to line the sphenoid opening may help in mucosal healing, and decrease the risk of restenosis by preventing cicatricial scarring.[26]

It is advisable to always preserve the superior turbinate while opening the sphenoid sinus as the superior turbinate is lined by olfactory epithelium. The turbinate, if left behind, can also serve as a landmark in case there is a need for further surgery.

Image Guidance

Image guidance may be used intraoperatively, if necessary. The American Academy of Otolaryngology—Head and Neck Surgery (AAO–HNS) policy on intraoperative use of computer-aided surgery includes the following indications:[27]
- Revision sinus surgery
- Distorted sinus anatomy of developmental, postoperative, or traumatic origin
- Extensive sinonasal polyposis
- Pathology involving the frontal, posterior ethmoid and sphenoid sinuses
- Disease abutting the skull-base, orbit, optic nerve, or carotid artery

- CSF rhinorrhea or conditions where there is a skull-base defect
- Benign and malignant sinonasal neoplasms.

POSTOPERATIVE CARE

Postoperative management plays an important role in achieving optimal outcomes following sinus surgery, more so in revision cases. Nasal saline irrigation, regular debridement as required, topical and oral steroids, and antibiotics help in promoting healing and achieving good postoperative results. Middle meatal spacers such as absorbable gelatin sponges and synthetic polyvinyl alcohol foam polymer sponges may help in preventing adhesions and middle turbinate lateralization.

Complications similar to those that can occur following a primary endoscopic sinus surgery may occur following a revision surgery. Revision surgery however, has a higher risk on account of obscured landmarks, scarring and potentially dehiscent structures. Steroid-eluting stents may improve local drug delivery, thus reducing postoperative adhesions, recurrence of polyposis, middle turbinate lateralization (by acting as spacers), the need for postoperative oral steroids and the need for additional postoperative interventions.[28,29]

CONCLUSION

Revision endoscopic sinus surgery has been shown to benefit patients who fail maximum medical therapy and prior sinus surgery for chronic rhinosinusitis.[30] Revision endoscopic sinus surgery serves as a challenge to the operating surgeon, mainly because it frequently involves dealing with the sinuses without any landmarks to serve as a roadmap. A detailed preoperative study of the CT scan images and a good knowledge of anatomy are invaluable in such cases. Understanding the principles and techniques of sinus surgery and following them during the primary surgery itself, would go a long way in reducing the need for revision surgeries.

REFERENCES

1. Cohen NA, Kennedy DW. Revision Endoscopic Sinus Surgery. Otolaryngol Clin N Am. 2006;39:417-35.
2. Kountakis S, Jacobs J, Gosepath J. Revision Sinus Surgery. Verlag-Berlin Heidelberg. Springer, 2008.
3. Kennedy DW, Senior BA, Gannon FH, et al. Histology and histomorphometry of ethmoid bone in chronic rhinosinusitis. Laryngoscope. 1998;108:502.
4. Moriyama H, Yanagi K, Ohtori N, et al. Healing process of sinus mucosa after endoscopic sinus surgery. Am J Rhinol. 1996;10:61.
5. Perloff JR, Gannon FH, Bolger WE, et al. Bone involvement in sinusitis: An apparent pathway for the spread of disease. Laryngoscope. 2000;110:2095.
6. Lee JM, Grewal A. Middle meatal spacers for the prevention of synechiae following endoscopic sinus surgery: A systematic review and meta-analysis of randomized controlled trials. Int Forum Allergy Rhinol. 2012;2(6):477-86.
7. Hanna BM, Kilty SJ. Middle turbinate suture technique: A cost-saving and effective method for middle meatal preservation after endoscopic sinus surgery. J Otolaryngol Head Neck Surg. 2012;41(6):407-12.
8. Bolger WE, Kuhn FA, Kennedy DW. Middle turbinate stabilization after functional endoscopic sinus surgery: The controlled synechiae technique. Laryngoscope. 1999;109(11):1852-3.
9. Lalwani A, Pfister M. Recent Advances in Otolaryngology. Head and Neck Surgery, April 2014; Volume 3.
10. Taskin U, Yigit O, Bilici S, et al. Efficacy of the combination of intraoperative cold saline-soaked gauze compression and corticosteroids on rhinoplasty morbidity. Otolaryngol Head Neck Surg. 2011;144(5):698-702.
11. Stankiewicz JA. Advanced Endoscopic Sinus Surgery. Mosby, 1995.
12. Kirihene RK, Rees G, Wormald PJ. The Influence of size of the maxillary sinus ostium on the nasal and the sinus nitric oxide levels. Am J Rhinol. 2002;16(5):261-4.
13. Luukkainen A, Myller J, Torkkeli T, Rautiainen M, Toppila-Salmi S. Endoscopic Sinus Surgery with Antrostomy has Better Early Endoscopic Recovery in Comparison to the Ostium-preserving Technique. ISRN Otolaryngology. Volume 2012 (2012), Article ID 189383.
14. Nada I, El-Sharnouby M, Abo-El-Ezz T. The role of local rotational flaps in minimizing sphenoidal and maxillary sinuses ostium stenosis. Egyptian Journal of Ear, Nose, Throat and Allied Sciences. 2014; 15(2):93-7.
15. Huang BY, et al. Failed Endoscopic sinus surgery: Spectrum of CT findings in the frontal recess. Radiographics journal. 2009; 29(1).
16. Friedman M, Landsberg R, Schults RA, Tanyeri H, Caldarelli DD. Frontal sinus surgery: Endoscopic technique and preliminary results. Am J Rhinol. 2000;14(6):393-403.
17. Draf W. Endonasal micro-endoscopic frontal sinus surgery: The Fulda concept. Op Tech Otolaryngol Head Neck Surg. 1991;2:234-40.
18. Citardi MJ, Javer AR, Kuhn FA. Revision endoscopic frontal sinusotomy with mucoperiosteal flap advancement: The frontal sinus rescue procedure. Otolaryngol Clin North Am. 2001;34(1):123-32.
19. Kuhn FA, Javer AR, Nagpal K, et al. The frontal sinus rescue procedure: Early experience and three-year follow-up. Am J Rhinol. 2000;14(4):211-6.
20. Philpott C, Mckiernan D, Javer A. Selecting the Best Approach to the Frontal Sinus. Ind J Otolaryngol Head Neck Surg. Jan 2011;63 (1):79-84.
21. Rains BM. Frontal sinus stenting. Otolaryngol Clinics of North America. 2001;34:101-10.

22. Weber R, Mai R, Hosemann W, et al. The success of 6 months stenting in endonasal frontal sinus surgery. Ear Nose Throat J. 2000;79:930-2.

23. Perloff JR, Palmer JN. Evidence of bacterial biofilms on frontal recess stents in patients with chronic rhinosinusitis. Am J Rhinol. 2004;18(6):377-80.

24. Musy PY, Kountakis SE. Anatomic findings in patients undergoing revision endoscopic sinus surgery. Am J Otolaryngol. 2004;25:418-22.

25. Khalil HS, Eweiss AZ, Clifton N, et al. Radiological findings in patients undergoing revision endoscopic sinus surgery: A retrospective case series study. BMC Ear Nose Throat Disord. 2011;11:4.

26. Thompson C, DeConde A, Chiu A, et al. Mini-nasoseptal flap for recalcitrant sphenoid sinusitis. Am J Rhinol Allergy. 2013; 27 (2):144-7.

27. American Academy of Otolaryngology–Head and Neck Surgery (AAO-HNS), AAO-HNS policy on intra-operative use of computer-aided surgery. Approved 2005 Sept. Available at: http://www.entlink.net/practice/rules/image-guiding.cfm.

28. Dautremont JF, Mechor B, Rudmik L. The role of immediate postoperative systemic corticosteroids when utilizing a steroid-eluting spacer following sinus surgery. Otolaryngol Head Neck Surg. 2014 Apr;150(4):689-95.

29. Campbell RG, Kennedy DW. What is new and promising with drug-eluting stents in sinus surgery? Curr Opin Otolaryngol Head Neck Surg. 2014 Feb;22(1):2-7.

30. McMains KC, Kountakis SE. Revision Functional Endoscopic Sinus Surgery: Objective and Subjective Surgical Outcomes. Am J Rhino. 2005;19(4):344-7.

CHAPTER 26

Balloon Sinuplasty

Nishit J Shah

INTRODUCTION

Chronic sinusitis affects millions of people worldwide. Whilst sinusitis may be bacterial, viral or fungal, over 100 million or 10% of the population has experienced sinusitis in India. A large percent continue to have persistent symptoms as a result of chronic sinusitis. What is underestimated is the impact on the quality of life in sinusitis sufferers. It is likely that more people have disruption of normal life as a result of sinusitis than diabetes mellitus and congestive heart failure put together. Various factors lead to the development of chronic sinusitis, including microbial immune, mucosal, bony structural, genetic and allergic factors.

The large majority of patients (about 80%) will respond to medical therapy, while about 20% may require surgical intervention. Of these, many will refuse surgery, as they are averse to surgery, unfit or have heard from others that results are not good. These will relapse into medical treatment and only get operated when symptoms worsen and there is no option. This is where Balloon sinuplasty™ (BSP) may be an acceptable option as it offers a surgical solution whilst being minimally invasive ensuring a quick return to work with no significant complications.

Endoscopic sinus surgery (ESS) has clearly scored over the traditional open procedures of Caldwell-Luc and ethmoidectomies, but some concerns still remain. There is considerable removal of bone and tissue which could lead to postoperative pain, scarring and bleeding. The possibilities of surgical complications remain, and there is an increased hospital stay and uncomfortable nasal packing. BSP was introduced in 2005 and underwent extensive multicenter testing for the next 2 years to confirm efficacy, safety and practicality of use.

It consisted of a guidewire, which could be navigated into the frontal, maxillary or sphenoid sinus through the ostium that could then be dilated using a sinus balloon.

Balloon sinuplasty helps with all these issues yet keeping in mind the goals of surgery which are to clear the blocked sinuses, restore normal sinus drainage and function whilst preserving normal anatomical structures and mucosa as much as possible. BSP is able to do this by widening the sinus ostia and transitional spaces by microfracturing surrounding bone so that the results are long lasting and yet no resection of tissue is required. The BSP technology is used as a stand-alone procedure, but could also be combined with ESS as an additional tool in cases where there is more extensive disease, instrumentation is difficult or identification of the sinus (especially frontal) could be challenging.

BALLOON SINUPLASTY SYSTEM

Balloon sinuplasty consists of many parts:
- Sinus guidewire (luma with light cable)
- Sinus guide catheter
- Sinus balloon catheter
- Inflation device
- Sidekick
- Vortex irrigation cannula
- Stratus

Guidewire (Fig. 26.1)

The guidewires are firm yet extremely flexible. Therefore, it is not possible to penetrate bone as the guidewire bends with any resistance. Hence, on entering a cell, the wire will bend and come back, but will smoothly enter a natural drainage pathway. This makes it very safe. The lighted tip at the end can be seen to move in the sinus due to transillumination, confirming its entry into the sinus.

Cannula (Fig. 26.2)

There are different cannulas that can be used in the sinuses. When dilating the sphenoid sinus, it is recommended to use the 0 or 30 cannula. For the frontal sinus, the 70 cannula is used. The maxillary sinus may be dilated with either the 90 or 110 cannula. These angles have been decided after extensive testing and provide the most appropriate angle for guiding the wire.

Balloon (Fig. 26.3)

Balloon Sizes

Balloons are available in various sizes (Fig. 26.4). For pediatric use, 12 mm length by 3.5 mm diameter balloon is used. For adults, balloons are available in lengths of 16 and 24 mm and diameters of 5, 6 and 7 mm. If you are using C-arm or fluoroscopy, then a 16 mm balloon can be used, as it can be accurately placed across the ostium and drainage pathway. When using the luma guidewire, it is better to use the 24 mm as it will cover a longer part of the drainage pathway. The 5 mm is the minimal size and one can decide the size based on anatomy and experience.

Relieva® Stratus (Fig. 26.5)

The stratus stents were made to deal with the ethmoid sinus. Since there was criticism that BSP did not address the crucial ethmoid area, the stratus was designed as a drug-eluting stent, which could be used with steroid or antibiotic. The stent was introduced with a deployment guide and kept in place for 6 weeks, during which time the drug slowly exuded and dealt with the pathology.

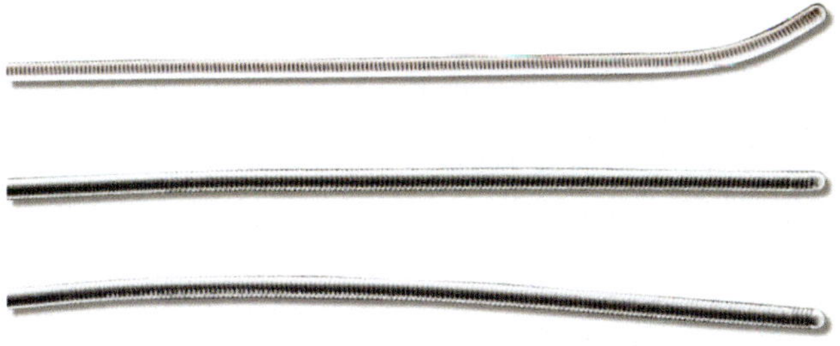

Fig. 26.1: Guidewire

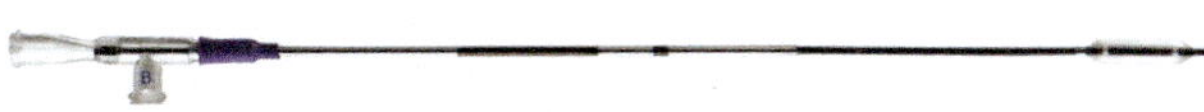

Fig. 26.3: Balloon

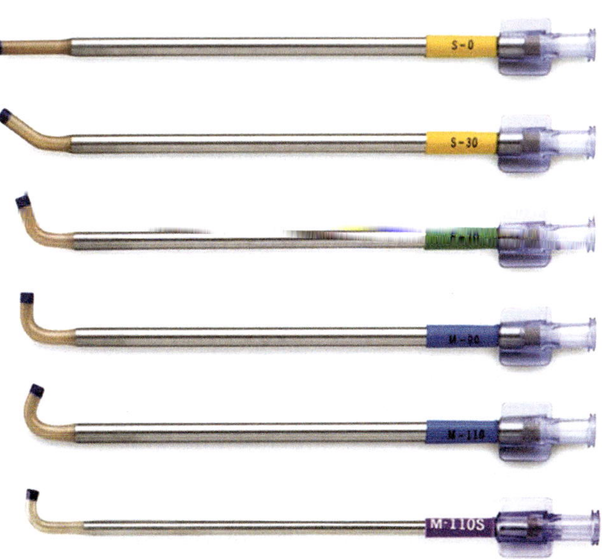

Fig. 26.2: Cannula

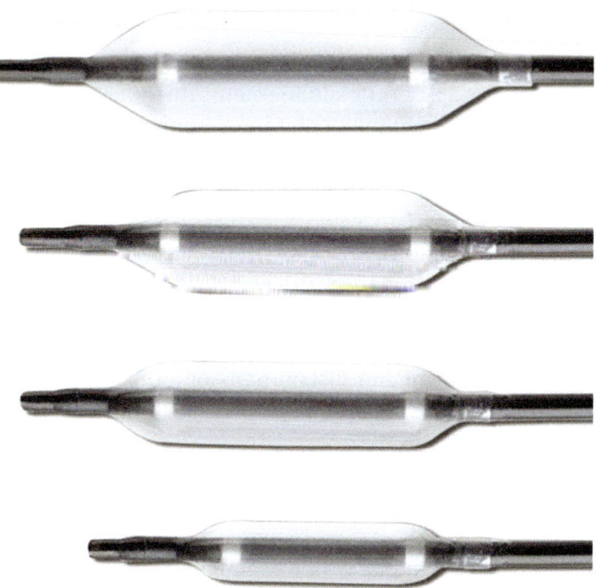

Fig. 26.4: Various sizes of balloon

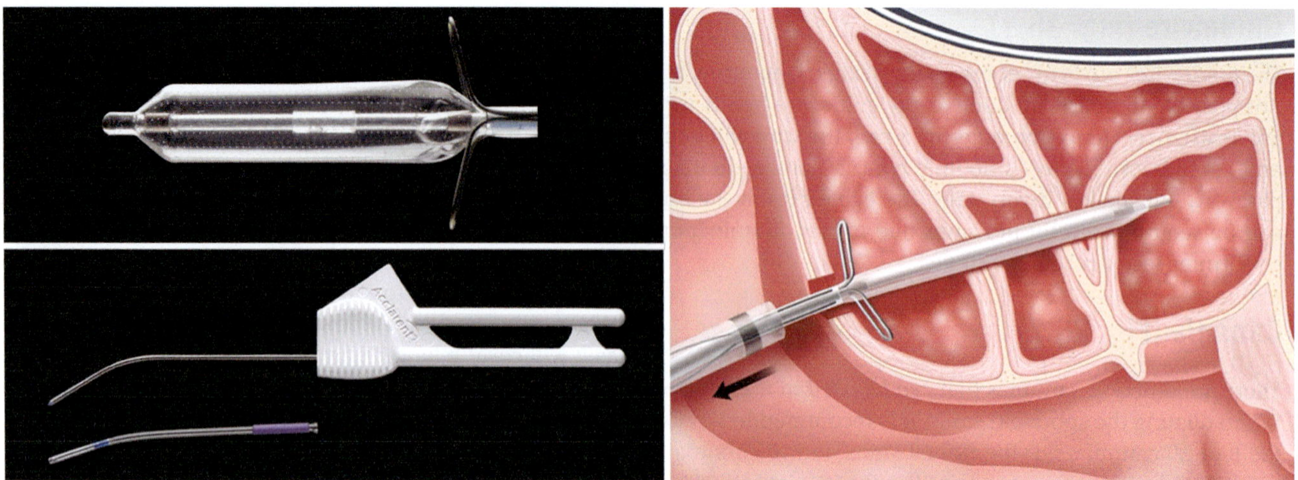

Fig. 26.5: Relieva® stratus

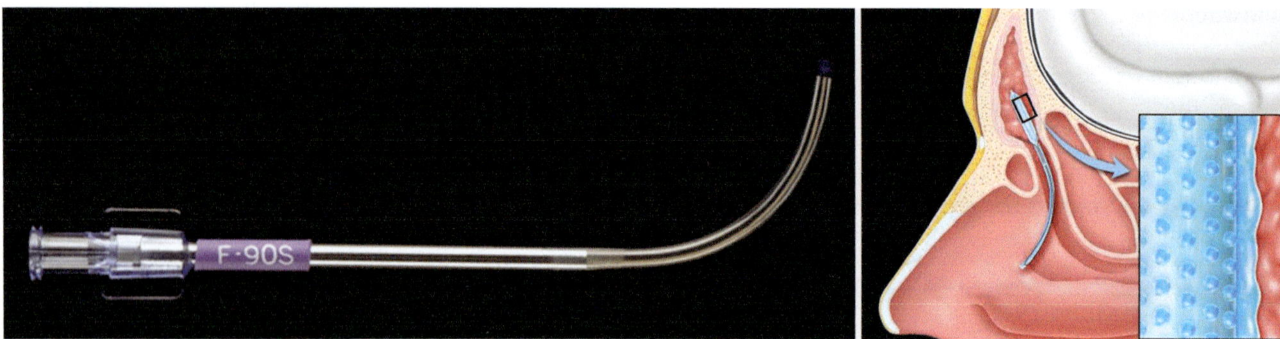

Fig. 26.6: Frontal deployment guide

Frontal Deployment Guide (Fig. 26.6)

Like the ethmoid stratus, the frontal stent can be kept for 6 weeks and is a drug-eluting stent. The difference being, it is introduced after the frontal sinus ostium has been dilated. The wings of the stent will keep it in place until removal.

Vortex (Fig. 26.7)

Vortex is the irrigation device used to clear the sinuses after dilatation. It has openings on the side as well. This ensures that all walls of the sinus get well irrigated. It can also be used to irrigate lateral and distant parts of the sinus that cannot be reached with suction, or as part of a hybrid (BSP + ESS) procedure.

PROCEDURE

CT images should be reviewed in all planes, similar to what one would do for an endoscopic sinus surgery (ESS). The agger nasi cells, uncinate attachment and configuration of the frontal recess should be noted. Supraorbital ethmoid cells, superior and lateral extent of frontal sinus, and presence of any septations should be looked for. Any asymmetries that could prove difficult to get the guidewire into the frontal sinus are also noted. There is no shortcut to knowing anatomy, and it is essential that the surgeon is experienced in conventional ESS and has a thorough understanding of reading scans and drainage pathways.

Balloon Introduction

Before introducing the balloon, the tip of the guide catheter should not be too far from the frontal recess and should be coaxial with it. At the same time, it is important not to bury the guide in the recess. The advancement of the balloon catheter will follow the direction of the frontal sinus guide and not the LUMA™ wire. When resistance is met, the system will buckle from the misaligned forces. It is important to identify potential sinus drainage pathways on the CT scan and openings via endoscopy (if possible). The sinus guide catheter is placed at the frontal recess, and the guidewire is

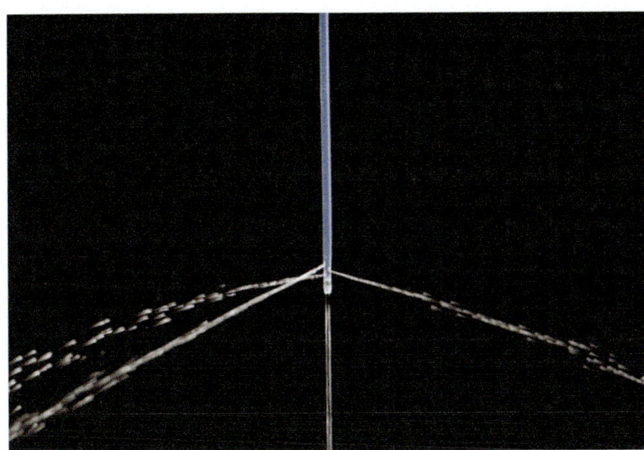

Fig. 26.7: Vortex

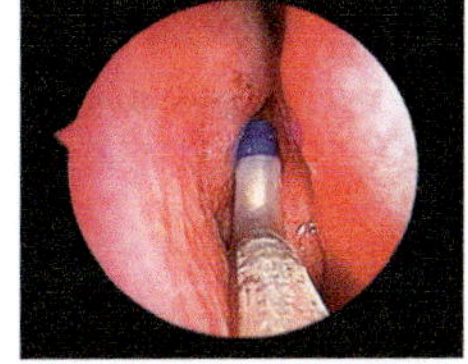

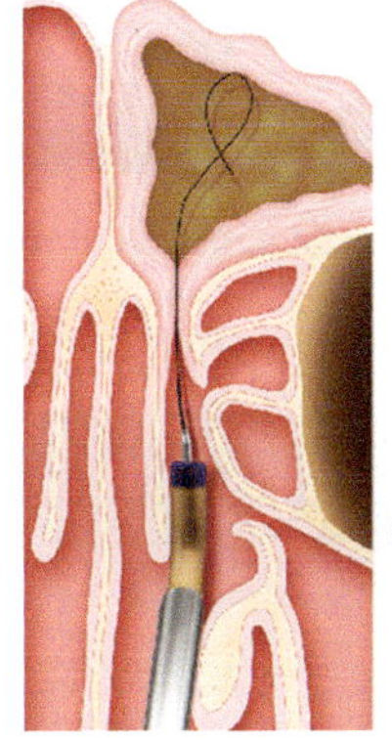

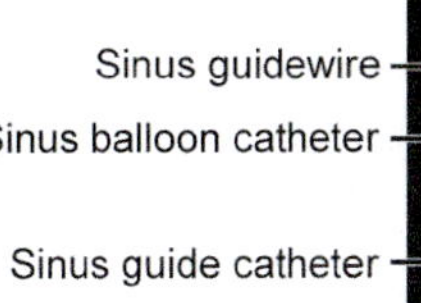

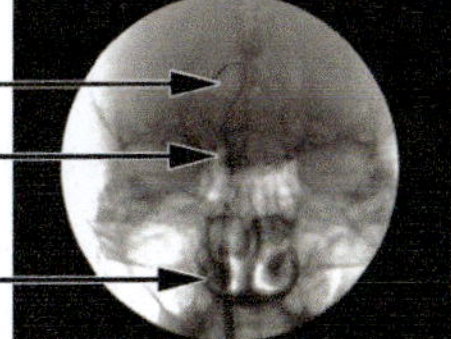

Fig. 26.8: Step 1

advanced in a systematic fashion to probe the infundibular space. The guide catheter is slowly rotated from medial to lateral while advancing the guidewire and the guide is filtered forward or backward to change angle of entry and medial-to-lateral rotation of guide catheter is repeated. It is confirmed that the guide is in the sinus by moving the LUMA, and seeing a light point moving in the sinus, as against a diffuse light. The appropriate balloon is then introduced over the guide and dilated. The dilation is done using the inflation device with saline and not air. Usually, 8–10 atmosphere pressure is enough, but one could go up to 12 atm. The vortex is then used to irrigate the sinus and collect mucus for culture, if required. This is done for the frontal, maxillary and sphenoid sinuses as required.

Hybrid Procedure

Balloon sinuplasty could also be used in conventional ESS as an additional instrument. This is done to facilitate sinus opening when it may be structurally difficult, especially in the frontal sinus. It is also useful when widening of the sinus is difficult because of instrumentation or tear of mucosal damage. Another area, it is useful in is, irrigating the distal areas of the sinus with the vortex, which are otherwise difficult to clear.

Procedure

Step 1: Place the loaded cannula and insert guidewire into the sinus (Fig. 26.8).
Step 2: Inflate the balloon to dilate the sinus (Fig. 26.9).
Step 3: Remove balloon and irrigate, if required (Fig. 26.10).

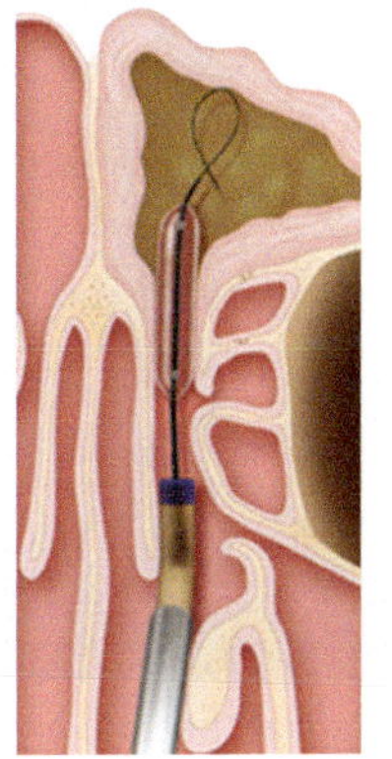

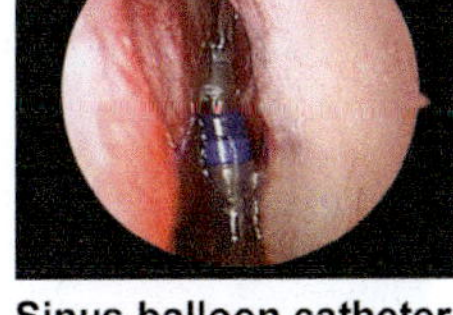

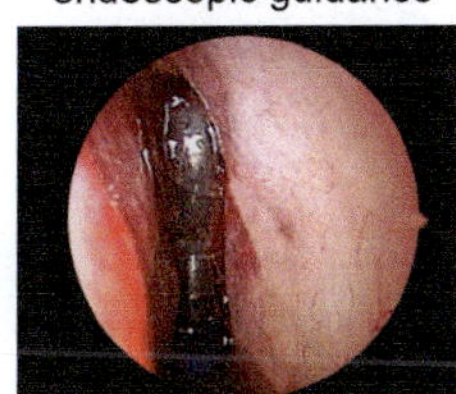

Fig. 26.9: Step 2—endoscopic view

Frontal Sinus

Procedure for the treatment of frontal sinus is shown in Figures 26.11 to 26.15.

Maxillary Sinus

Procedure for the treatment of maxillary sinus is shown in Figures 26.16 to 26.18.

Sphenoid Sinus

Procedure for the treatment of sphenoid sinus is shown in Figures 26.19 to 26.21.

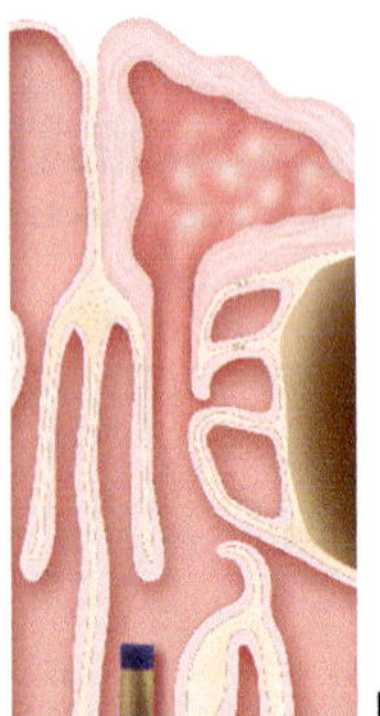

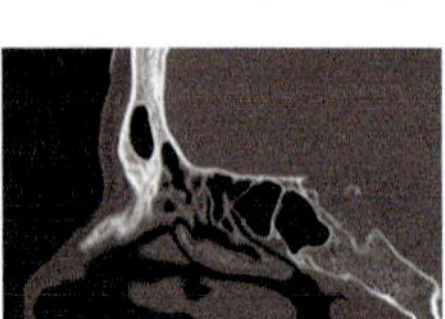

Frontal sinus dilation

Final endoscopic image

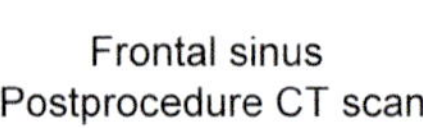

Frontal sinus
Postprocedure CT scan

Fig. 26.10: Step 3

CLINICAL STUDIES FOR SAFETY AND EFFICACY

The clinical evaluation to confirm safety and efficacy of sinuplasty in the paranasal sinuses (CLEAR) study is an international, multicenter, nonrandomized, prospective evaluation for tracking safety and efficacy of the Relieva® BSP system. Data has been published at 6 months, 1 year, and 2 years.

No serious adverse events occurred during the study.

Patient outcomes: Sinonasal outcome test (SNOT-20) scores demonstrated clinically and statistically significant difference from baseline at all time points.

Levine et al. did a multicenter center study across the US involving 1,036 patients from December 1995 to May 1997

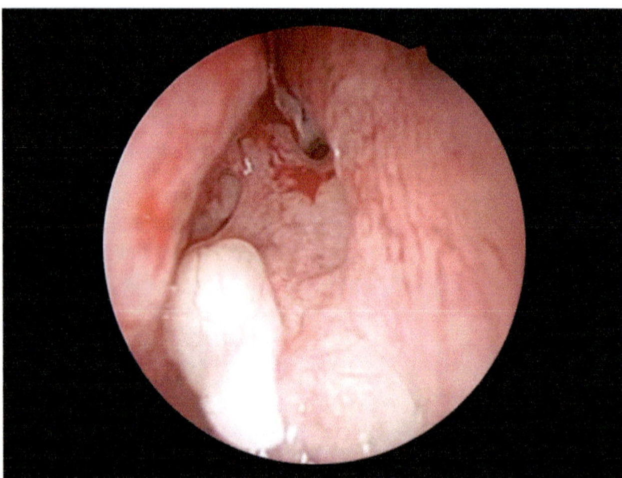

Fig. 26.11: In the left frontal recess, identify potential openings and drainage pathways on endoscopy

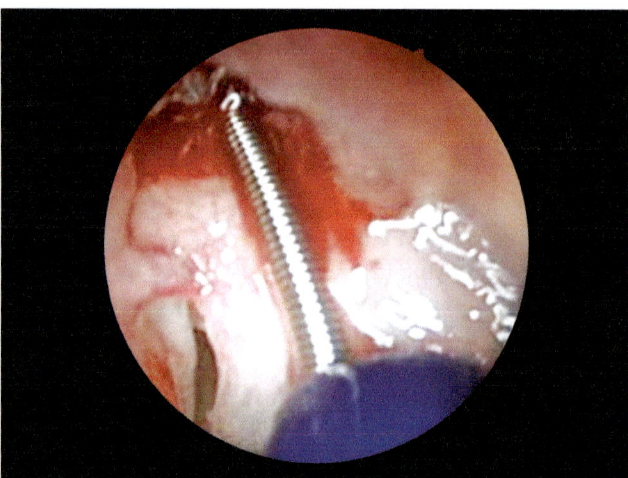

Fig. 26.12: Using the 70° cannula, insert the guidewire into the most likely opening to locate the frontal sinus

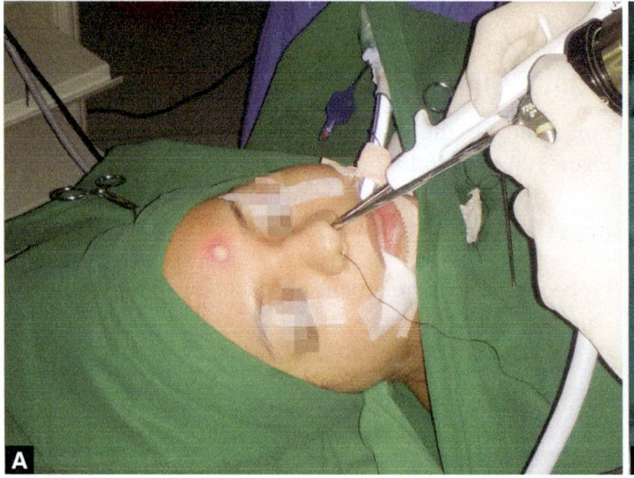

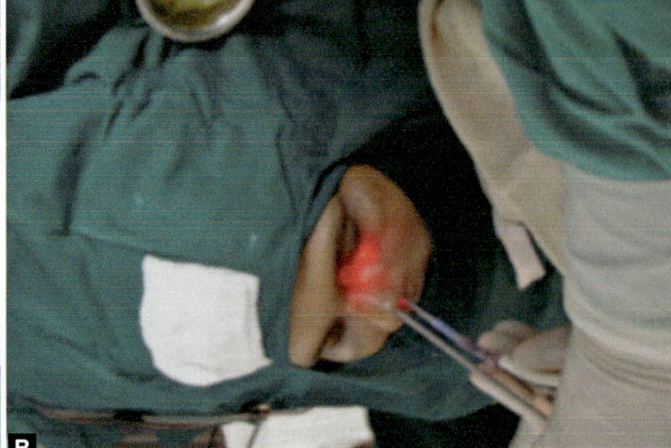

Figs 26.13A and B: Confirm guide in frontal sinus: (A) Pinpoint light in sinus and (B) Diffuse light

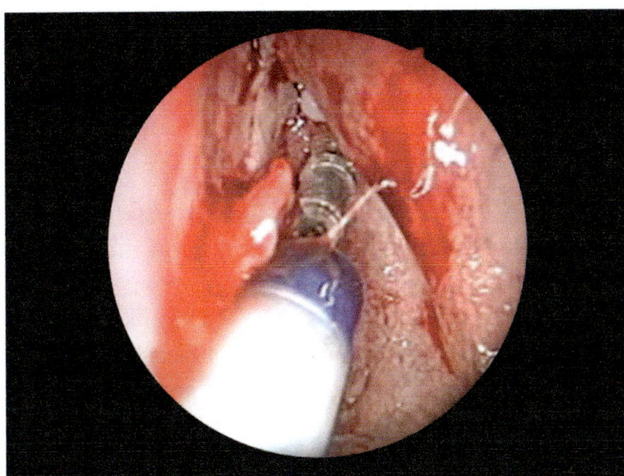

Fig. 26.14: Insert and inflate the appropriate balloon to widen the drainage pathway

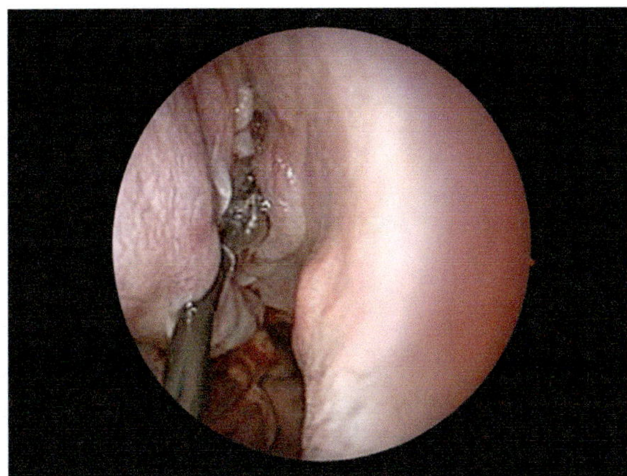

Fig. 26.17: Inflate the balloon after withdrawing the cannula out of the infundibulum to enable vision of the balloon end. The uncinate should move medially to confirm widening of the ostium and infundibulum as against an accidental widening of the posterior fontanelle

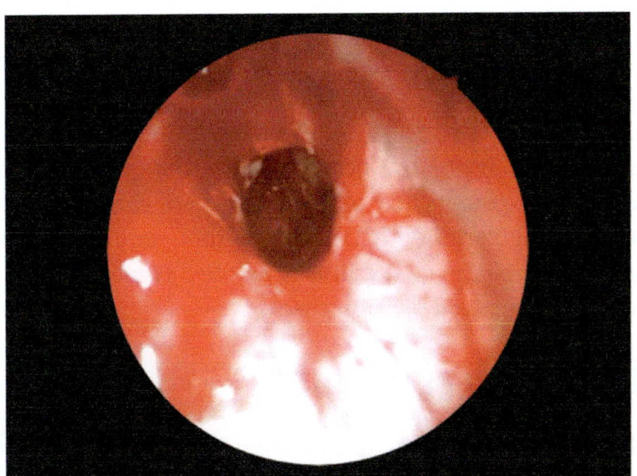

Fig. 26.15: View of widened frontal ostium after removal of balloon

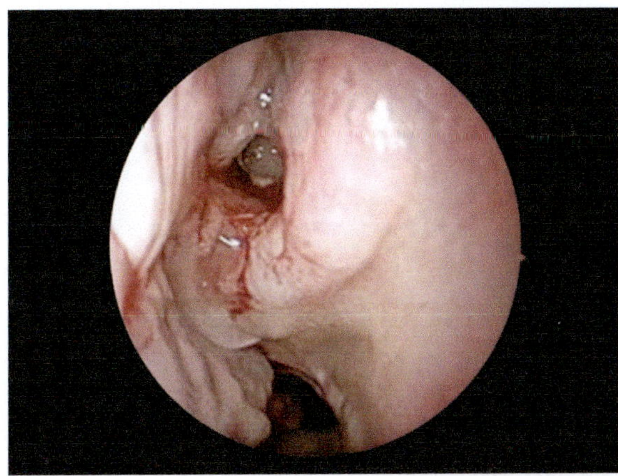

Fig. 26.18: Remove the balloon and irrigate, if required. The ostium may not always be easily visible

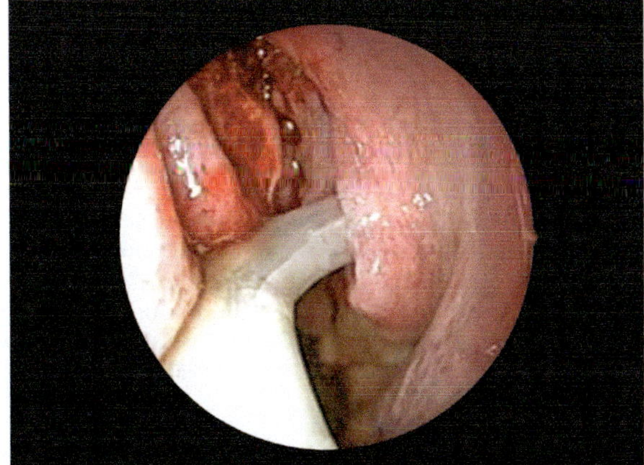

Fig. 26.16: Using the 90° or 110° cannula enter into the left infundibulum and introduce guidewire into maxilla to see the light probe in the sinus

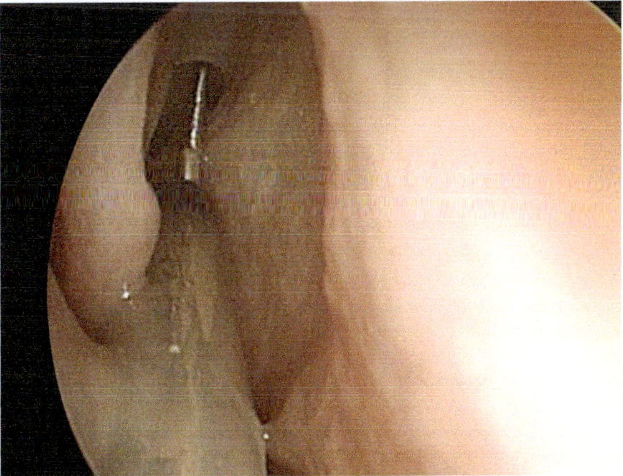

Fig. 26.19: Probing the right sphenoethmoidal recess about 1.5 cm above the choanal arch until the guidewire easily slips in. Fluoroscopy may be used to confirm the position of guide in sphenoid, if required. Usually this is not necessary

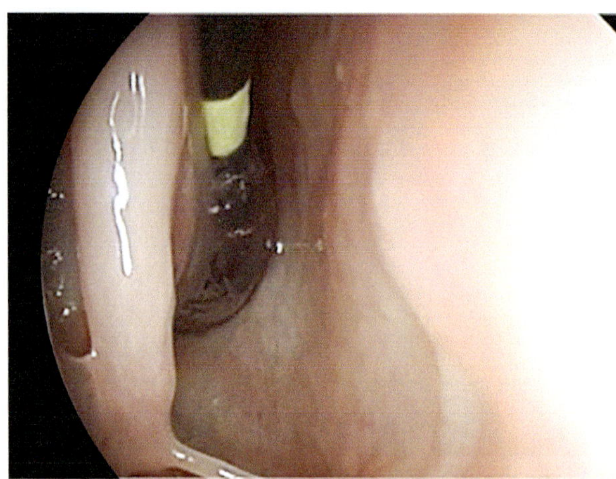

Fig. 26.20: Inflating the balloon to dilate the sinus opening

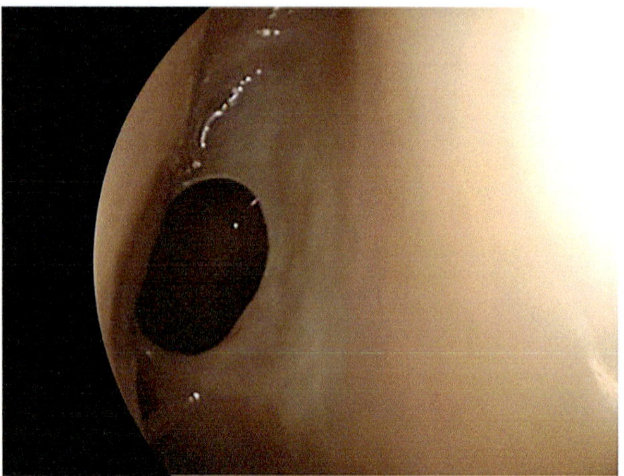

Fig. 26.21: Balloon removed to show the widened sphenoid ostium

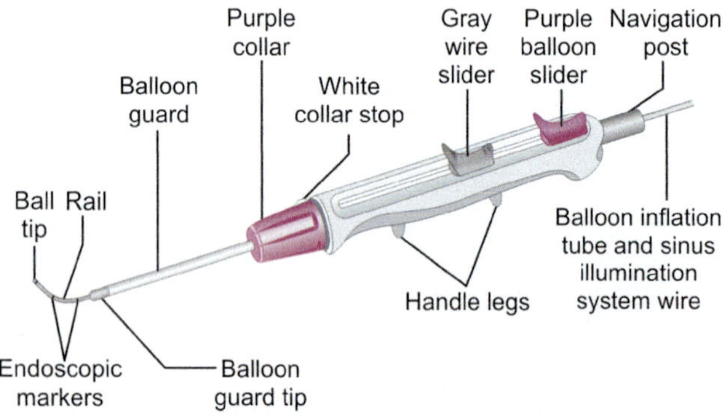

Fig. 26.22: SCOUT™ sinus dilation system

that demonstrated 95.2% symptom improvement at 40 weeks with no serious adverse events.

RECENT ADVANCES

The Relieva® spin comes as a preloaded system with control for the guidewire and balloon insertion on the hand device itself.

The latest is the SCOUT™ sinus dilation system which is for the frontal sinus and comes with a firm frontal seeker in front of the spin system. This allows for probing of the frontal sinus and then insertion of guidewire and balloon over the seeker (Fig. 26.22).

SUMMARY

Balloon sinuplasty™ technology offers a novel, endoscopic catheter-based approach, which is minimally invasive, safe and effective. There is reduced bleeding, shorter recovery time and better patient compliance. It does not limit treatment options and could be done along with conventional FESS. Balloon sinuplasty provides a valuable training and learning tool, especially for the frontal sinus. It efficacy and safety is clinically established and is of further value in patients on anticoagulants or ICU patients that require minimally invasive sinus directed culture samples. Finally, it may also be used in selected revision cases.

ACKNOWLEDGMENTS

My thanks to Acclarent and Johnson & Johnson for providing some of the images and material.

I am grateful to Dr Jordan Pritikin (MD) from the Chicago Nasal and Sinus Center, who has been kind to share his material and experience.

BIBLIOGRAPHY

1. Bolger WE, Brown CL, Church CA, et al. Otolaryngol Head Neck Surg. 2007;137:10-20.
2. Kuhn FA, Church CA, Goldberg AN, et al. Otolaryngol Head Neck Surg. 2008;139:S27-37.
3. Levine HL, Sertich AP, Hoisington DR, et al. A multi-center registry of balloon catheter sinusotomy outcomes for 1036 patients. Ann Otol Rhinol Laryngol. 2008;117:263-70.
4. Weiss RL, Church CA, Kuhn FA, et al. Long-term outcome analysis of balloon catheter sinusotomy: two-year follow-up. Otolaryngol Head Neck Surg. 2008;139:S38-46.

CHAPTER 27

Pediatric Endoscopic Sinus Surgery

Hetal Marfatia Patel

INTRODUCTION

Professor Messerklinger's work on sinus mucosa and ciliary movement has changed the whole concept of treatment of paranasal sinus (PNS) inflammation.[1] This was implemented as better illumination in nasal cavity was possible with the help of nasal endoscope. The term "Functional Endoscopic Sinus Surgery" (FESS) was introduced by Professor David Kennedy.[2] To begin with, it was used to improve drainage and ventilation of paranasal sinuses, mainly for adults. With the result of its applications in the adult population, the same was applied for the pediatric population and development of pediatric telescope and miniaturization of instruments was encouraged.

As far as the pediatric age group is concerned, the main objective is to treat conservatively and avoid surgery. However, there are situations where surgical intervention is inevitable. For example, complications of sinusitis, choanal atresia (CA), meningoencephalocele, foreign body removal, antrochoanal polyp, etc.

In pediatric sinusitis, like any other sinusitis, anterior ethmoid is a reservoir of infection.[2] However, endoscopic sinus surgery for pediatric age group is performed very conservatively.[3] Acute sinusitis with complication is one of the main indications. As far as chronic sinusitis is concerned, surgery is performed only when maximal medical therapy fails and other trigger factors are taken care off.[4,5] Even if the surgery is planned, only minimal intervention is done to retain the normal physiology of sinuses, e.g. in a child with persistent maxillary sinusitis great relief can be obtained by removing just a part of the uncinate process at the junction of the horizontal and vertical portion of the uncinate process. It is done by using the Ostrum's reverse cutting forceps. The Parson's window thus created allows drainage of secretions and ventilation of the maxillary sinus (Figs 27.1 and 27.2).[3]

ANTROCHOANAL POLYP

Another common intervention is antrochoanal polyp. The etiology is not well understood but it is thought to be secondary to inflammation[6], or arises from the intramural

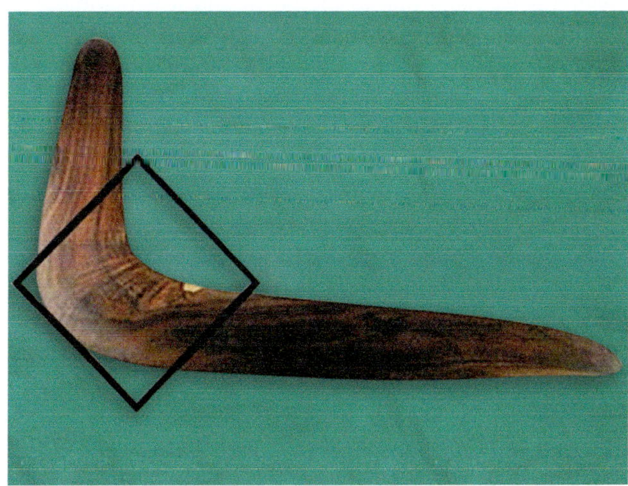

Fig. 27.1: Boomerang showing the site for Parson's window

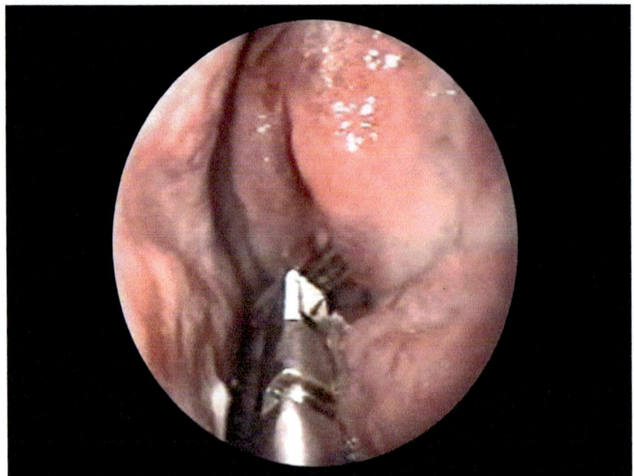

Fig. 27.2: Ostrum's reverse cutting forceps being used at the junction of vertical and horizontal part of uncinate process

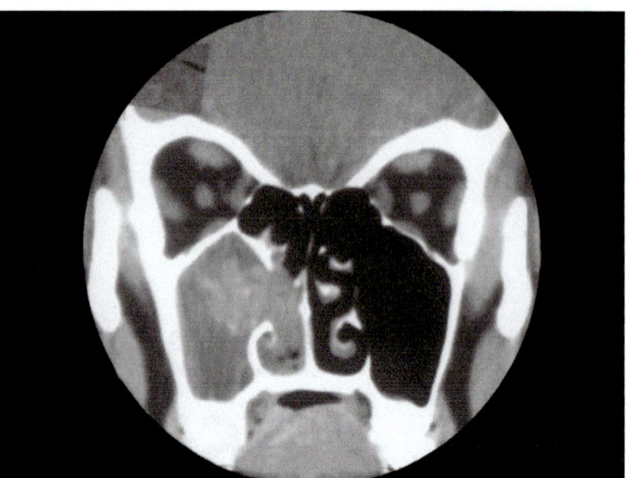

Fig. 27.3: CT scan showing widening of right maxillary ostium due to an antrochoanal polyp

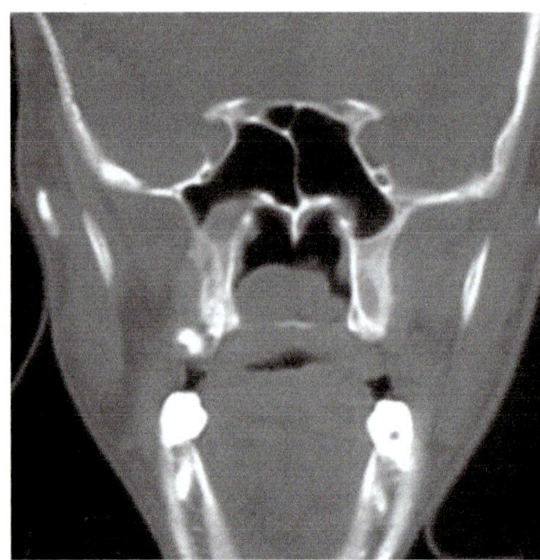

Fig. 27.4: CT scan showing choanal part of antrochoanal polyp

Thornwaldt's cyst in the wall of maxillary sinus.[7] This is usually unilateral. The patient presents with a pearly white mass in the nasal cavity, nasal block, rhinitis, headache and mouth breathing. The nasal obstruction may be unilateral or bilateral depending on the size of nasopharyngeal extension. If there is an oropharyngeal extension, there may be difficulty in swallowing and speech. As the name suggests, it arises from the maxillary antrum and grows backward to reach the choana. This trifoliate polyp has three parts, namely the antral part, the nasal part and the choanal part. The antral part is often cystic arising from the posterior or anterolateral wall (Figs 27.3 and 27.4).[8] Computed tomography (CT) scan shows a polyp occupying the maxilla, exiting through the widened ostium and occupying the nasopharynx. After the uncinotomy is done the anterior ethmoids are cleared and the maxillary ostium is widened. This polyp often exits through an accessory ostium in the posterior fontanelle,[9] which is widened due to the polyp and it is mandatory to join this accessory ostium to the natural ostium to prevent recirculation of the mucus. It is necessary to remove the maxillary attachment to prevent recurrence.[10] One may require 45° or 70° telescopes, angled forceps, viz. Heuweiser forceps or even the angled microdebrider blade (Rad 60) to facilitate its complete removal. When the choanal part is huge or there is an oropharyngeal extension, the polyp which is dissected all around is pushed backwards and delivered from the oral cavity. To facilitate its removal, Boyle Davis mouth gag may be used.

ETHMOIDAL POLYPI

Ethmoidal polypi are rare in the pediatric age group. They may be associated with chronic rhinosinusitis, which may be eosinophil dominated, or non-eosinophil dominated. More likely this polyposis may be associated with ciliary dysfunction, cystic fibrosis and asthma.[10] These polyps are difficult to treat and preventing their recurrence may also be difficult. Due to ciliary dysfunction their clearance must be combined with inferior meatal antrostomy for drainage purpose.

MENINGOCELE

At times, one sees a polypoidal lesion medial to the middle turbinate, arising from the roof. This should not be mistaken for a mass and biopsied, but a possibility of a meningocele should be kept in mind.[11] These patients often present with nasal block and recurrent attacks of meningitis. High resolution CT scan of PNS shows the defect in the cribriform area, and MRI will confirm the diagnosis of meningoencephalocele (Figs 27.5 and 27.6). Here, the base is cauterized with the help of a

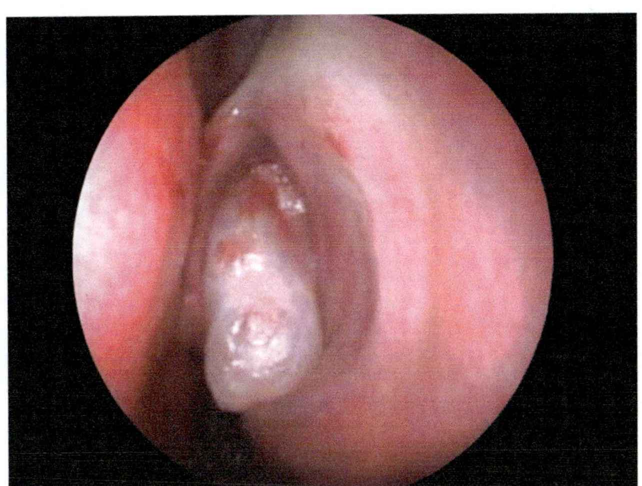

Fig. 27.5: Meningocele in left middle meatus

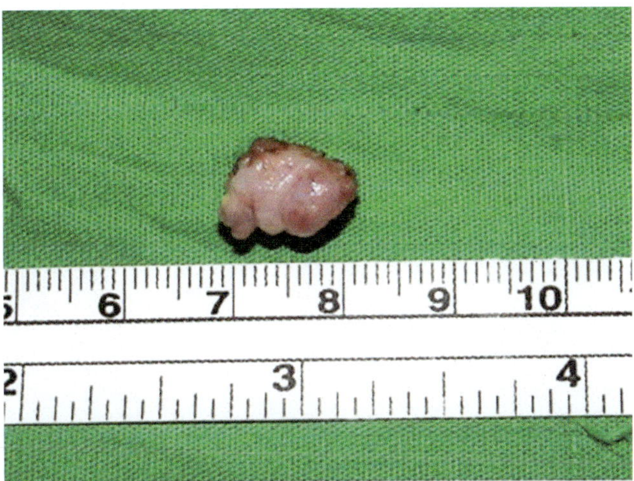

Fig. 27.6: Excised specimen of meningocele

bipolar cautery. The prolapsed encephalocele is excised and a surrounding raw area is created for the graft to be placed. If there is an active cerebrospinal fluid leak a bath plug[12] may be used. Larger defects may be reinforced using a piece of septal cartilage harvested endoscopically from the opposite nostril. The area of the defect is covered using fascia lata graft, which is kept in place using tissue glue. The area is covered with gelatin sponge and a piece of polyvinyl oxycellulose is used as a tamponade.

DEVIATED NASAL SEPTUM

In pediatric patients, correction of deviated nasal septum (DNS) is avoided as far as possible. In case of marked DNS with severe obstruction limited septoplasty may be done with preservation of bone, as further growth need not be affected.[13]

CONGENITAL DACRYOCYSTOCELE

Congenital nasolacrimal drainage system impatency is relatively common, occurring in approximately 20% of children within the first year of life. Most of them are treated conservatively by massage and hot fomentation. Figure 27.7 shows a left congenital dacryocele, which recovered on conservative treatment. If no recovery is seen, lacrimal probe or forced syringing may be required. Dacryocystocele is thought to result from obstruction at both, the proximal Rosenmüller's valve and distal Hasner's valve. If it gets infected, then emergency endoscopic dacryocystorhinostomy may be required to prevent fistula formation.[14] Figure 27.8 is a coronal CT scan showing a right-sided infected congenital dacryocele and endoscopic DCR in such cases may be

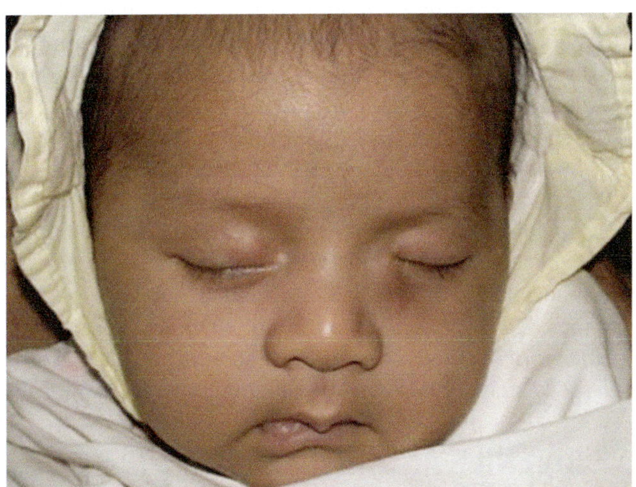

Fig. 27.7: Left congenital dacryocele which recovered on conservative treatment

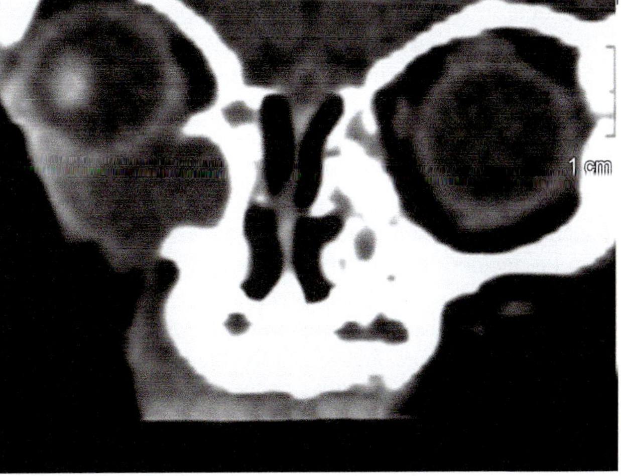

Fig. 27.8: Coronal CT scan showing right infected congenital dacryocele

theoretically easy as the lacrimal bone is very thin. However, the narrow space and presence of inflammation pose a challenge of the same patient. However, challenges are due to narrow space and presence of inflammation. Adequate decongestion is done and 4 mm scope is used for better visualization (Fig. 27.9).[15] This can be used at the cost of miniaturization of instruments by using an otology set.

CHOANAL ATRESIA (CA)

It is a rare congenital condition, incidence being 1 in 5,000. It may be bilateral or unilateral. Bilateral CA presents as an acute emergency as children are obligatory nose breathers. It presents as difficulty in breathing, difficulty in feeding, cynosis, severe hypoxia. It may be associated with other anomalies, e.g. CHARGE (Coloboma, Heart disease, Renal anomalies, Growth retardation, Ear defects).[16] It may be due to persistent buccopharyngeal membrane or incomplete resorption of nasopharyngeal mesoderm. CT scan is performed in both axial and coronal view, to confirm the presence of either bony or membranous atresia, narrowing of the posterior nasal cavity and bony septal deviation (Fig. 27.10). Transnasal endoscopic approach for the repair of CA has gained favor in recent years.[17] LASER may be used to prevent the bleeding while incising the mucosa. Correction of associated posterior septal deviation may also be done to increase the space. Canalization of the CA is done at the expense of the posterior part of the septum, and care is taken to prevent creation of raw areas to minimize granulation.

JUVENILE ANGIOFIBROMA

It is a benign highly vascular tumor occurring exclusively in pediatric or adolescent males.[18] It presents with painless profuse bleeding without any precipitating cause and nasal obstruction. There may be facial dysmorphism depending on the size and extent of the tumor. It classically arises from the sphenopalatine foramen and may be confined to the nose, nasopharynx or can extend along the pterygopalatine fissure to the infratemporal fossa, or can extend to the parasellar region, or to the infraorbital fissure, supraorbital fissure and orbital apex. At times, there can be intracranial extradural extension. Depending upon the size, extent, vascularity, it can be decided whether it can be dealt with endoscopically or not.[19] Preoperative embolization is a must for a better surgical field and to decrease intraoperative bleeding, thereby decreasing mortality. Figure 27.11A CT scan (axial) shows left-sided angiofibroma involving pterygomaxillary fissure and Figure 27.11B shows the same lesion in coronal plane. Figure 27.12 shows the in toto specimen of angiofibroma removed endoscopically.

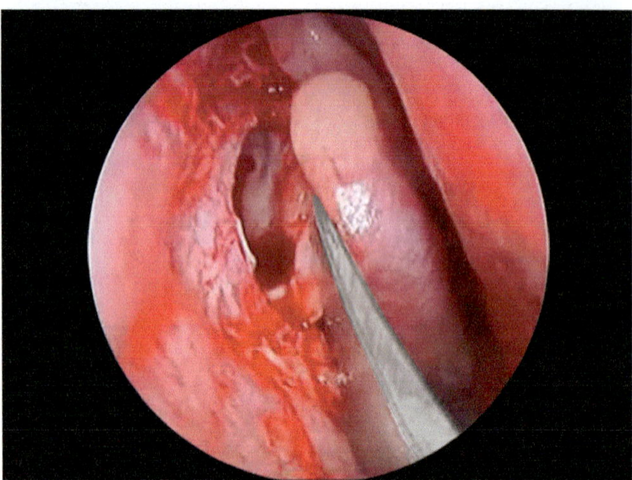

Fig. 27.9: Endoscopic view of an opened lacrimal sac in a 40-day-old child with a right sided dacrocystocele

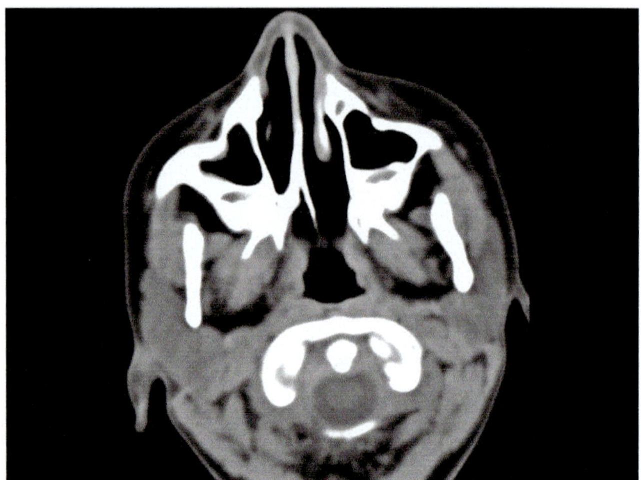

Fig. 27.10: CT scan showing right bony choanal atresia

HEMANGIOMA

It is a benign lesion presenting as recurrent epistaxis and causes nasal obstruction. Usually, it is a capillary hemangioma, which may be sessile or pedunculated attached to the nasal septum. It needs to be removed completely and its base is cauterized.[20]

NASAL GLIOMA

Nasal glioma is a glial hamartoma that is extremely rare. It is a benign developmental abnormality of neurogenic origin, where the glial tissue gets separated from the brain due to abnormal fusion of the nasal and frontal bones. Thus, it is an ectopic neuroglial tissue. Histologically, it has glial cells and

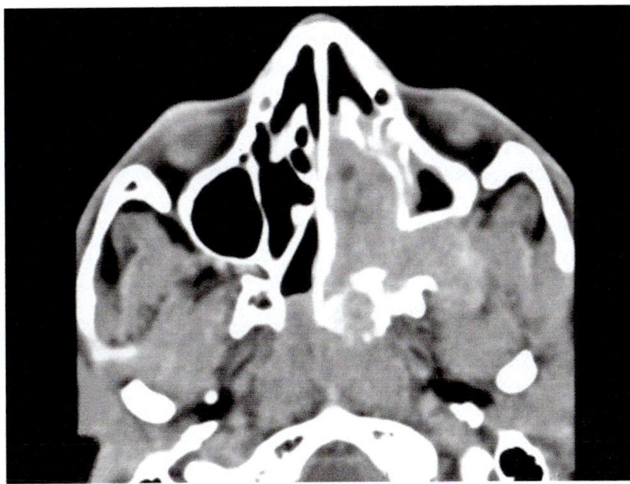

Fig. 27.11A: CT scan (axial) showing left-sided angiofibroma involving pterygomaxillary fissure

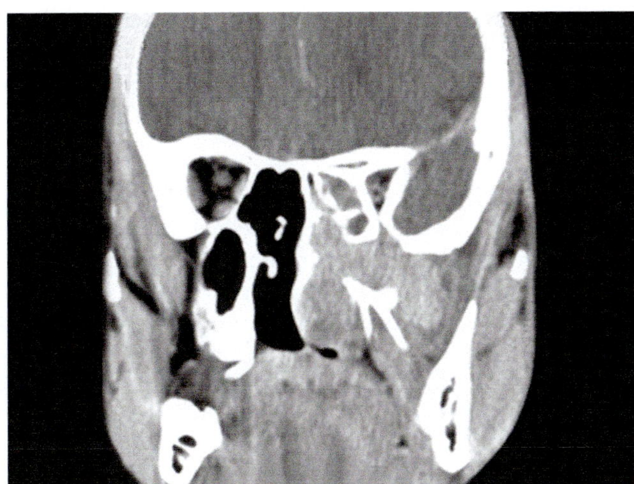

Fig. 27.11B: CT scan (coronal) showing left-sided angiofibroma involving pterygomaxillary fissure

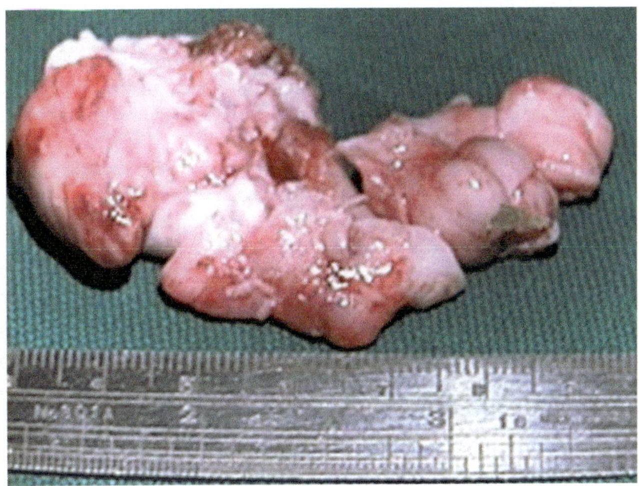

Fig. 27.12: *In toto* specimen of angiofibroma removed endoscopically

connective tissue. It may or may not be connected to the dura. It may be intranasal, or extranasal; where it is covered by the skin. Intranasal glioma can be easily removed endoscopically if there is no dural connection. If there is a dural connection then it is treated similar to a meningoencephalocele.[21]

PREOPERATIVE WORK-UP

Preoperative work-up is similar to that of adults. Preoperative CT PNS is a must, as it serves as a road map during the surgery. Patient must be prepared with antibiotics and decongestants, and in cases of polyposis, even preoperative steroids should be given so that the surgical field is good.

ANESTHESIA

Pediatric endoscopic sinus surgery is always performed under general anesthesia. Adequate meticulous decongestion is performed using 4% lignocaine and adrenaline solution (1:1,00,000), to which 0.5% xylometazoline may be added for better decongestion.

INSTRUMENTS

- 2.7 mm or 4 mm (0°, 45° and 70° scopes) endoscope
- 1–1.5 mm upward and straight forceps
- 1.5–2 mm through cut forceps
- 2.9 mm microdebrider blade
- If the child is very small then otology sickle knife, side knife, crocodile forceps may be used. A malleus head nipper could be used as a punch.

TIPS AND PEARLS

- After meticulous decongestion, 4 mm scope may be used for better visualization and larger field of surgery.
- Uncinotomy must be done using a small reverse cutting forceps and care must be taken not to enter the orbit.
- Care must be taken to prevent any injury to middle turbinate, thereby preventing adhesions.
- To do minimum surgery; if the frontal recess is not involved, do not dissect in that area to prevent iatrogenic disease.
- Pediatric blade with debrider helps in preserving mucosa, decreases instrumentation due to inbuilt suction, provides clearer vision, minimizes surgical time and allows early recovery due to minimal raw area.

- Absorbable nasal packs, such as biodegradable synthetic polyurethane foam may be used to avoid the discomfort during pack removal. Precise atraumatic surgery gives the best results.

CONCLUSION

Endoscopic technique provide excellent visualization and its use can be extended to perform pediatric sinus surgery safely by an experienced surgeon as it demands more delicate and steady hands to perform precise surgery in a narrow space.

REFERENCES

1. Messerklinger W. Endoscopy of the nose. Germany: Urban and Schwarzenberg; 1978.
2. Kennedy DW, Zinreich SJ, Rosenbaum AE, et al. Theory and diagnostic evaluation. Arch Otolaryngol. 1985;111(9):576-82.
3. Parsons DS, Phillips SE. Functional endoscopic surgery in children: a retrospective analysis of results. Laryngoscope. 1993;103(8):899-903.
4. Ramadan HR. Adenoidectomy vs. endoscopic sinus surgery for the treatment of pediatric sinusitis. Arch Otolaryngol Head Neck Surg. 1999;25:1208-11.
5. Rosenfeld RM. Pilot study of outcomes in pediatric rhinosinusitis. Arch Otolaryngol Head Neck Surg. 1995;121:729-36.
6. Kladzien J, Litwin JA, Nowogrodzka-Zagórska M, et al. Morphological and clinical characteristics of antrochoanal polyps: comparison with chronic inflammation-associated polyps of the maxillary sinus. Auris Nasus Larynx. 2001;28(2):137-41.
7. Berg O, Carnfelt C, Silfversward C, et al. Origin of the choanal polyp. Arch Otolaryngol Head Neck Surg. 1988;114(11):1270-1.
8. Lee TJ, Huang SF. Endoscopic sinus surgery for anterochoanal polyps in children. Otolaryngol Head Neck Surg. 2006;135(5):688-92.
9. Frosini P, Picarella G, De Campora E. Antrochoanal polyp: analysis of 200 cases. Acta Otorhinolaryngol Ital. 2009;29(1):21-6.
10. Stammberger H. Surgical treatment of nasal polyps: past, present, and future polyps: past, present, and future. Allergy. 1999; 54(53):7-11.
11. Van Den Abbeele T, Elmaleh M, Herman P, et al. Transnasal endoscopic repair of congenital defects of the skull-base in children. Arch Otolaryngol Head Neck Surg. 1999;125(5):580-4.
12. Wormald PJ, McDonogh M. Bath-plug' technique for the endoscopic management of cerebrospinal fluid leaks. J Laryngol Otol. 1997;111(11):1042-6.
13. Christophel JJ, Gross CW. Pediatric septoplasty. Otolaryngol Clin North Am. 2009;42(2):287-94.
14. MacEwen CJ, Young JDH. Epiphora during the first year of life, Eye. 1991;5:596-600.
15. Berlucchi M, Staurenghi G, Rossi Brunori P, et al. Transnasal endoscopic dacryocystorhinostomy for the treatment of lacrimal pathway stenoses in pediatric patients. Int J Pediatr Otorhinolaryngol. 2003;67(10):1069-74.
16. Demerath T, Krüger M, Meckel S. CHARGE-syndrome: pictorial review of cranial malformations. Rofo. 2013;185(8):683-8.
17. Durmaz A, Tosun F, Yldrm N, et al. Transnasal endoscopic repair of choanal atresia: results of 13 cases and meta-analysis. J Craniofac Surg. 2008;19(5):1270-4.
18. Beham A, Kainz J, Stammberger H, et al. Immunohistochemical and electron microscopical characterization of stromal cells in nasopharyngeal angiofibromas. Eur Arch Otorhinolaryngol. 1997;254(4):196-9.
19. Boghani Z, Husain Q, Kanumuri VV, et al. Juvenile nasopharyngeal angiofibroma: a systematic review and comparison of endoscopic, endoscopic-assisted, and open resection in 1047 cases. Laryngoscope. 2013;123(4):859-69.
20. Hochman M, Mascareno A. Management of nasal hemangiomas. Arch Facial Plast Surg. 2005;7(5):295-300.
21. Bonne NX, Zago S, Hosana G, et al. Endonasal endoscopic approach for removal of intranasal nasal glial heterotopias. Rhinology. 2012;50(2):211-7.

CHAPTER 28

Imaging of Paranasal Sinuses Pathologies

Abhijit A Raut, Prashant S Naphade

INTRODUCTION

Cross-sectional imaging has become integral part of diagnosis and management of sinonasal disease. In the era of endoscopic sinus surgery CT paranasal sinuses (PNS) is used as a road map by the endoscopic sinus surgeons. Magnetic resonance imaging (MRI) enjoys better soft tissue resolution and characterization without radiation. When intracranial and intraorbital spread of the PNS pathology is suspected MRI has an edge over CT. Disadvantages of MRI include limitation in evaluating bony details, long acquisition time and higher cost. In this chapter we will briefly discuss imaging of PNS pathologies.

GENERAL CONSIDERATIONS

CT Scan

CT has a unique capability to differentiate fat, calcification, blood, soft tissue and sinus pneumatization. It provides accurate assessment of bony sinus anatomy, drainage pathways, normal and dangerous variants of PNS.

Modern multidetector CT scanners allow volumetric data acquisition with axial, coronal and sagittal reconstruction of PNS. Plain coronal CT scan of PNS is a gold standard for evaluation of inflammatory sinonasal disease. Axial images demonstrate sphenoethmoid recess and posterior wall of sinuses. Sagittal images show nasofrontal recess and its relation to agger nasi cell.

Osseous erosions are well demonstrated on CT scan. Aggressive erosions are frequent with malignant neoplasms (Fig. 28.1) and invasive fungal diseases. Neoplasms like lymphoma, sarcoma and metastases less commonly show bone erosions. Bony erosions in benign tumors like polyps and inverted papilloma and inflammatory sinonasal disease like allergic fungal sinusitis and mucocele are less aggressive (Fig. 28.2). Skull-base erosion is common in carcinomas, sarcomas, lymphoma, and esthesioneuroblastoma. Bone erosion with sclerosis on CT scan is often seen in chronic

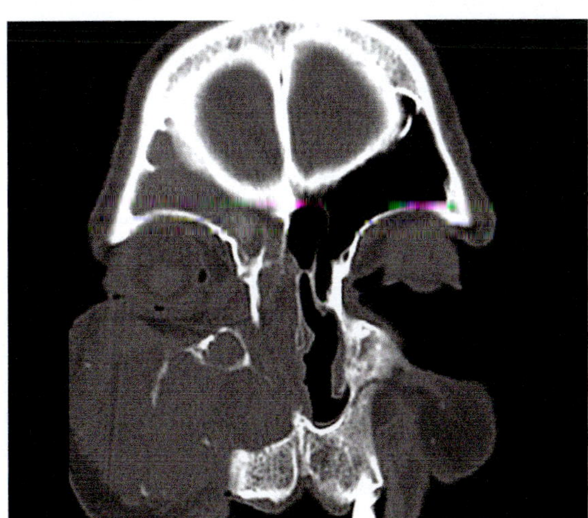

Fig. 28.1: Coronal CT bone window reveals aggressive bone destruction of right maxilla due to malignancy

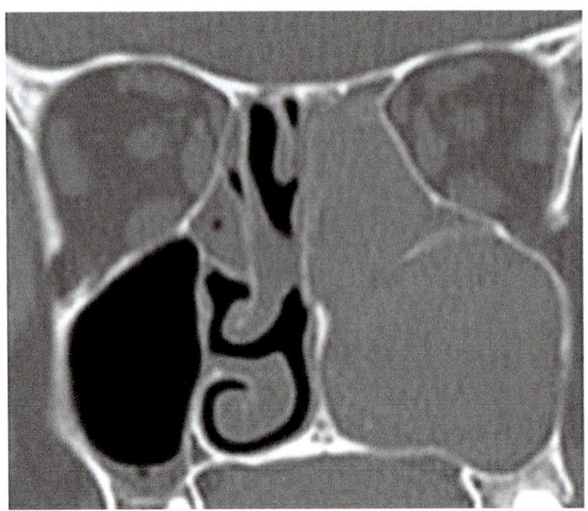

Fig. 28.2: Coronal CT bone window reveals benign bone remodeling of left maxillary and ethmoid sinuses

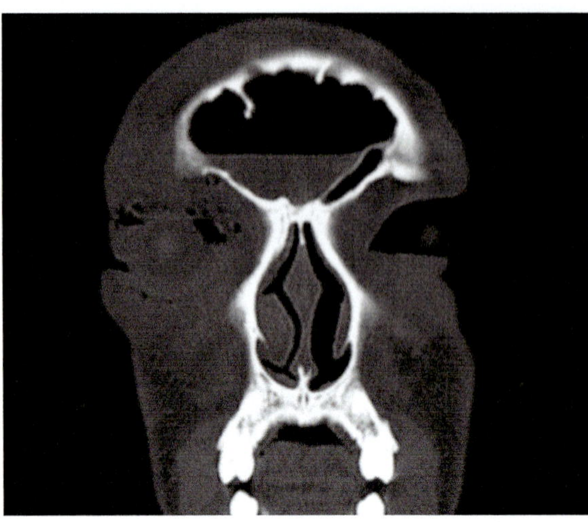

Fig. 28.4: Coronal CT bone window reveals post-traumatic air-fluid level in frontal sinus with entrapped air in right orbital soft tissues

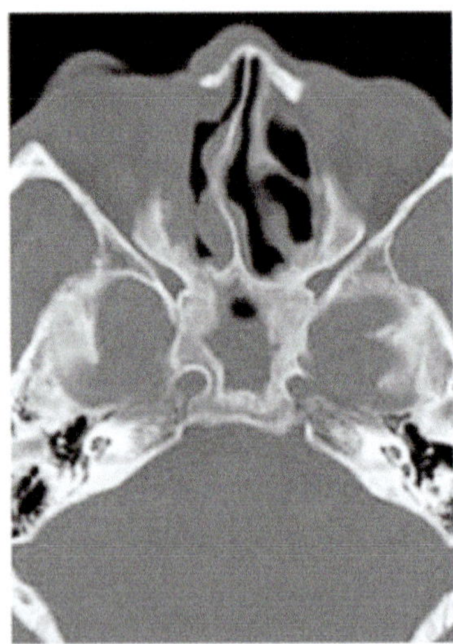

Fig. 28.3: Axial CT bone window reveals thickening and sclerosis of sphenoid sinus wall with mucosal thickening due to chronic sinusitis

osteomyelitis, Wegener's granulomatosis, fungal infections and malignancies superimposed on chronic sinusitis. Sinus wall sclerosis is uncommon among malignancies and commonly seen in chronic sinusitis (Fig. 28.3).

Focal calcification or antrolith in the nasal cavity or maxillary sinus is diagnostic of fungal mycetoma. Antrolith is usually thought to arise from encrustation of either an endogenous (tooth, sequestrum, old blood products) or exogenous (dental material or intrasinus foreign body) nidus. Calcification may be associated with partially or treated lymphoma, metastasis and bone tumors like chondrosarcoma or osteosarcoma.

Air-fluid levels in the maxillary frontal and ethmoid sinuses are seen in acute bacterial sinusitis or due to obstruction of the sinus ostium. An air-fluid level in the sinuses may suggest acute bacterial sinusitis. Sphenoid sinus air-fluid level may be secondary to acute sinusitis or nasal cavity obstruction. In post-traumatic patients air-fluid level may suggest cerebrospinal fluid (CSF) leak or hemosinus (Fig. 28.4).

MRI

MRI enjoys superior contrast resolution and can easily differentiate benign inflammatory sinonasal disease from tumor (Figs 28.5A and B). Sinus secretions have variable appearance on MRI imaging depending upon protein content and duration. As the protein content of the secretions increases they appear as an intermediate to hypointense signal on T2-weighted images. Sinonasal inflammatory disease and secretions appear hyperintense, while tumors appear as an intermediate to hypointense signal. Postcontrast scan shows heterogeneous to solid enhancement of the tumors while inflammatory sinonasal disease shows peripheral enhancement. MRI has an edge over CT when intracranial or intraorbital spread of the disease or marrow invasion is suspected. In adults, normal marrow is hyperintense on T1-weighted images. Marrow invasion by the tumor appears hypointense on T1-weighted images; although bone marrow edema and hematopoietic marrow also may appear hypointense on T1-weighted images. Correlation with T2 and postcontrast images can differentiate these conditions.

Diffusion weighted images are used for better characterization, especially in neoplasm. The apparent diffusion coefficient (ADC) value varies depending upon aggressiveness of neoplasm and cellularity. Thus, ADC values can differentiate malignant tumors from benign conditions. It can be also useful in grading the malignant tumors and assessing the response to the therapy.

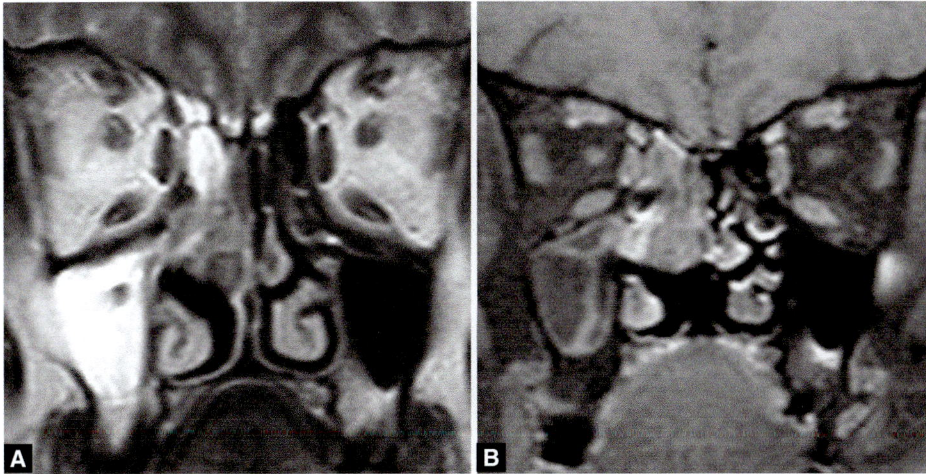

Figs 28.5A and B: Coronal T2 (A) and postcontrast T1 (B) weighted images demonstrate differentiation of tumor and impacted secretions. Tumor appears iso- to hypointense on T2-weighted images with homogeneous postcontrast enhancement. Impacted sinus secretions/benign sinonasal disease appear hyperintense on T2-weighted images with peripheral postcontrast enhancement

PET CT

Positron emission tomography CT (PET CT) has special ability to detect increased glucose metabolism of the malignant cells. Currently [18F] fluorodeoxyglucose (FDG) PET is widely used in the clinical oncology practice. Localization, delineation of tumor border and differentiation of tumor from postoperative changes can be detected with confidence on PET CT. It is helpful in accurate staging, focused treatment and early detection of the recurrence. PET CT is more accurate in nodal staging and can detect unsuspected metastatic deposits elsewhere; however only 10–15% of head and neck malignancies have distinct metastasis at the time of presentation.

FDG PET has suboptimal spatial resolution compared to endoscopy, CT and MRI. Small and superficial lesions and low grade tumors may be missed on PET CT scan. Asymmetric uptake can lead to diagnostic dilemma. Inflammatory/infectious lesions, radiation-induced inflammation and osteoradionecrosis may have increase uptake and may mimic neoplasm.

COMMON PATHOLOGICAL CONDITIONS

Silent Sinus Syndrome

Silent sinus syndrome is spontaneous painless enophthalmos associated with involution of maxillary sinus secondary to infundibular stenosis or occlusion. On imaging, opacification of the sinus is seen with complete occlusion of infundibulum and inward retraction of sinus walls secondary to negative pressure. Downward retraction of the orbital floor into the maxillary sinus results in facial asymmetry.

Acute Sinusitis

Acute sinusitis often accompanies viral or systemic infections and is frequently observed in patients with allergy. Secondary bacterial infection may occur. More severe infections like invasive fungal infections are frequent among diabetic, immunosuppressed and patients with systemic illness.

CT scan often shows air-fluid levels, mucosal thickening, and soft-tissue secretions mixed with air in acute sinusitis (Figs 28.6A and B). These findings are not specific and may be seen in trauma, recent antral lavage, barotrauma, postsurgical procedures, or mucociliary dysfunction secondary to intubation. Intraorbital and intracranial extension of the infection is a usual complication.

Intraorbital extension is seen more often among children and usually spreads by direct extension or through the valveless venous channels between orbit and sinuses. On CT scan inflammatory edema, orbital periostitis, subperiosteal or orbital phlegmon or abscess formation and facial cellulitis may be evident. Cavernous sinus or superior ophthalmic vein thrombosis, meningeal infection and epidural or subdural empyema or collections suggest intracranial extension (Figs 28.7A to C). MRI has an edge over CT in detecting intracranial spread of infection.

Chronic Rhinosinusitis (CRS)

Multiple factors predispose to CRS, which include nasal allergy, ASA (asprin sensetivity, nasal polyps or asthma) syndrome, dental infections, anatomic variants, immunodeficiencies, mucociliary dysfunction and iatrogenic factors (mechanical

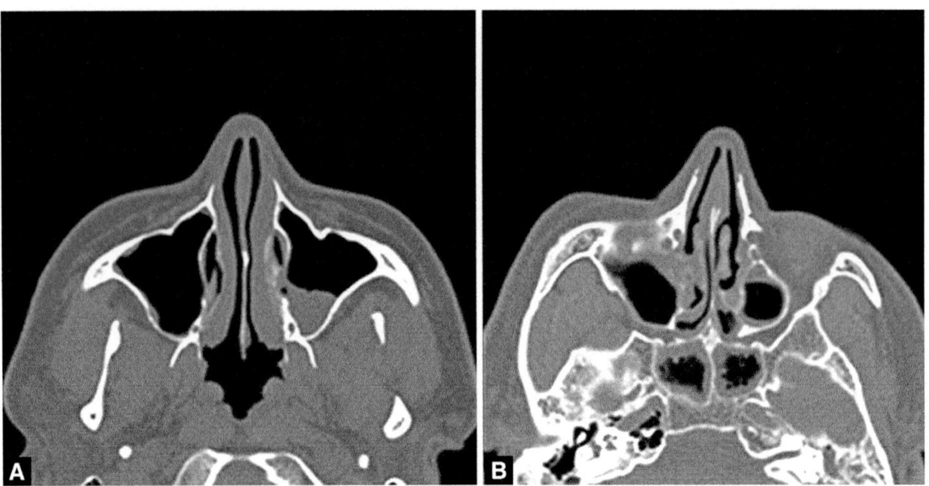

Figs 28.6A and B: Axial CT bone windows reveal fluid level in left maxillary sinus (A) and entrapped air foci in sphenoid sinus secretions (B) suggestive of acute sinusitis

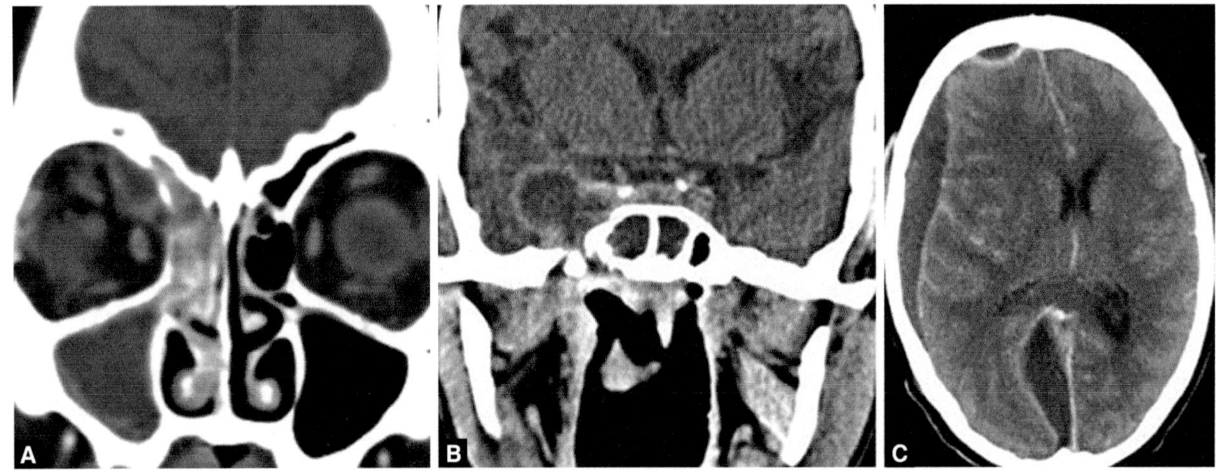

Figs 28.7A to C: Postcontrast coronal and axial CT images reveal complication of acute sinusitis—intraorbital abscess (A), right cavernous sinus thrombosis with intracranial abscess formation (B) and right subdural empyema (C)

ventilation, nasogastric tubes, nasal packing, postoperative scarring in the osteomeatal complex).

Plain CT PNS is the modality of choice for investigation of CRS. Postcontrast evaluation is performed when complications of CRS are suspected. CT provides vital information about mucociliary drainage pathway, predisposing anatomical variants and endoscopic approach.

Depending upon the level of and pattern of obstruction, different patterns of CRS have been described.

Infundibular Pattern

Obstruction at the level of maxillary infundibulum, secondary to mucosal thickenings, or isolated polyps or anatomical variants like infraorbital cells, uncinate process variations or hypoplasia of the maxillary sinus can lead to infundibular pattern of sinusitis. On CT scan, inflammatory changes of maxillary sinus mucosa can be seen with obstruction at the level of infundibulum (Fig. 28.8A).

Ostiomeatal Unit Pattern

Ostiomeatal unit (OMU) is the final pathway of drainage for maxillary, frontal, and anterior ethmoid sinuses. Obstruction at the level of OMU due to mucosal thickening or nasal polyps, or anatomical variations as concha bullosa or marked septal deviation may lead to OMU pattern of sinusitis. Rarely, lesions at the level of lateral nasal wall like inverted papilloma can lead to OMU pattern of sinusitis (Fig. 28.8B).

Sphenoethmoid Recess Pattern

Sphenoethmoid recess drains sphenoid and posterior ethmoid sinuses. Obliteration of this recess by inflammatory mucosal thickening or polyp or bony lesion can lead to sphenoethmoid pattern of sinusitis (Fig. 28.8C).

Nasal Polyposis Pattern

Nasal polyposis arises from the sinus outflow tract from the mucosa investing ostia, clefts, recesses and the uncinate process. They are often bilateral and involve middle meati, ethmoid infundibula and nasal cavity.

Polyposis appears as lobulated soft tissue attenuation lesions filling the sinus cavity on plain CT scan (Figs 28.9A and B). Often it is hyperdense due to trapped inspissated secretions. Bone remodeling may be seen due to pressure erosion. Thinning and displacement of bone structures (such as ethmoid labyrinth and lamina papyracea) or sclerosis of sinus walls may also be seen. Widening of ethmoid infundibulum and truncation of the more distal, bulbous part of the middle turbinate may also be seen. On MRI images polyps appear hyperintense on T2-weighted images and show smooth peripheral enhancement of the mucosa.

Antrochoanal polyp, a variant of sinonasal polyp arises in the maxillary sinus and protrudes in the middle meatus through the maxillary infundibulum or through an accessory ostium reaching the choana (Figs 28.8D and E). The intramaxillary portion of the polyp is typically cystic while the intranasal portion is solid. As the sinochoanal polyps pass through the narrow ostia they are subjected to vascular compromise, which may lead to dilatation and stasis of the vessels. These polyps show brilliant postcontrast enhancement and are often called as angiomatous polyps. Prolonged vascular compromise may lead to necrosis of polyp.

Sporadic Pattern

A wide variety of conditions like isolated sinusitis, retention cyst, mucocele, postsurgical changes are included in this group.

Isolated sinusitis presents as partial or complete obliteration of a sinus cavity secondary to low attenuated thickened mucosa having smooth or lobulated margins without bone changes on CT scan. It is seen in maxillary and sphenoid sinuses. On T2-weighted images the thickened mucosa appears bright and shows thin peripheral enhancement on postcontrast scan.

Retention cysts are commonly seen in the maxillary sinus. They are secondary to obstruction of mucosal or minor salivary glands. On imaging, retention cysts are of fluid attenuation with smooth convex free margin (Fig. 28.8F).

Blockage of sinus ostium results in accumulation of secretions, desquamation, and inflammation within the sinus with mucocele formation. Postoperative mucoceles are due to postsurgical compartmentalization. Expansion of the sinus results in mass effect on the adjacent vital structures with subsequent extension of the mucocele into the orbit, anterior cranial fossa or optic nerve canal. Mucoceles are more common in frontal sinus (60–65%), followed by ethmoid (25%), maxillary (5–10%) sinuses. They are rarely found in sphenoid (2–5%) sinuses. They are often painless and if associated with pain mucopyocele should be suspected. On CT images the sinus is airless and filled with mucoid density secretions. Expansion of the sinus is seen with thinning of the wall (Figs 28.10A and B). Pressure erosion at few places can be seen. The MRI appearance of mucocele varies depending upon the protein content of the secretions. On postcontrast evaluation, peripheral enhancement may be evident.

Aggressive Inflammatory Lesions

Fungal sinusitis is an infection of PNS caused by fungi and classified into noninvasive and invasive forms depending upon mucosa, submucosa and bone involvement.

Non-invasive forms: Fungus ball and allergic fungal rhinosinusitis.

Invasive forms: Acute fulminant rhinosinusitis, chronic invasive fungal rhinosinusitis and granulomatous invasive fungal rhinosinusitis.

Fungal ball or mycetoma: It is a noninvasive chronic fungal rhinosinusitis confined to a single sinus; usually affecting the maxillary sinus. It is common among immunocompetent nonatopic hosts. Remodeling of sinus wall with reactive osteitis and mucosal thickening without bony erosion are common CT features. The mycetoma appears well-defined hyperdense/calcified mass surrounded by hypodense mucosal thickening (Figs 28.11A and B).

Allergic Fungal Rhinosinusitis

Allergic fungal rhinosinusitis (AFS) is a noninvasive fungal infection frequently seen in atopic individuals. Patients present with recurrent sinusitis affecting multiple sinuses. Allphin's diagnostic criteria for diagnosis of allergic fungal rhinosinusitis include: (1) allergic mucin identified at

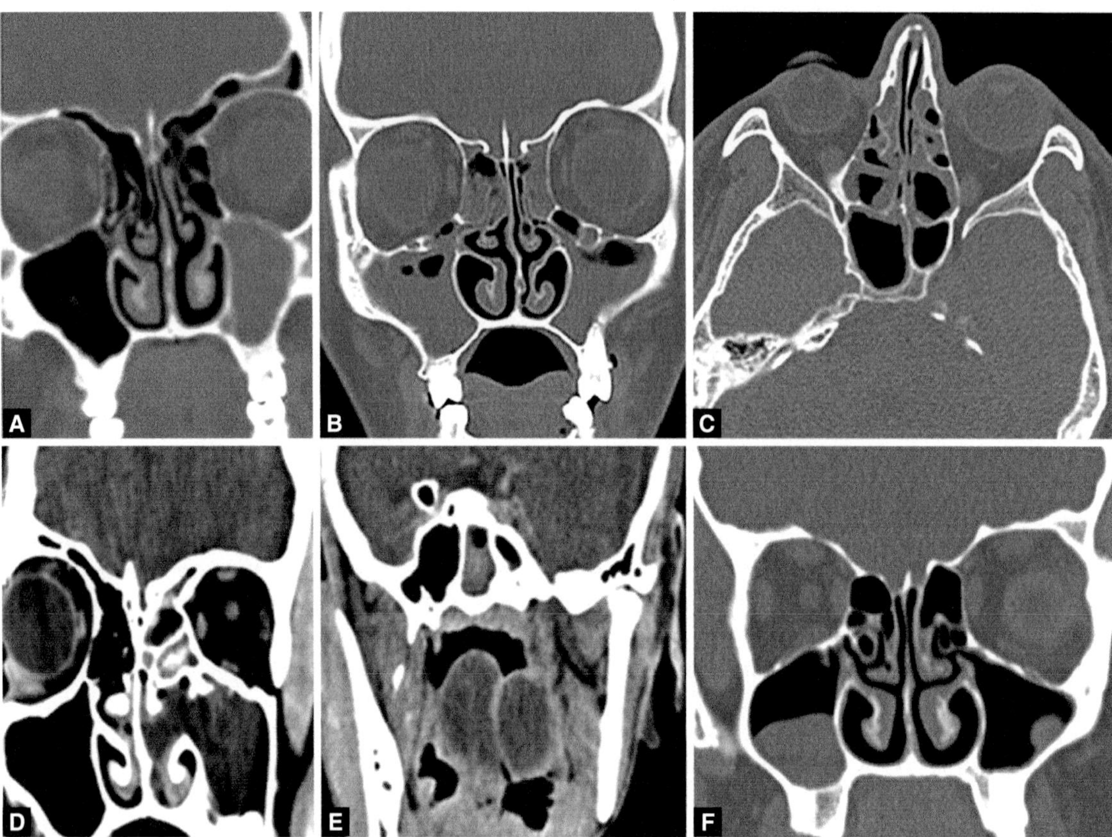

Figs 28.8A to F: Coronal and axial CT bone windows reveal infundibular (A), ostiomeatal (B) and sphenoethmoidal pattern (C) of chronic sinusitis. Coronal CT soft tissue windows reveal hypodense left antrochoanal polyp extending in nasopharynx (D and E). Retention cysts with convex margins are seen in bilateral maxillary sinuses (F)

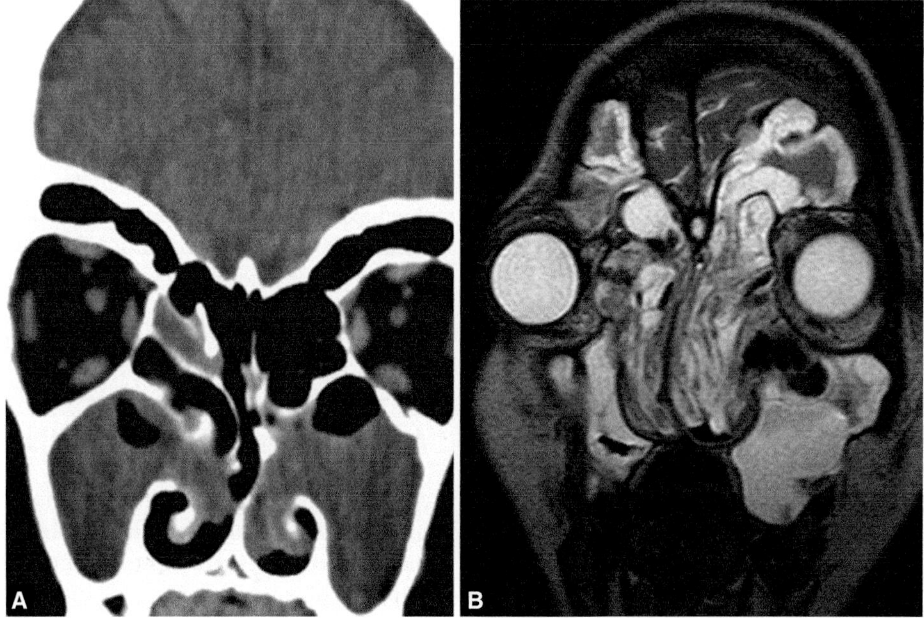

Figs 28.9A and B: Coronal CT soft tissue window (A) reveals hypodense polyposis in bilateral maxillary sinuses with widening of maxillary ostia. Polyposis appears hyperintense on T2-weighted images (B)

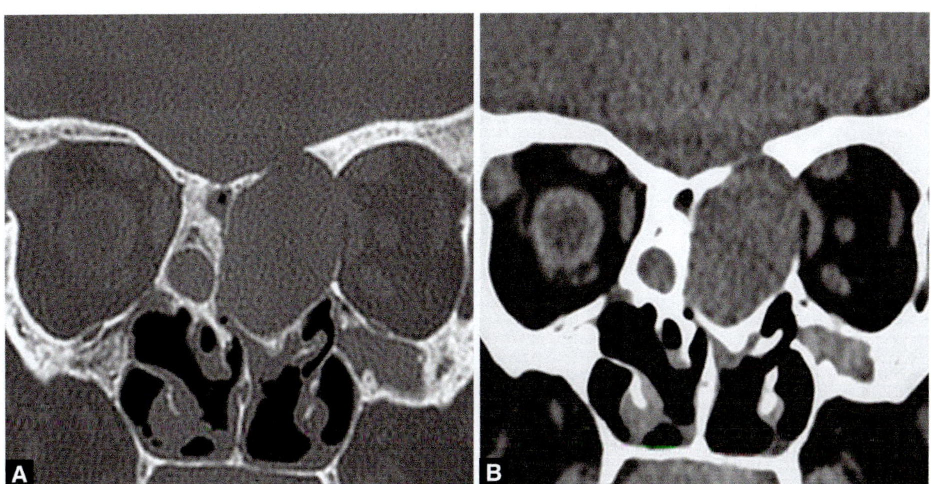

Figs 28.10A and B: Coronal CT bone (A) and soft tissue (B) windows reveal left ethmoidal mucocele with bone remodeling

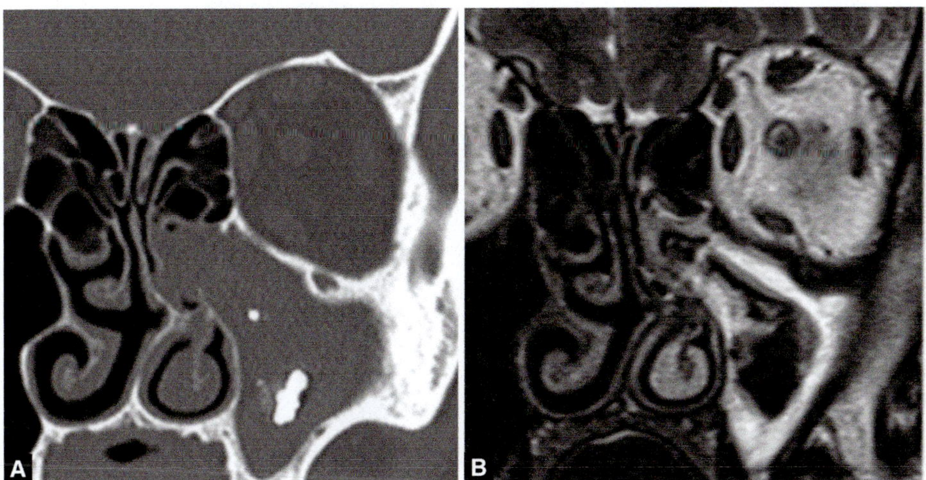

Figs 28.11A and B: Coronal CT bone window (A) and T2-weighted image (B) reveal mucosal thickening with central calcification in left maxillary sinus suggestive of fungal ball. Mucosal thickening appears hyperintense with central areas of T2 hypointensity

endoscopy, (2) fungal hyphae within the mucin, (3) lack of mucosal invasion, (4) characteristic CT findings, and (5) immunocompetence. Fungal hyphae are rich in calcium, iron and manganese. On plain CT scan (Fig. 28.12), fungal elements appear hyperdense. On T1- and T2-weighted MR images, they appear dark. Sometimes calcification may be detected within affected sinuses. Fungal calcification is typically central and has a fine configuration, whereas calcification detected in nonfungal sinusitis is usually peripheral and has an egg-shell configuration. Multiple sinus involvement is a rule with total opacification and expansion of the sinus wall. Remodeling and pressure erosion of the sinus wall may be observed. Mucosa lining is typically preserved. It appears hypodense on plain CT scan and hyperintense on T2-weighted images and shows postcontrast enhancement. If neglected intraorbital and intracranial extension may be seen. Dural and extradural space limits intracranial extension.

Acute Invasive Fungal Sinusitis

Acute invasive fungal sinusitis is a rapidly progressive lethal form of fungal sinusitis, commonly observed among immunocompromised hosts and patients with poorly controlled diabetes mellitus. Among poorly controlled diabetic patients *Zygomycetes* (*Rhizopus, Rhizomucor, Absidia, and Mucor*) are common while among immunocompromised hosts with severe neutropenia (chemotherapy patients, bone marrow and organ transplants, AIDS) *Aspergillus* is more frequent. Usually, the infection begins in the nose and spreads to the PNS.

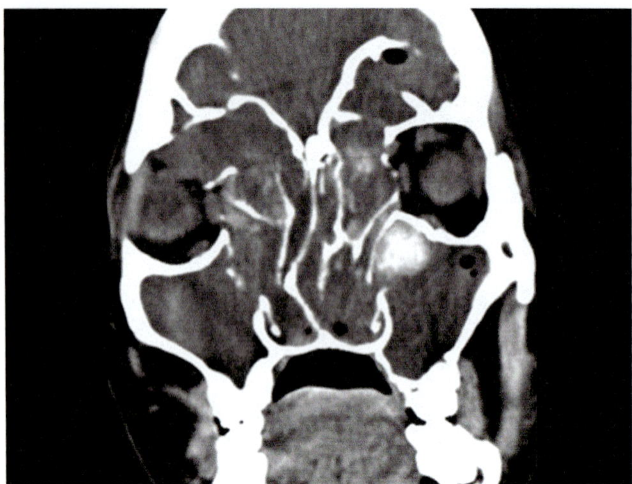

Fig. 28.12: Coronal CT soft tissue reveals panpolyposis with bone remodeling. Patchy hyperdensities are seen in paranasal sinuses suggestive of allergic fungal sinusitis

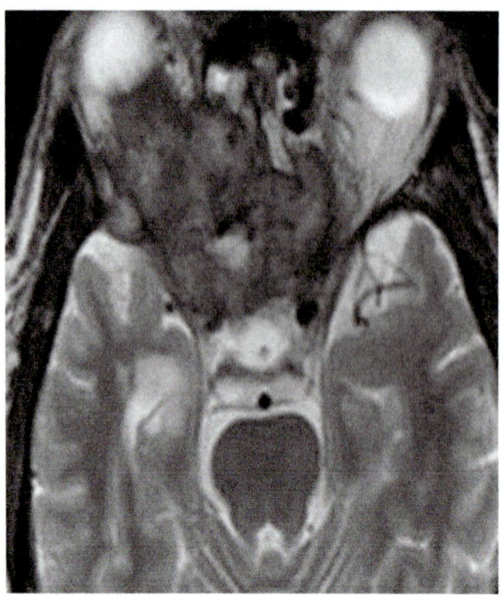

Fig. 28.13: T2 axial image reveals hypointense soft tissue in bilateral ethmoid sinuses with intraorbital and intracranial invasion suggestive of invasive fungal sinusitis

The maxillary, ethmoid or sphenoid sinuses are commonly involved with rare affection of the frontal sinus.

Soft tissues of cheek and adjacent nasal fossa show inflammatory soft tissue thickening. Normal retroantral fat plane along the posterior wall of the maxillary sinus in the infratemporal fossa is replaced by inflammatory soft tissue without obvious destruction of bone. This antral fat pad sign is an early sign detected on CT and MRI imaging. Other findings include nodular mucosal thickening and spotty, aggressive erosion of sinus wall. Unilateral involvement of sinuses is common (Figs 28.13 and 28.14).

The fungal hyphae invade the blood vessels and proliferate in the muscular wall with resultant arteritis, thrombophlebitis, vessel occlusion and subsequent arterial or venous infarction. Intracranial and intra-arterial extension of infection occurs via hematogenous route or direct invasion. Resultant cavernous sinus thrombosis, carotid artery invasion, occlusion, or pseudoaneurysm, subdural or epidural collections, meningitis and cerebral abscesses can occur.

Chronic Invasive and Granulomatous Invasive Fungal Sinusitis

These are slowly progressive infections of at least 12 weeks duration. Chronic invasive disease is common in immuno-compromised patients and often involves the ethmoid and sphenoid sinuses. Locally invasive fungal mass with occasional vascular involvement may be seen associated with minimal adjacent inflammation. Thus on imaging, they may resemble aggressive masses or neoplasm. Most of the cases present with chronic sinusitis, however, focal neurological or visual symptoms or facial soft tissue swelling may also be presenting

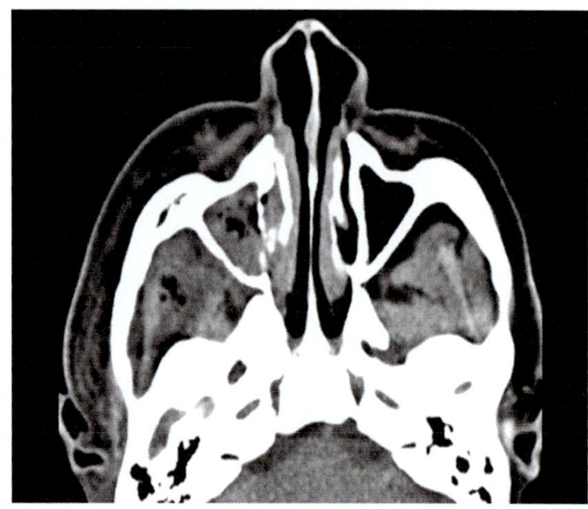

Fig. 28.14: Axial CT soft tissue window reveals hypodense soft tissue in right maxillary sinus with air foci within, spotty erosions of medial wall and positive antral fat pad sign in a proven case of mucormycosis. Inflammatory soft tissue is seen in right infratemporal fossa

symptoms. Plain CT scan shows hyperdense intrasinus mass lesion often associated with osseous erosion. On T2-weighted images the fungal masses show marked T2 shortening, as they are rich in iron, manganese, and magnesium and often associated with calcification and proteinaceous contents.

Granulomatous Disease of Sinonasal Cavities

A variety of granulomatous processes affect sinonasal cavities, which include infective and noninfective processes. Infective granulomatous processes include fungal infection, tuberculoma, actinomyces, nocardia, leprosy, syphilis and rhinosporidiosis. Noninfective varieties include sarcoidosis,

Wegener's granulomatosis, angiitis, and foreign body granulomas, etc.

Wegener's granulomatosis is a chronic necrotizing vasculitis affecting the upper and lower respiratory tract and the kidneys. Patients may present with nasal pain and stuffiness, rhinitis, and perforation or erosion of nasal septum. In early stage, imaging features are nonspecific sinonasal mucosal thickening similar to that found in chronic inflammatory sinonasal disease. In the advanced stage of the disease, extensive soft tissue with bone destruction may be seen. Submucosal granulomas appear hypointense on both T2-weighted and T1-weighted sequences seen in advanced phase and show variable postcontrast enhancement.

Actinomycosis classified as filamentous bacterium rather than a fungus is a commensal organism present around the teeth, especially carious teeth, and in tonsillar crypts. Post-traumatic spread of the infection can be seen. On imaging, soft tissue inflammatory thickening with abscess formation and draining fistulous tracts may be seen.

Rhinosporidium seeberi is endemic to South-East Asian countries. It most commonly affects the conjunctiva and nasal cavity. On imaging well-defined, lobulated, or irregular polypoidal soft tissue lesions are seen arising from the nasal cavity extending into the vestibule anteriorly and through the choana into the nasopharynx posteriorly. Moderate to intense postcontrast enhancement of the lesion is seen.

CT-MRI Cisternography

CSF rhinorrhea occurs when osseous and dural defects coexist and the results in communication of subarachnoid space and nasal cavity. It can be traumatic, nontraumatic (i.e. spontaneous), or postsurgical. Traumatic CSF leak is the most common variety of CSF rhinorrhea. Non-traumatic causes include congenital defects such as meningocele, meningoencephalocele, skull-base malformation, hydro-cephalus, and erosions secondary to skull-base infections or tumors. Patients with CSF rhinorrhea may present with intracranial infections or meningitis. For surgical repair of the CSF leak, precise identification of the location of CSF leak is essential. Various imaging techniques including high resolution CT and MRI of skull-base and CT and MRI cisternography are available for detection of CSF leaks. The most common site for a CSF leak rhinorrhea is at the cribriform plate, followed by anterior ethmoid, posterior ethmoid, sphenoid and frontal sinus.

High-resolution CT images through base skull can detect small osseous defects. With the advent of multidetector CT scanner, the sensitivity and specificity can be as high as 92% and 100% respectively. CSF leak is seen as skull-base bone defect, or an air-fluid level or opacification of the

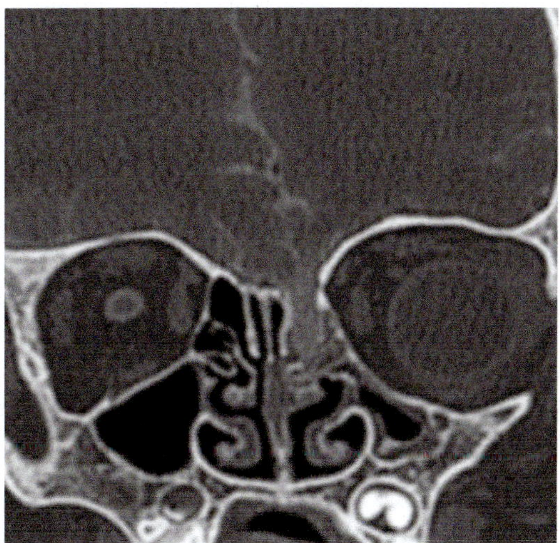

Fig. 28.15: Coronal CT cisternography images reveal osseous defect with resultant CSF leak through roof of ethmoid sinuses

contiguous sinus on HRCT PNS (Fig. 28.15). On plain CT scan, intracranial or skull-base tumor or meningocele and/or meningoencephalocele can be detected. CT PNS provides intraoperative "road map" for endoscopic sinus surgery in repair of CSF leak.

CT cisternography is highly sensitive for active leaks, but is a relatively time consuming and invasive procedure. During active leak sensitivity of CT cisternography is as high as 92% and it falls down to around 40% in intermittent CSF leak. Pre- and post-cisternography CT scans are looked at for skull-base defect and corresponding opacification of sinus or nasal cavity. CT-MRI cisternography is contraindicated in patients with meningitis or elevated intracranial pressure.

Skull-base tumors and cephalocele or meningo-encephalocele are better detected by MRI. High resolution fat saturated T2-weighted images are used to detect fistulous tract, or CSF column. Additional high resolution T1-weighted and FLAIR images may be useful to detect the site of CSF leak more precisely. MRI has limited role in defining osseous details and skull-base fractures.

Sinonasal Tumors

Sinonasal neoplasms are often detected in advanced course of the disease. In addition, associated infections may delay the diagnosis. Cross-sectional imaging plays crucial role in tumor mapping, staging, planning the treatment and in follow-up of these patients. It detects intraorbital and intracranial extent which influences the treatment, and predicts prognosis. Imaging can differentiate infections from neoplasm; although histopathological diagnosis is often difficult on imaging and biopsy gives final diagnosis.

Special Issues

Orbital Invasion

Orbital extension by the malignant neoplasm is associated with bad prognosis. Periorbita is periosteum along the orbital walls, which is continuous with the dura at the superior orbital fissure and the optic canal. When periorbital invasion of tumor occurs, orbital exenteration is indicated. Orbital fat stranding is a strong indicator for orbital invasion; with sensitivity of 40% on MRI and 60% on CT scan. Nodularity at the tumor-periorbita interface, extraocular muscle enlargement, signal abnormality, distortion, or displacement and the integrity of the orbital walls adjacent to tumor can be evaluated with CT and MRI. When thin smooth hypointense signal is detected on T2-weighted images between neoplasm and orbital fat interface, the periorbita is considered preserved. Many times MRI and CT are complementary to each other when orbital invasion is suspected. When the results are equivocal, the surgeons have to depend on the intraoperative findings and intraoperative frozen section histopathology.

Perineural Spread

Perineural spread of the tumor is often associated with adenoid cystic and squamous cell carcinomas. Basal cell carcinoma, mucoepidermoid carcinoma, lymphoma, rhabdomyosarcoma, and desmoplastic melanoma can also show perineural spread. Patients with perineural spread may be asymptomatic or may present with cranial nerve palsy. Pterygopalatine fossa, foramen rotundum and vidian canal must be carefully evaluated to rule out perineural spread. On CT scan, widening or erosion of the affected foramina may be seen. Often fat within these structures is lost, suggesting perineural spread. Postcontrast fat saturated T1-weighted MRI can easily detect enhancing tumor along the course of cranial nerves (Fig. 28.16).

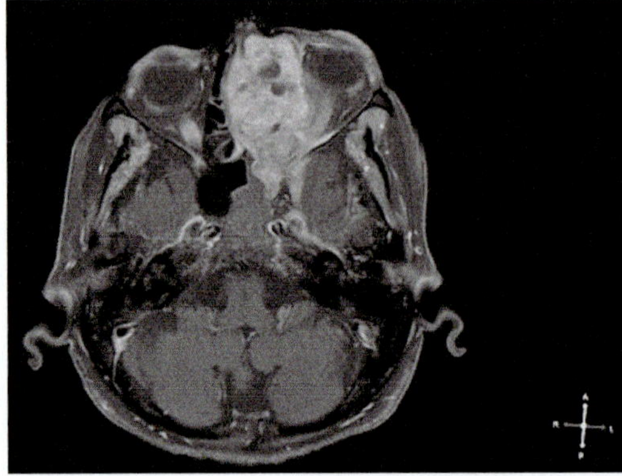

Fig. 28.16: Postcontrast axial T1-weighted image reveals intensely enhancing soft tissue mass in left ethmoid sinus with intraorbital extension and perineural spread along the maxillary nerve in a case of adenoid cystic carcinoma

Lymphatic Spread

Lymphadenopathy is less common in PNS neoplasms and when present, carries a poor prognosis. The posterior nasal cavity, ethmoid, and sphenoid sinus masses drain to the retropharyngeal lymph nodes and subsequently to jugular chain. Maxillary sinus malignancies may metastasize to submandibular lymph nodes.

BENIGN SINONASAL NEOPLASMS

Juvenile Nasopharyngeal Angiofibroma

Juvenile nasopharyngeal angiofibroma (JNAF) is a highly vascular, uncapsulated fibrous tumor. The term "nasopharyngeal" is a misnomer as the tumor actually starts in the nose at the sphenopalatine foramen. It occurs almost exclusively in adolescent males presenting with unilateral nasal obstruction and epistaxis.

On imaging, the epicenter of mass is seen in the posterior nasal cavity at the sphenopalatine foramen with early involvement of pterygopalatine fossa. On CT scan, JNAF appears as a soft tissue density mass with intense postcontrast enhancement causing widening of posterior nasal cavity, sphenopalatine foramen and pterygopalatine fossa. Bowing of posterior wall of maxillary sinus is also seen. Bony remodeling is characteristic of JNAF. On MRI, it appears as intermediate intensity on T1 and hyperintense on T2-weighted images with multiple flow voids within suggestive of vascularity (Figs 28.17 and 28.18).

JNAF can extend in middle cranial fossa via vidian canal and foramen rotundum. It extends into the orbit via inferior orbital fissure. Posteriorly, it extends into the nasopharynx. Extension in the PNS occurs most commonly in sphenoid sinus secondary to erosion of its floor. Maxillary sinus extension can occur due to destruction of its posterior wall. The mass extends into the masticator space via pterygomaxillary fissure.

Cross-sectional imaging plays an important role in the diagnosis of JNAF. JNAF is commonly supplied by branches of external carotid arteries. Additional supply from internal carotid artery branches can be seen in cases with skull-base and intracranial extension. Surgical resection after preoperative embolization is treatment of choice. Radiotherapy is used for residual unresectable tumor.

Schneiderian Papillomas

These tumors arise from Schneiderian mucosa lining the nose and PNS probably secondary to human papilloma virus infection. These tumors reveal male predominance and present with unilateral nasal obstruction, epistaxis and symptoms of secondary sinusitis due to ostiomeatal obstruction.

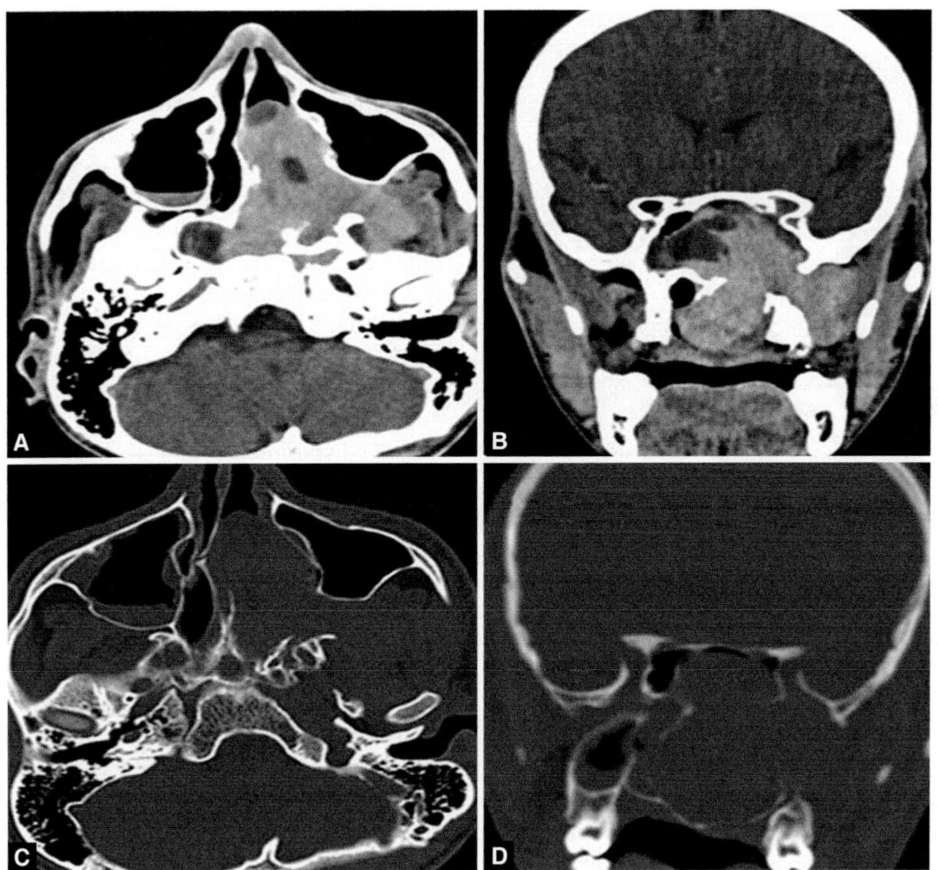

Figs 28.17A to D: Postcontrast soft tissue (A and B) and bone window (C and D) images reveal intensely enhancing soft tissue mass centered at left sphenopalatine foramen with extension in nasal cavity and nasopharynx suggestive of juvenile nasopharyngeal angiofibroma. The mass extends in left pterygopalatine fossa with its resultant widening. The mass extends in left infratemporal fossa through widened infratemporal fossa

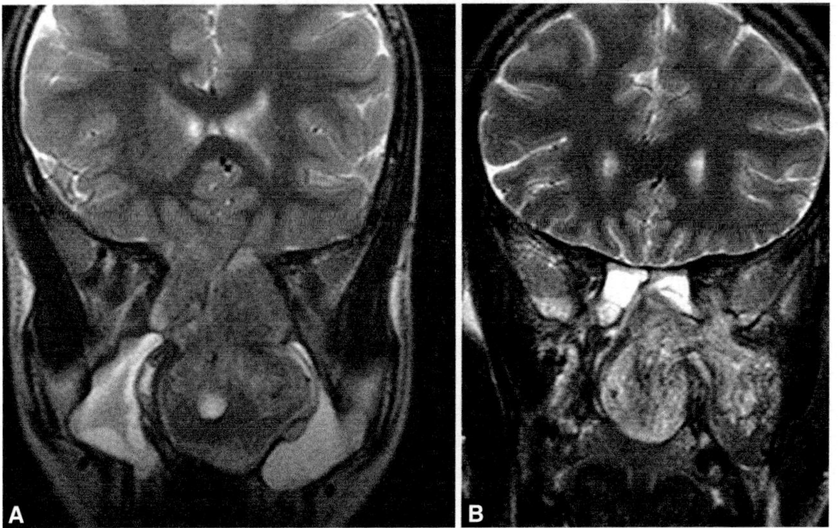

Figs 28.18A and B: Coronal T2-weighted images reveals intermediate to hyperintense juvenile nasopharyngeal angiofibroma with intracranial extradural (A) and masticator space extension (B)

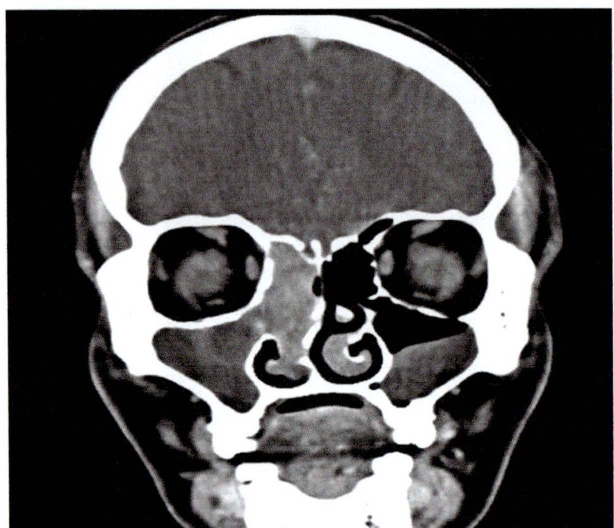

Fig. 28.19: Postcontrast coronal soft tissue CT reveals heterogeneously enhancing mass in right nasal cavity with extension in the right maxillary osteum in a proven case of inverted papilloma. Hypodense nonenhancing secretions are seen in right maxillary sinus due to outlet obstruction

More than 90% tumors are of fungiform and inverted varieties. Fungiform papillomas arise from the nasal septum in young males. Inverted and oncocytic papillomas occur in older males (40 to 70 years) arising classically from the lateral nasal wall near the attachment site of the middle turbinate. Inverted papillomas can extend into the maxillary and ethmoid sinuses secondary to bone remodeling.

On CT scan, they appear as an unilateral soft tissue density mass centered at the lateral nasal wall or nasal septum. These tumors reveal homogeneous or heterogeneous postcontrast enhancement (Fig. 28.19). Extension into adjacent PNS and orbits can occur secondary to bony remodeling. Intratumoral calcifications actually represent residual bone rather than tumoral calcification. Papillomas appear as intermediate intensity on T1, and heterogeneous hyperintense on T2-weighted images with heterogeneous enhancement on postcontrast images. These tumors may demonstrate convoluted cerebriform pattern of alternate hypo and hyperintensities on T2 and postcontrast T1-weighted images. The necrotic areas within the tumor and obstructive sinusitis component do not enhance on postcontrast images.

Complete surgical excision is the treatment of choice. Papillomas are locally aggressive tumors and can recur postoperatively. Five to ten percent patients have associated squamous cell carcinoma (SCC) and possibility of associated SCC should be considered in cases of aggressive bony destruction.

Hemangioma

Capillary hemangiomas are more common in infancy and typically occur in anterior nasal septum. Cavernous hemangiomas occur along the lateral nasal wall in adolescent age group. They usually present with epistaxis and nasal obstruction. Primary involvement of PNS is very rare. Infantile and pregnancy related hemangioma typically regress over time. They present as soft tissue density lesions (usually less than 2 cm) on plain CT in nasal septum/lateral nasal wall without any bone destruction with diffuse (capillary type) or heterogeneous (cavernous type) postcontrast enhancement. Intermediate intensity on T1-weighted images and hyperintensity of T2-weighted images is typically seen. Tiny T1 hyperintense and T2 hypointense foci within the lesion represent hemorrhagic foci. Flow voids can be seen occasionally.

Osteoma

Osteomas are slow growing tumor composed of mature bone and are usually asymptomatic. They commonly occur in PNS and skull vault in adults. Majority of tumors occur in frontal sinus followed by ethmoid, maxillary and sphenoid sinuses. Symptoms can occur secondary to sinus drainage pathway with resultant sinusitis and mucocele formation. On CT scan, osteoma appears as a well-defined high density mass projecting into the sinus lumen with broad base attachment to the sinus wall (Figs 28.20A and B). Pneumocephalus and CSF leak can be seen secondary to erosion of inner wall and dura. Osteoma appears as hypointense mass on both T1 and T2-weighted images and can be confused with air. These tumors do not reveal any postcontrast enhancement and postcontrast scan is reserved for detecting the complication of subdural empyema and abscess formation. MRI is useful for involvement of intracranial structures. Multiple osteomas involving facial bones and calvarium are seen in Gardner's syndrome.

Ossifying Fibroma

Ossifying fibroma is a benign fibro-osseous tumor commonly seen in the mandible and maxilla. It commonly occurs in young adult population with female predominance. Common presenting features include post-obstructive sinusitis and cosmetic deformity. It appears as a well demarcated expansile mass with radiolucent fibrous center and peripheral well defined thick ossified rim (Fig. 28.21). It can appear as an ossified mass with interspersed soft tissue areas. On postcontrast scan, it shows inhomogeneous enhancement. On MRI, fibrous component shows intermediate signal on

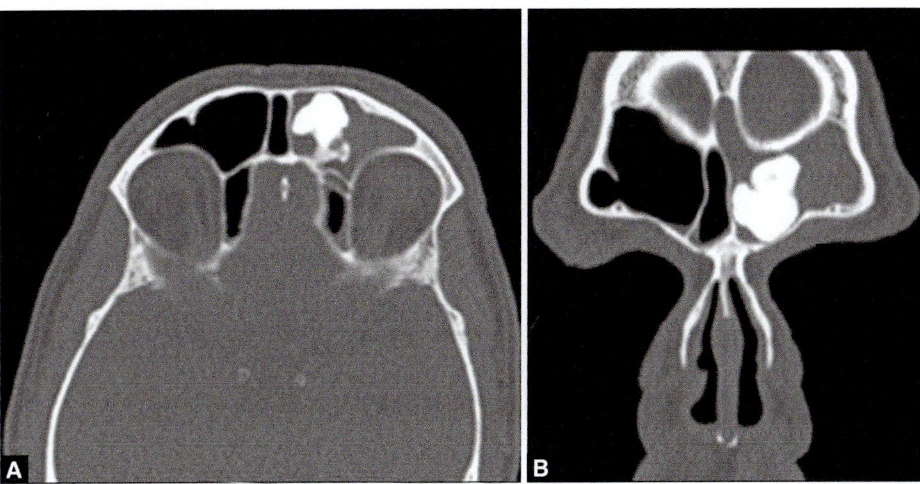

Figs 28.20A and B: Axial (A) and coronal (B) CT bone window images reveal a well-defined hyperdense osteoma in frontal sinus attached by a thin pedicle to posterior wall of left frontal sinus

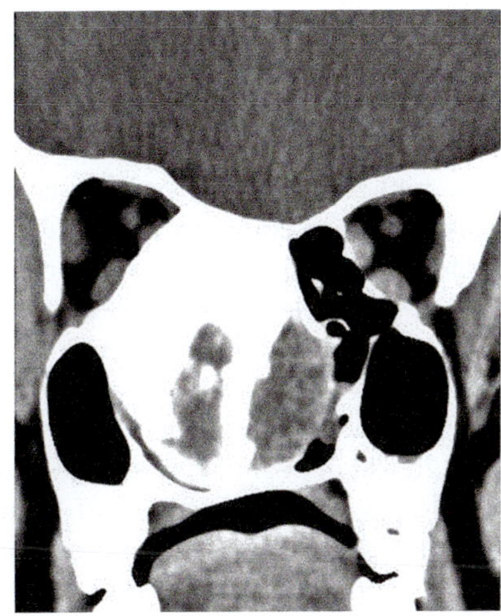

Fig. 28.21: Coronal CT soft tissue window image reveals a large rounded expansile soft tissue mass lesion involving right ethmoid sinus and nasal cavity with thick ossified rim suggestive ossifying fibroma

T1 and hyperintense signal on T2-weighted images. The ossified component appears as low signal intensity on both T1 and T2-weighted images. Surgical excision is treatment in symptomatic cases. Imaging plays an important role in describing the extent of the lesion and mass effect on orbits and intracranial structures.

Fibrous Dysplasia

Fibrous dysplasia is a benign intramedullary fibro-osseous lesion characterized by replacement of normal bone by immature woven bone. It commonly occurs in patients less than 30 years with female predominance. On CT scan, it appears as ill-defined expansion of bone with loss of corticomedullary differentiation and ground glass appearance (Figs 28.22A and B). Cystic areas appear more lucent and represent active lesions. On MRI, it appears heterogeneous with intermediate to low signal on T1 and intermediate to hyperintense signal on T2-weighted images. Postcontrast scan shows heterogeneous enhancement. Thus fibrous dysplasia can be confused with malignant tumors and correlation with CT findings is required to prevent unnecessary biopsies.

Peripheral Nerve Sheath Tumors

Peripheral nerve sheath tumors are uncommon tumors in sinonasal region. They commonly occur in the nasal cavity, maxillary and ethmoid sinuses presenting with a unilateral painless polypoidal mass. These tumors appear as soft tissue density oval lesions on plain CT with homogeneous or heterogeneous postcontrast enhancement depending upon the cystic component (Fig. 28.23). Neurofibroma may contain fatty areas within. These tumors cause bony remodeling without any destruction. Bone destruction should suggest either squamous cell carcinoma or malignant degeneration of neurofibroma. Schwannoma appears as homogeneous T2 hyperintense and T1 intermediate intensity mass with usually homogeneous postcontrast enhancement. Neurofibroma appears as a heterogeneous T2 hyperintense and T1 intermediate intensity mass with usually heterogeneous postcontrast enhancement.

Midline Nasofrontal Masses in Children

During the embryonic development, frontal and nasal bones are separated by fonticulus nasofrontalis. Nasal bones are separated from underlying cartilaginous nasal capsule by

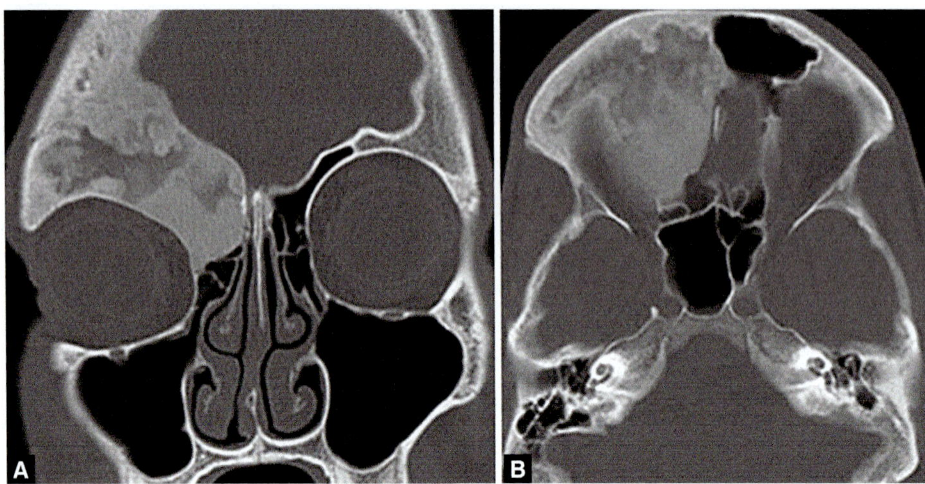

Figs 28.22A and B: Coronal (A) and axial (B) CT bone window images reveal expansion of right frontal bone involving frontal sinus with loss of corticomedullary differentiation and ground-glass appearance suggestive of fibrous dysplasia

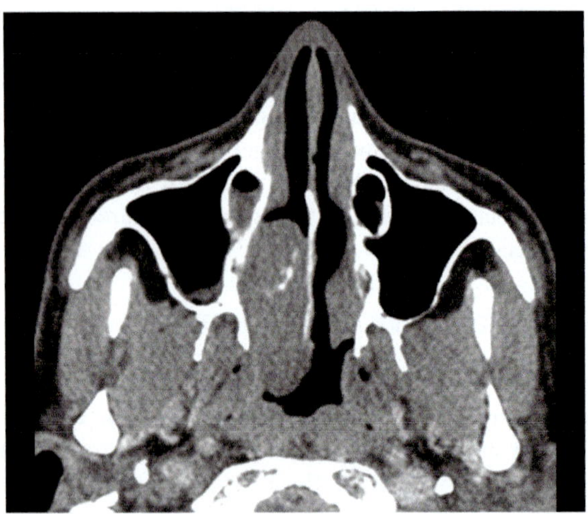

Fig. 28.23: Axial CT soft tissue window image reveals a well-defined intermediate density mass in right nasal cavity with extension in nasopharynx in a proven case of neurofibroma

prenasal space. Dural diverticula project into these spaces and later retract intracranially before the bony fusion. Depending upon the variation in this normal developmental process; nasal dermal sinuses with dermoid/epidermoid cysts, nasal cephalocele and glial heterotopia can occur. Nasal dermal sinus occurs when the dural diverticulum retracts along with the surface ectoderm and can reach up to the falx though the canal in the frontonasal suture or widened foramen cecum. External opening of sinus tract is seen at the glabella or the nose. Epidermoid and/or dermoid cysts can form along the course of dermal sinus tract. Cephalocele forms if the dural diverticulum persists, containing meninges, cerebrospinal fluid and brain parenchyma. Constriction of dura causes the formation of glial heterotopia.

Nasal dermoid and epidermoid cysts appear as midline cystic lesions without any intracranial communication. Dermoid cysts are more common along the bridge of the nose while the epidermoid cysts are common at glabella and nasion junction. Presence of intralesional fat raises the possibility of dermoid cyst while presence of restriction of diffusion on diffusion weighted MR favors epidermoid cyst. Fat appears as hypodense on plain CT scan with average HU of -60 to -120. Fat appears hyperintense on both T1 and T2-weighted images with suppression of signal on T1 fat saturated sequences. Sagittal T2 and postcontrast T1 fat saturated sequences are important in differentiating between nasal cephalocele and glial heterotopia. High resolution thin T2-weighted images can demonstrate the continuity of nasal cephalocele with brain parenchyma. Glial heterotopia is a benign midline nasal mass without any intracranial extension of CSF filled subarachnoid space and reveals heterogeneous postcontrast enhancement. They may be connected to brain parenchyma by glial tissue without any leptomeningeal CSF filled sheath.

MALIGNANT SINONASAL NEOPLASMS

Squamous Cell Carcinoma

Squamous cell carcinoma is an aggressive malignant neoplasm arising from surface epithelium of nose and PNS. It is the most common sinonasal malignancy. More than two-third cases occur in PNS, predominantly involving maxillary and ethmoid sinuses. Primary involvement of frontal and sphenoid sinuses is very rare. Less than one-third cases occur in nasal cavity, common sites being nasal septum and middle turbinate. They commonly present in elderly patients with male predominance. Nasal cavity masses present earlier with symptoms of nasal obstruction and epistaxis. Maxillary sinus carcinoma usually presents late with chronic sinusitis symptoms, facial asymmetry, or with a protruding mass in the nasal or oral cavity.

Classically these tumors present as a soft tissue mass involving the sinonasal region with aggressive bone destruction. Tumors anteroinferior to Ohgren's line (line from medial canthus to angle of mandible on lateral view) have better prognosis as compared to those posterosuperior to it. On CT scan, these appear as soft tissue density masses with homogeneous/heterogeneous postcontrast enhancement and destruction of adjacent bony walls. These tumors appear as intermediate intensity on T1 and intermediate to hyperintense intensity on T2-weighted images. Obstructed secretions appear hyperintense as compared to tumor on T2-weighted images. As compared to other sinonasal tumors, squamous cell carcinomas demonstrate less T2 hyperintensity due to their high cellularity (Figs 28.24 and 28.25).

Imaging plays an important role in detecting the spread of malignancy. Maxillary sinus carcinoma extends anterolaterally to involve the cheek, superiorly to involve the orbit, inferiorly to involve the maxillary alveolar ridge/ hard palate and posteriorly to involve the buccal fat pad and pterygopalatine fossa. Perineural spread of the malignancy occurs along the branches of maxillary nerve with intracranial extension through foramen rotundum (with resultant widening) into the cavernous sinus. Perineural tumor is best detected by T1 fat saturated postcontrast sequence. Complete surgical excision followed by radiotherapy is the usual treatment.

TNM Staging of Sinonasal Carcinomas

Maxillary sinus carcinoma: T1-Tumor limited to maxillary sinus mucosa without erosion or destruction of bone. *T2*-Tumor causing bone erosion or destruction including involvement of hard palate and/or middle nasal meatus. *T3*-Tumor invasion any of the following: bony posterior wall of maxillary sinus, subcutaneous tissues, medial wall/floor of orbit, pterygopalatine fossa, or ethmoid sinuses. *T4a*-Tumor invasion of anterior orbital contents, skin of cheek, pterygoid plates, infratemporal fossa, cribriform plate or sphenoid/ frontal sinus. *T4b*-Tumor invasion of orbital apex, dura, brain, middle cranial fossa, cranial nerves other than maxillary division of trigeminal nerve (V2), nasopharynx or clivus.

Nasal Cavity and Ethmoid Sinus Carcinoma

T1-Tumor limited to any one subsite, with or without bony invasion. *T2*-Tumor invading two subsites in a single region or extending to involve an adjacent region within the nasoethmoidal complex, with or without bony invasion. *T3*-Tumor invasion of medial wall/floor of the orbit, maxillary sinus, palate, or cribriform plate. *T4a*-Tumor invasion of anterior orbital contents, skin of nose or cheek, minimal extension to anterior cranial fossa, pterygoid plates or sphenoid/frontal sinus. *T4b*-Tumor invasion of orbital apex, dura, brain, middle cranial fossa, cranial nerves other than (V2), nasopharynx or clivus.

Metastatic Regional Lymph Node Staging

Single ipsilateral lymph node less than or equal to 3 cm is N1. Any regional lymph node greater than 6 cm is N3.

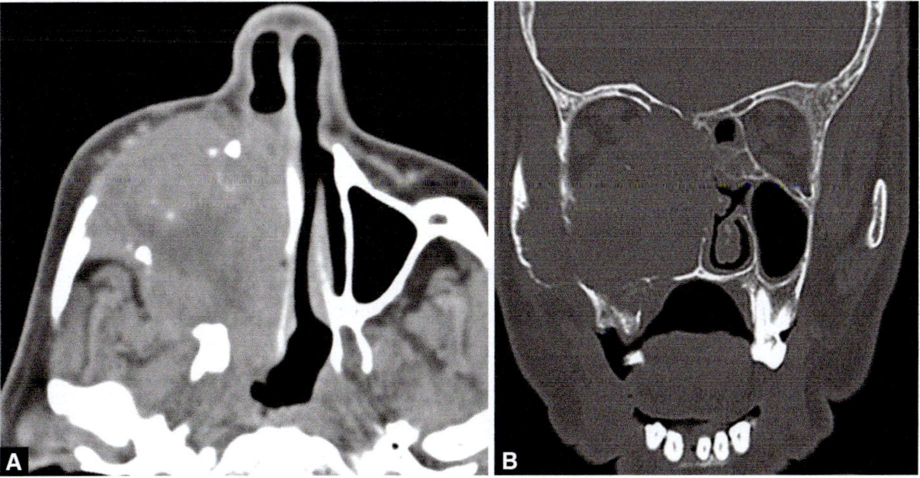

Figs 28.24A and B: Postcontrast axial (A) and coronal bone window (B) CT images reveal heterogeneously enhancing mass lesion in right maxillary sinus with irregular bone destruction suggestive of carcinoma. Extension of the mass is seen into right nasal cavity, ethmoid sinus and masticator space

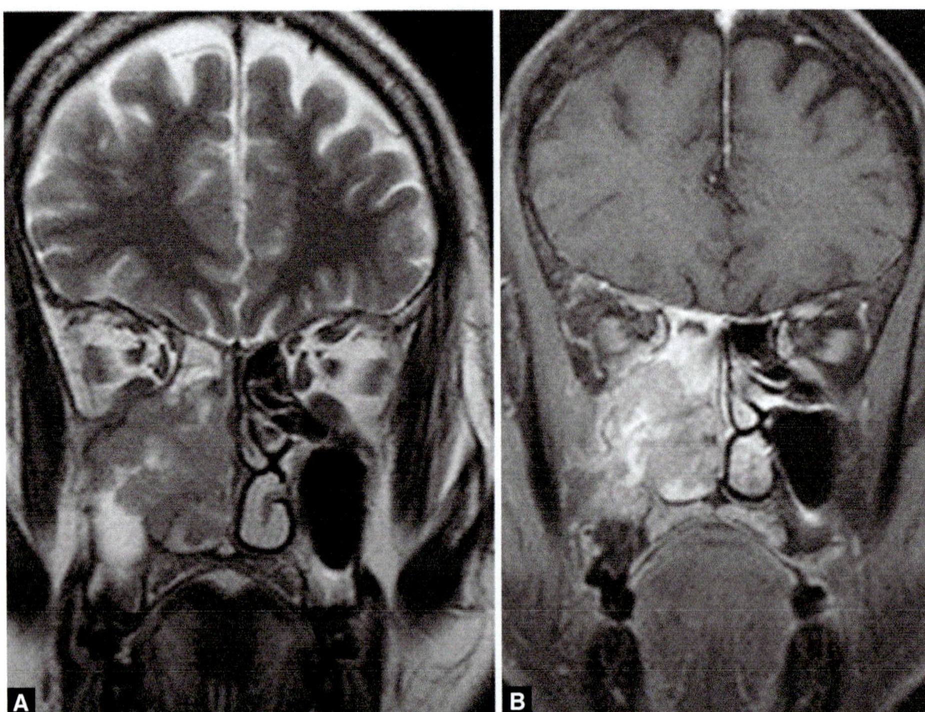

Figs 28.25A and B: T2 coronal (A) and postcontrast T1 coronal (B) images reveal intermediate intensity intensely enhancing mass lesion in right maxillary sinus, nasal cavity and ethmoid sinus in a known case of carcinoma maxilla

N2 comprises single ipsilateral lymph node greater than 3 cm but less than or equal to 6 cm, multiple ipsilateral/single or multiple contralateral or bilateral lymph nodes; each of which is less than or equal to 6 cm.

Adenocarcinoma

Adenocarcinoma comprises less than 10% malignancies of sinonasal region. Adenoid cystic carcinoma is the most common type followed by mucoepidermoid, malignant pleomorphic adenoma and intestinal type adenocarcinoma. These tumors also occur in elderly patients and imaging characteristics are usually similar to squamous cell carcinoma. Adenoid cystic tumor occurs in maxillary sinus and has a strong propensity for perineural spread (Fig. 28.26). Adenoid cystic and mucoepidermoid carcinomas may cause bone remodeling rather than aggressive bone destruction.

Olfactory Neuroblastoma

Olfactory neuroblastoma is a neural crest tumor arising from olfactory mucosa in the superior meatus. Bimodal age distribution is seen with peaks in second and fifth/sixth decades and mild female predominance. In early stages, the tumor is localized to the superior meatus. In advanced cases, spread to

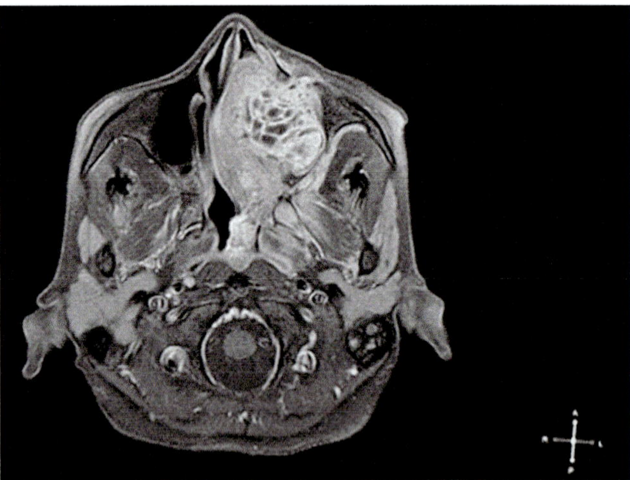

Fig. 28.26: Postcontrast axial T1 weighted image reveal heterogeneously enhancing mass in left maxillary sinus in a proven case of adenoid cystic carcinoma. The mass extends into left nasal cavity, nasopharynx, pterygopalatine fossa and masticator space

adjacent nasal cavity, PNS (ipsilateral ethmoid and maxillary sinuses) and intracranial extension is seen. A superior nasal fossa mass which bleeds on biopsy is an usual presentation.

On CT scan, it presents as a homogeneously enhancing mass centered at the superior nasal wall with remodeling of adjacent bone. Intracranial extension is seen through

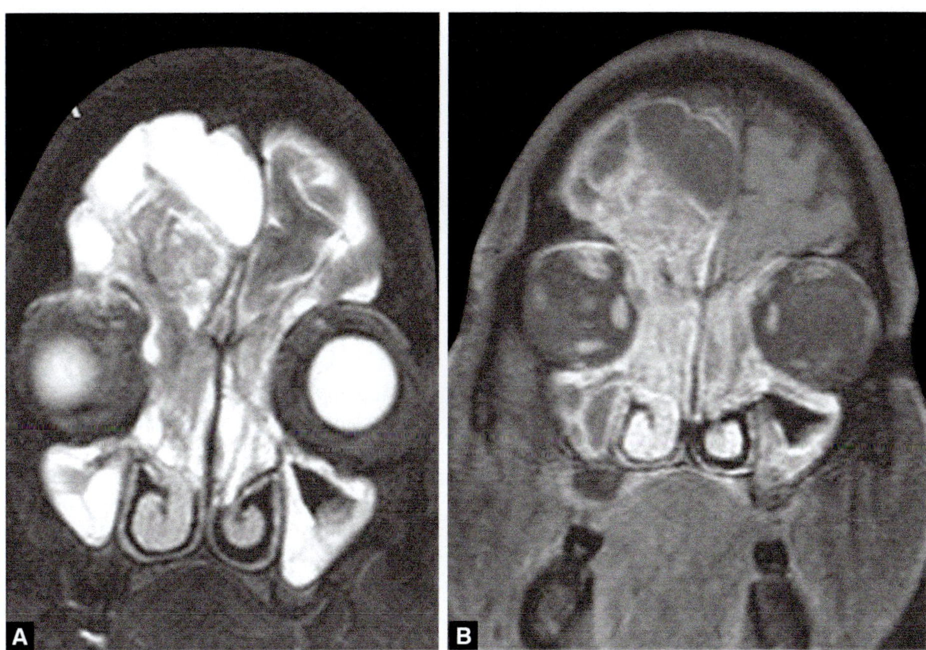

Figs 28.27A and B: Coronal MR images (A and B) reveal T2 intermediate heterogeneously enhancing soft tissue mass in bilateral nasal cavities with intracranial extradural extension in a case of esthesioneuroblastoma. Few large T2 hyperintense cysts are seen at the interface between the mass and brain parenchyma

the defect in cribriform plate. Dumbbell shape mass due to intranasal and intracranial component is classic presentation of advanced tumor. On MRI, solid component of the tumor appears intermediate on T1 and intermediate to hyperintense on T2 weighted images. Cystic areas appear T2 hyperintense without any postcontrast enhancement. Multiple T2 hyperintense cysts at the brain tumor interface are usually diagnostic of olfactory neuroblastoma. Intense heterogeneous postcontrast enhancement is common (Figs 28.27A and B). Metastatic cervical lymphadenopathy may be present. Complete surgical excision followed by radiotherapy is treatment of choice. Late recurrences are common with olfactory neuroblastoma.

Lymphoma

Sinonasal lymphoma represents extra nodal form of head and neck lymphoma, other sites being tonsil and thyroid. Majority of the tumors occur in nasal cavity followed by maxillary and ethmoid sinuses. Three types of sinonasal lymphoma include B-cell, T-cell and T/NL cell forms. B-cell lymphoma occurs in elderly patients involving the PNS. Involvement of orbit is common in these tumors. T cell lymphomas occur in the nasal cavity with destruction of nasal septum due to angioinvasive growth. T cell lymphomas are aggressive tumors occurring in younger patients. On CT scan, homogeneously enhancing mass in sinonasal area is seen with bony remodeling.

Aggressive bone destruction is uncommon. On MRI, lymphoma displays intermediate signal on both T1 and T2-weighted images with moderate postcontrast enhancement. Diagnostic clues may include bulky cervical lymph nodes, hypertrophy of Waldeyer's ring and sinonasal mass in a known case of systemic lymphoma. Further evaluation with CT neck, chest and abdomen should be performed to detect systemic spread of disease. Chemoradiotherapy is the treatment of choice.

Melanoma

Melanoma is more common in the nasal cavity than PNS, common sites being nasal septum, inferior turbinate and maxillary sinus. They commonly occur in elderly patients presenting with nasal obstruction and epistaxis. On CT scan, melanoma appears as a homogeneously enhancing mass in sinonasal area with bony remodeling. T1 hyperintense mass is a characteristic finding on MRI. However, not all melanomas are T1 hyperintense. They display hypointense to intermediate signal on T2-weighted images. Postcontrast enhancement of melanoma is usually difficult to perceive on MRI due to inherent T1 hyperintensity. Wide surgical resection followed by radiotherapy is the treatment of choice. Melanoma has poor prognosis and a majority of patients present with early local recurrence or lung, liver and lymph nodal metastasis.

Metastasis

Metastasis to sinonasal region is uncommon. Common malignancies with sinonasal metastasis include renal cell carcinoma, lung/breast/testis/prostate carcinoma and gastrointestinal carcinoma. Metastasis usually presents as soft tissue mass with irregular bone destruction. Presence of multiple lesions can provide a clue to metastatic etiology. Renal cell carcinoma can present as expansile hypervascular metastasis with bone destruction, and often with epistaxis. Prostate carcinoma can present as expansile sclerotic lesion in the sinonasal area without any soft tissue mass.

Sarcomas

Primary osteosarcoma commonly occurs in the first two decades of life, while secondary osteosarcoma occurs in elderly patients secondary to radiation or Paget's disease. Chondrosarcoma occurs in fourth/fifth decades with secondary causes being Ollier's disease, Maffucci syndrome and radiation therapy. Osteosarcoma occurs in the maxilla and mandible presenting with a bone destruction, dense intratumoral bone and perpendicular periosteal reaction. These tumors appear predominantly hypointense on T1 and T2-weighted images. Chondrosarcoma appears as T2 hyperintense mass involving maxillary/ethmoid sinus, nasal septum and mandible. Multiple discrete punctate intratumoral calcifications on CT are characteristic of chondrosarcoma.

Rhabdomyosarcoma

It is the most common soft tissue sarcoma in children arising from skeletal muscles. Orbital rhabdomyosarcoma is the most common site in head and neck region. Sinonasal tumors are uncommon presenting with nasal obstruction. On imaging, these tumors can be indistinguishable from more common squamous cell carcinomas. These tumors display homogeneous intermediate signal on both T1 and T2-weighted images, with or without bone destruction. Homogeneous postcontrast enhancement is usually seen.

CONCLUSION

Imaging plays an important role in the diagnosis and management of the sinonasal diseases. Further imaging has vital role in mapping the extent of the disease, in deciding operability, predicting prognosis and in follow up evaluation. CT scan of PNS is the modality of choice in inflammatory sinonasal disease. MRI has better soft tissue resolution and has added advantages over CT when neoplastic etiology is suspected and intracranial or intraorbital extent of the disease is anticipated.

BIBLIOGRAPHY

1. Allphin AL, Strauss M, Abdul-Karim FW. Allergic fungal sinusitis: problems in diagnosis and treatment. Laryngoscope. 1991;101:815-20.
2. Amol M Takalkar, Ghassan El-Haddad, David L Lilien. FDG-PET and PET/CT - Part II. Indian J Radiol Imaging. 2008;18(1):17-36.
3. Aygun N, Zinreich SJ. Imaging for functional endoscopic sinus surgery. Otolaryngol Clin North Am. 2006;39(3):403-16.
4. Brooks I, Gooch WM, Jenkins SG, et al. Medical management of acute bacterial sinusitis. Recommendations of a clinical advisory committee on pediatric and adult sinusitis. Ann Otol Rhinol Laryngol Suppl. 2000;182:2-20.
5. Chakrabarti A, Denning DW, Ferguson BJ, et al. Fungal rhinosinusitis: a categorization and definitional schema addressing current controversies. Laryngoscope. 2009;119:1809-18.
6. Harnsberger HR, Wiggins RH, Hudgins PA, et al. Diagnostic imaging. Diagnostic Imaging: Head and Neck, 1st edition, Salt Lake City: Amirsys; 2004.
7. Lanza DC, Kennedy DW. Adult rhinosinusitis defined. Otolaryngol Head Neck Surg. 1997;117:S1-S7.
8. Madani G, Beale TJ. Differential diagnosis in sinonasal disease. Semin Ultrasound CT MR. 2009;30:39-45.
9. Muhle C, Reinhold-Keller E, Richter C, et al. MRI of the nasal cavity, the paranasal sinuses and orbits in Wegener's granulomatosis. Eur Radiol. 1997;7(4):566-70.
10. Peter MS, Hugh DC. Head and Neck Imaging, 4th edition, Mosby, 2003.
11. Romett J, Newman R. Aspergillosis of the nose and paranasal sinuses. Laryngoscope. 1982;92:764-6.
12. Shetty PG, Shroff MM, Sahani DV, et al. Evaluation of high-resolution CT and MR cisternography in the diagnosis of cerebrospinal fluid fistula. AJNR. 1998;19: 633-9.
13. Sonkens JW, Harnsberger HR, Blanch GM, et al. The impact of screening sinus CT on the planning of functional endoscopic sinus surgery. Otolaryngol Head Neck Surg. 1991;105(6): 802-13.

Index

Page numbers followed by *f* refer to figure and *t* refer to table